RGUHS

Rajiv Gandhi University of Health Sciences

Solved Papers in

Oral Medicine and Radiology

Second Edition

Other CBS Books in Dental Sciences...

- BDS & CBS India Exam-Oriented Series Physiology & Biochemistry: Questions & Answers (PB) — Bansal
- Biochemistry by Target Educare: Topic wise arranged MCQs of AIIMS & All India Postgraduate Entrance Exam (With Explanatory Answers) — Bansal
- Clinical Manual for Oral Diagnosis — Beena Verma
- COMEDK Previous Years Solved Papers — Reddy/Murugesh
- Comprehensive Review of Dental Postgraduate Entrance Examinations: By Target Educare — Bichu
- Conservative Dentistry Including Endodontics: Questions & Answers (PB) — Bansal
- Concise Oral Radiology, 2e — Umarji HR
- Dental Materials: Questions & Answers (PB) — Bansal
- Evolving Trends in Oral & Maxillofacial Surgery — Taware
- General Pathology & Microbiology Questions & Answers (PB) — Bansal
- KCET Previous Years Solved Papers — Reddy/Murugesh
- Manipal Manual of Medicine for Dental Students (PB) — Shastry
- Manipal Textbook of Biochemistry for Dental Students — Nayak
- Manual of Oral Histology & Oral Pathology: Colour Atlas and Text — Jose Maji
- Materials in Restorative Dentistry — Karthikeyan
- Medicine for Dental Students, 2e — Khosla/Khosla
- Notes on Operative Dentistry and Endodontics, 2e — Reddy/Vanitha
- Oral History, Oral Physiology and Dental Anatomy — Reddy/Murugesh
- Oral Pathology Medicine and Radiology by Target Educare (PB) — Gupta Ambika
- Orban's Oral Histology & Embryology, 10e — Bhaskar
- Practical Guide to Oral and Maxillofacial Surgery (PB) — Taware
- Pre-Clinical Conservative Dentistry (PB) — Sikri Vimal K
- Pre-Clinical Operative Dentistry & Endodontics: Including Viva Voce Questions (PB) — Reddy/Vanitha
- Pre-Clinical Prosthodontics (PB) — Reddy/Vanitha
- Prosthodontics: Questions & Answers (PB) — Bansal
- Public Health Dentistry — Sikri Poonam
- Science of Dental Materials Clinical Applications — Bhatt S
- Short Notes for Dental PG Entrance Examinations, Vols 1–5: BDS I–V — Goyal Sandeep
- Target Educare's COMEDK-KCET PG Dental Entrance Examinations Question Bank with Explanatory Answers and References — Bansal
- Textbook of Complete Denture Prosthodontics — George Binu
- Textbook of Operative Dentistry, 2e (HB) — Sikri Vimal K
- Textbook of Oral Microbiology (PB) — Masthan KMK
- Textbook of Removable Partial Prosthodontics (PB) — Gupta Sharad
- Viva Voce in Orthodontics — Goyal Sandeep

RGUHS

Rajiv Gandhi University of Health Sciences

Solved Papers in

Oral Medicine and Radiology

Second Edition

Sumathi S Narsapur BDS
Bengaluru

Editor-in-Chief
Narendranatha Reddy P MDS
Founder-Director
Brihaspathi Academy
Bengaluru

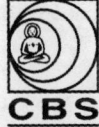

CBS

CBS Publishers & Distributors Pvt Ltd

New Delhi • Bengaluru • Pune • Kochi • Chennai

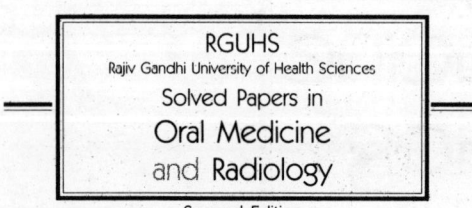

RGUHS
Rajiv Gandhi University of Health Sciences
Solved Papers in
Oral Medicine
and Radiology

Second Edition

ISBN: 978-81-239-2041-2

Second Edition: 2011

First Edition: 2005

Published by Satish Kumar Jain and produced by Vinod K. Jain for
CBS Publishers & Distributors Pvt Ltd
4819/XI Prahlad Street, 24 Ansari Road, Daryaganj,
New Delhi 110 002, India.
Ph: 23289259, 23266861, 23266867
Fax: 011-23243014

Website: www.cbspd.com
e-mail: delhi@cbspd.com
cbspubs@airtelmail.in.

Branches

- Bengaluru: Seema House 2975, 17th Cross, K.R. Road, Banasankari 2nd Stage, Bengaluru 560 070, Karnataka
  Ph: +91-80-26771678/79   Fax: +91-80-26771680   e-mail: bangalore@cbspd.com

- Pune: Bhuruk Prestige, Sr. No. 52/12/2+1+3/2 Narhe, Haveli (Near Katraj-Dehu Road Bypass), Pune 411 051, Maharashtra
  Ph: 020-64704058, 64704059, 32342277 Fax: +91-020-24300160   e-mail: pune@cbspd.com

- Kochi: 36/14 Kalluvilakam, Lissie Hospital Road, Kochi 682 018, Kerala
  Ph: +91-484-4059061-65   Fax: +91-484-4059065   e-mail: cochin@cbspd.com

- Chennai: 20, West Park Road, Shenoy Nagar, Chennai 600 030, Tamil Nadu
  Ph: +91-44-26260666, 26208620   Fax: +91-44-45530020   email: chennai@cbspd.com

Printed at India Binding House, Noida, UP

to
___
Parents

Preface to the Second Edition

The second edition of *RGUHS Solved Papers in Oral Medicine and Radiology* has been adequately revised and updated in response to the felt need among the students of dentistry.

In this edition, solutions to the oral medicine and radiology from August 2005 to December 2010 have been added to the earlier papers.

This book is not to be considered as a guide as the solutions have been compiled after referring to more than one standard book.

It is sincerely hoped that this edition will be as helpful as the first title in aiding the students to prepare well for the examination.

Sumathi S Narsapur
Narendranatha Reddy P

Acknowledgements

At the very outset I bow my head to thank God the almighty, whose kind grace has made it possible for me to bring out the second edition of *RGUHS Solved Papers in Oral Medicine and Radiology*.

At the beginning, I would like to give a sweet thanks to my husband Dr Shirish M. Narsapur who has spent his precious time in editing the contents, typing the answers, and helping me in bringing this edition.

A thanks my brother Ramchandra Koty for motivating me to come out with an idea of writing the solutions to previous years question papers for the first time.

I take the opportunity to express my great sense of gratitude to my friend Dr Narendranatha Reddy MDS (Oral Pathology) who has contributed unselfishly his time, knowledge and effort in editing the contents and helped me in the publication of this edition.

I am greatly indebted to my parents Mrs Kusuma and Mr Jayateerth Koty and my in-laws Dr Malati and Dr Madhusudan Narsapur.

It is a great pleasure for me to acknowledge the moral support from my elder sister Mrs Shalini and brother-in-law Mr Venkatesh Rao, Mrs Aruna, Mrs Snehal and Mr Punit. I would like to acknowledge names of my loved ones, my daughter Shasta and nephews Pranshu and Pratyay.

I am thankful to my friends and cousins Vijay Vittal, Priya Dixit, Vidya Rao, Tanmay Tiwari, Dr Sandya BM, Dr Madhumati, Dr Ragesh and Mohit for their technical help.

I sincerely thank Mr YN Arjuna, Senior Director, Editorial and Publishing, Mr SK Jain, Managing Director, and other staff of CBS Publishers & Distributors for bringing out the second edition of this book.

Sumathi S Narsapur

Contents

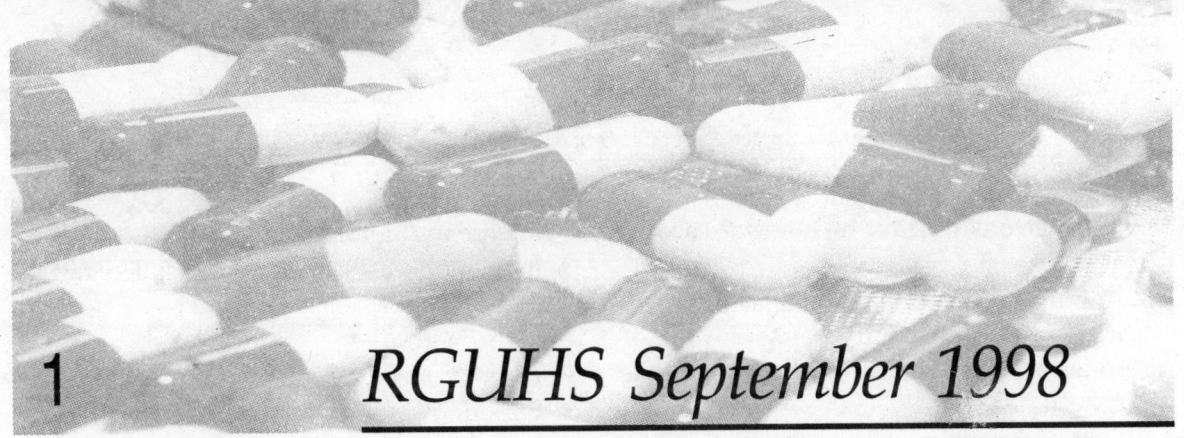

RGUHS September 1998

1

QUESTION PAPER

PART A

1. Define Trigeminal Neuralgia. Mention etiopathological causes and a note on its management.
2. Describe various types of Anemias. Mention the oral manifestations of Anemia.
3. Short notes
   i. Lichen planus
   ii. Vincent's infection (ANUG; Trench mouth)

PART B

4. What are the general defects in radiographs and how do you prevent them?
5. Describe in detail the procedure of taking periapical radiograph of maxillary central incisor.
6. Write short notes on
   i. Occlusal film
   ii. Fixer and developer

SOLUTIONS

PART A

Q1 Define Trigeminal Neuralgia. Mention etiopathological causes and a note on its management.

Ans.

Definition

Trigeminal neuralgia is defined as sudden, usually unilateral severe, brief, stabbing, lancinating, recurring pain in the distribution of one or more branches of trigeminal nerve.

Etiopathological Causes

1. *Vascular factors:* Transient ischemia and autoimmune hypersensitivity responses leads to demyelination of nerve
2. *Idiopathic causes:* The defect in the sensory nucleus of 5th cranial nerve
   • Trigeminal Gasserian ganglion
   • Any nerve may lose myelin sheath
3. *Secondary causes*
   • Trauma   • CNS lesions

4. *Mechanical factors:* Pressure of aneurysm of intrapetrous portion of internal carotid artery

5. Anomaly of superior cerebellar artery as it lies in contact with sensory root of trigeminal neuralgia and its elevation has reduced pain

6. *Dental cause:* Stress or local anesthetics may initiate the pain

7. Infection

8. Jaw bone cavities

9. Multiple sclerosis

10. Petrous ridge compression

11. Post traumatic neuralgia

12. Intracranial tumor

13. Intracranial vascular abnormality

14. Viral etiology—post herpetic neuralgia.

Clinical Features

Signs

- Trigeminal neuralgia occurs in late middle-aged persons with no abnormal neurological deficit as loss of corneal reflex, anesthesia, paresthesia and muscular atrophy/weakness
- Intermittent paroxysmal, lancinating shock like pain, elicited by slight touching superficially
- Trigger points are there depending on the division of nerve is involved:
  - V1–Supraorbital ridge of affected side
  - V2–Skin of upper lip, ala of nose/cheek of upper gums
  - V3–Trigger points are on lower lip, teeth/gums
- Pain rarely cross the midline
- Refractory period is there between attacks but dull aching persists
- The paroxysms occur in cycles, each cycle lasting for weeks or months and with time, cycle appears closer and closer

- With each attack pain seems to become more intense and intolerable
- In extreme cases frozen or mask like face is seen.

Symptoms

- Patient complains of sudden, unilateral intermittent paroxysmal, sharp, shooting pain, elicited suddenly by touching or cold breeze or while brushing
- Patient always complains of dull aching pain.
- During an attack of 1–10 min, the patient grimaces with pain, clutches his hands over affected side of the face, avoids touching the area
- Oral hygiene is poor
- Patient will lead a poor quality of life, as he will always be scared of getting pain.

Medical Treatment

- Carbamazapine 100 mg TID for 1–5 weeks
- Sodium valproate 600 mg/day + Phenytoin
- Clonazepam 1.5 mg/day if carbamazapine is contraindicated
- Phenytoin 100 mg TID (side effects: slurred speech, abnormal movements, gingival hypertrophy)
- Valproic acid 600 mg/day.

Surgical Treatment

The interruption of pain pathways between center and periphery.

Extracranially

- Alcohol block in peripheral nerve
- Nerve section avulsion
- Electrosurgery
- Cryosurgery
- Thermocoagulation.

Intracranially

- Alcohol block at gasserian ganglion

- Retrogasserian rhizotomy
- Medullary tractomy
- Midbrain tractomy
- Intracranial nerve decompression.

Physiologic Inhibition

- TENS—transelectrical nerve stimulation
- Acupuncture
- Biofeedback
- Psychiatric counseling.

Q2 Describe various types of Anemias. Mention the oral manifestation of Anemia.

Ans.

Definition

Anemia is defined as reduction of hemoglobin level or hematocrit in the blood below the lower limit of normal for the age and sex of an individual.
Normal 13–18/dl or % for males
          11–12 gm or % for females.

Types of Anemia

Classification

According to Robins

1. Etiological
   A. Blood loss
      - Acute blood loss
      - Chronic blood loss
   B. Increased rate of destruction leading to hemolytic anemia
      1. Intrinsic causes
         - Acquired membrane defects
           Paroxysmal nocturnal hemoglobinemia.
      2. Hereditary
         a. Red cell membrane defect
            Hereditary spherocytosis
         b. Red cell enzyme defect
            G-6 phosphate dehydrogenase enzyme deficiency

      c. Disorder of hemoglobin
         Thalassemia
         Sickle cell anemia
      2. Extrinsic causes
         a. Disorder of hemoglobin
         b. Immune mediated
            Autoimmune hemolytic anemia
            ABO and Rh incompatibility
         c. Mechanical destruction of RBC
            March hemoglobinuria
         d. Miscellanous
            Parasitic malaria
            Burns
   C. Impaired red cell production
      1. Disturbance in proliferation
         a. Differentiation in impairment of stem cell.
            Aplastic anemia
            Anemia of renal failure
         b. Impairment in maturation of erythroblast
            Deficiency of vitamin B12 and folic acid.
      2. Defective hemoglobin synthesis
         Globin synthesis impairment
         Heam synthesis impairment
      3. Miscellaneous
         Sideroblastic anemia
         Anemia of chronic disease
2. Morphological classification
   a. Microcytic hypochromic
      - Iron deficiency anemia
      - Sideroblastic anemia
      - Thalassemia
   b. Normocytic normochromic
      - Acute blood loss
      - Hemolytic anemia
      - Bone marrow failure
      - Anemia of chronic disorder
   c. Macrocytic megaloblastic anemia
      - Deficiency of vitamin B_{12}.

Oral Manifestation of Anemia

1. *Pernicious anemia* (primary or) glossitis, painful and burning lingual sensations which may be so annoying that the dentist is often consulted first for local relief. Tongue is inflamed, beefy red in color, either entirely or in patches scattered. In some cases small shallow ulcers are seen. Characteristically, with the glossitis, glossodynia and glosso-pyrosis, there is a gradual atrophy of the papillae of the tongue that eventuates in a smooth or "bald" tongue which is often referred to as Hunter's glossitis or Moeller's Glossitis. Inflammation and burning sensation may extend to the entire oral mucosa.

2. *Iron deficiency anemia*
   Plummer-Vinson syndrome
   - Cracks and fissures at corners of mouth
   - A lemon tinted pallor of skin
   - A smooth, red, painful tongue with atrophy of filliform and later fungiform papillae
   - Dysphagia resulting from an esophageal strincture or web
   - The mucous membrane of oral cavity and esophagus are atrophic and show loss of normal keratinization which may predispose to carcinoma
   - Koilonychia (spoon–shaped fingernails) or nails that are brittle and break easily
   - Splenomegaly has been reported.

3. *Aplastic anemia:* Petechiae, purpuric spots or frank hematomas of the oral mucosa may occur at any site, spontaneous gingival hemorrhage is common. Due to neutropenia there is generalized lack of resistance to infection. This is manifestated by the ulcerative lesions of the oral mucosa.

4. *Thalassemia (Cooley's anemia, erythroblastic anemia):* Unusual prominence of the premaxilla. Oral mucosa will be pallor.

5. *Sickle cell anemia:* There will be alterations in the bone in the dental roentgenograms. These alterations consist of a mild to severe generalized osteoporosis and a loss of trabeculation of the jaw bones with the appearance of the large, irregular marrow spaces. The trabecular changes is predominant in the alveolar bone.

Q3(i) Lichen planus

Ans.

Lichen planus is the dermatologic disease which manifests in the oral cavity. It is the common chronic immunologic inflammatory disorder which varies in appearance from keratotic to erythematous and ulcerative.

Classification

Lichen planus may be divided into the following types

1. Configuration
   - Annular lichen planus
   - Linear lichen planus.

2. Morphology of Lesion
   - Hypertrophic lichen planus
   - Atrophic lichen planus
   - Vesiculobullous lichen planus
   - Ulcerative lichen planus
   - Follicular lichen planus
   - Actinic lichen planus
   - Lichen planus pigmentosus.

3. Site of involvement
   - Lichen planus of the palms and soles (palmoplantar lichen planus)
   - Mucosal lichen planus
   - Lichen planus of the nails
   - Lichen planus of the scalp
   - Inverse lichen planus.

4. Special Forms

- Drug-induced lichen planus
- Lupus erythematosus-lichen planus overlap syndrome
- Lichen planus pemphigoides
- Keratosis lichenoides chronica
- Lichenoid reaction of graft-versus-host disease
- Lichenoid keratosis
- Lichenoid dermatitis.

Causes

It is not contagious and does not involve any known *pathogen*. Lichen planus has been reported as a complication of chronic *hepatitis C* virus infection and can be a sign of chronic *graft-versus-host disease* of the skin. It has been suggested that true lichen planus may respond to *stress*, where lesions may present on the mucosa or skin during times of stress in those with the disease. Lichen planus affects women more than men (at a ratio of 3:2), and occurs most often in middle-aged adults.

Nervous, high strung person, malnutrition and infection.

Grinspan's syndrome – Diabetes millitus, Lichen planus and hypertension.

Clinical Features

The typical rash of lichen planus is well-described by the "5 P's": well-defined pruritic, planar, purple, polygonal papules. The commonly affected sites are near the wrist and the ankle. The rash tends to heal with prominent blue-black or brownish discoloration that persists for a long time. Besides the typical lesions, many morphological varieties of the rash may occur. The presence of cutaneous lesions is not constant and may wax and wane over time. Oral lesions tend to last far longer than cutaneous lichen planus lesions.

Oral lichen planus (OLP) may present in one of three forms.

- The reticular form is the most common presentation and manifests as white lacy streaks on the mucosa (known as *Wickham's striae*) or as smaller papules (small raised area). The lesions tend to be bilateral and are asymptomatic. The lacy streaks may also be seen on other parts of the mouth, including the gingiva (gums), the tongue, palate and lips.
- The bullous form presents as fluid-filled vesicles which project from the surface.
- The erosive form presents with erythematous (red) areas that are ulcerated and uncomfortable. The erosion of the thin epithelium may occur in multiple areas of the mouth, or in one area, such as the gums, where they resemble *desquamative gingivitis*. Wickham's striae may also be seen near these ulcerated areas. This form may undergo malignant transformation.

The microscopic appearance of lichen planus is pathognomonic for the condition

- *Hyperparakeratosis* with thickening of the granular cell layer
- Development of a "saw-tooth" appearance of the *rete pegs*
- Degeneration of the *basal cell layer*
- Infiltration of *inflammatory cells* into the subepithelial layer of connective tissue.

Lichen planus may also affect the genital mucosa-vulvovaginal-gingival lichen planus. It can resemble other skin conditions such as *atopic dermatitis* and *psoriasis*.

Rarely, lichen planus shows esophageal involvement, where it can present with erosive esophagitis and stricturing. It has also been hypothesized that it is a precursor to squamous cell carcinoma of the esophagus.

Clinical experience suggests that Lichen planus of the skin alone is easier to treat as compared to one which is associated with oral and genital lesions.

Treatment

Care of OLP is within the scope of *Oral medicine* speciality. Currently there is no cure for lichen planus but there are certain types of medicines used to reduce the effects of the inflammation. Lichen planus may go into a dormant state after treatment. There are also reports that lichen planus can flare up years after it is considered cured.

Medicines used to treat lichen planus include:
• Oral and topical steroids.
• Oral retinoids
• Immunosuppressant medications
• Hydroxychloroquine
• Tacrolimus
• Dapsone
• Aloe vera.
Non-drug treatments: UVB narrow band phototherapy.

Other Methods

• Hydrogen peroxide mouthwash 2–3 times daily
• Ulcerated areas are dried with a sterile sponge and a corticosteroid ointment or cream rubbed gently into lesions several times daily
• Topical anesthetics to relieve pain
• Intralesional steroids are injected in severe cases
• Topical/Systemic costicosteroids reduce inflammation
  – 0.05% flurocinonide and 0.005% clobestol in form of paste or gel
  – Prednisone 40–80 mg daily for less than 10 days with out tapering (systemically)
  – Retinoids are also useful
  – Topical application of cyclosporine.

Q3(ii) Vincent's infection (ANUG; Trench mouth)

Ans.

ANUG (Acute Necrotizing Ulcerative Gingivostomatitis).

Clinical Features

Oral Signs

1. Characteristic lesions are punched out crater like depressions at the crest of the interdental papillae, subsequently extending to marginal gingival
2. The surface of gingival crater is covered by a gray, pseudomembranous slough demarcated from the remainder of the gingival mucosa by a pronounced linear erythema
3. Gingival hemorrhage or pronounced bleeding on the slightest provocation.

Oral Symptoms

1. Extremely sensitive to touch
2. Patient complains of constant radiating, gnawing pain that is intensified by spicy or hot foods and chewing
3. There is a metallic foul taste in the mouth
4. The patient is conscious of an excessive amount of pasty saliva.

Extraoral and Systemic Signs and Symptoms

1. Local lymphadenopathy
2. In mild cases there is slight elevation in body temperature
3. In severe cases there is marked systemic complications such as fever, increased pulse rate, leukocytosis, loss of appetite and general lassitude
4. Insomnia, constipation, GIT disorders, head ache and mental depression
5. In rare cases, severe sequelae of the ANUG is seen which are Noma, or gangrenous stomatitis, fusospirocheatal meningitis and peritonitis, pulmonary infections
6. *Clinical course:* Destruction of periodontium and denudation of roots, accompanied by an increase in severity of toxic systemic complications.

{Refered from Caranza Text}

Treatment Plan

A. The acutely involved areas are isolated with cotton rolls and dried
- A topical anesthetic is applied
- Supragingival scaling is done
- Patient is told to rinse mouth every 2 hours with a glassful of an equal mixture of warm water and 3% Hydrogen Peroxide
- Twice daily with 0.12% Chlorhexidine are also effective
- Patient is instructed to avoid tobacco, smoking, alcohol.

B. Patient with moderate or severe ANUG and local lymphadenopathy or other systemic symptoms are placed on an antibiotic regimen

1. Systemic antibiotics
   a. Penicillin 250/500 mg orally every 6 hours
   b. For penicillin–sensitive patients Erythromycin 250/500 mg every 6 hours
   c. Metronidazole–250/500 mg three times daily for 7 days
   - Contouring of gingiva as an adjunctive procedures in cases of severe gingival necrosis
   - Topical drug therapy is only an adjunctive measure
   - Escharotic drugs–phenol, silver nitrate and chronic acid should not be used as they may cause necrosis and destroy nerve endings.

2. *Oxygen liberating agents:* Hydrogen peroxide
3. *Mercurial derivatives:* Tincture nitromersol 1:200
4. *Spirocheticides:* Sodium Carbonate 10% aqueous solution
5. *Aniline dyes:* Gentian violet
6. *Others:* Vancomycin/Surgical pack.

Supportive Systemic Treatment

- Copious fluid consumption
- Administration of analgesics for relief of pain
- Bed rest is necessary for patients with toxic systemic complications.

Nutritional Supplements

- Intake of water soluble vitamin B and C
- Patient is placed on a balanced diet.

PART B

Q4 What are the general defects in radiographs and how do you prevent them?

Ans.

1. *Light radiographs*
   A. *Processing errors*
      These errors in radiograph are produced during the processing of X-ray film, i.e developing, fixing or exposing the film, directly into unsafe light. These errors are as follows:
      - Under development causes
         a. *Temperature too low:* When the temperature is too low, the developer contains élan + hydroquinone as reducing agent which is very sensitive to temperature changes. Developer becomes inactive at or below 60°F
         b. *Time too short:* If during processing film is not kept in developer or fixer for minimum time required to develop and fix the black silver halide crystals then light radiographs are produced. Developing time is 3–6 min between temperature of 65°F–76°F Fixing time is 10–15 min
         c. *Inaccurate thermometer:* This will give false reading of temperature and hence it may lead to under development or overdevelopment of film.
      - Depleted developer solution
         As the developer solution is kept for certain time period it may get oxidized

by atmospheric oxygen. Also it may get contaminated by various foreign agents so this leads to decrease in concentration of developer so it becomes impure. Developing X-ray film in this solution will lead to light radiograph since all the ionized metallic halide ions will not be converted to black metallic halide ions

- Diluted or contaminated developer
  Dilution or contamination of developer solution by any foreign matter like water, may lead to decrease in reducing agent per unit area of developing solution resulting in light radiograph

- Excessive fixation done for several hours removes some of the black metallic halide ions which leads to decreased density of film resulting in light radiograph.

B. *Under exposure:* Occurs during the process of taking radiograph. Causes are:

- Insufficient tube current (mA)
  The quantity of radiation produced by X-ray tube is directly related to tube current. Thus if tube current is very low then less quantity of radiation will be produced which will lead to less ionization of X-rays film during exposure which in turn lead to less black metal halide ions fixation causing light radiographs. Therefore less tube current leads to decreased no. of radiation per unit area leading to decreased ionization of metallic halide crystals which further leads to decreased conversion of metallic halide crystals into black metal halide ions thus increased fixing or washing of unionized crystals finally resulting in light radiographs

- Insufficient kVp or tube voltage. Tube voltage decreases causing energy of electrons when it strikes the target. This

decreases conversion of electron energy into X-ray photons. When there is decrease in no. of photons and energy of photon, the ionization will be less and light radiographs are produced

- *Insufficient exposure time:* Less number of photons are generated causing relatively less ionization

- *Excessive film–source distance:* X-ray produced is of divergent nature so when film-source distance increases X-ray per unit area decreases and also the intensity of X-ray beam or photon decreases. Intensity is inversely proportional to square of the distance.

2. *Dark radiographs*
A. *Overdevelopment*
If film gets overdeveloped then black metallic halide ions increase leading to increased fixation and dark radiograph.

Causes are:

- *Temperature too high:* As reducing agent hydroquinone is very sensitive to temperature, its activity increases as temperatures increases

- *Time too long:* If film is kept too long in developer then it will lead to over-development of film, as more number of black metallic halide ions will be formed causing dark radiographs

- *Developer concentration too high:* Freshly prepared developer has very high concentration of reducing agent in solution which is very reactive

- *Inadequate fixation:* Will leave unexposed metal halide crystals which causes films to opaque and resultant radiograph will be dark and non diagnostic

- *Accidental exposure to light:* There will be conversion of non-ionized silver halide crystals into ionized silver halide crystals, so when these are developed

all the ionized metallic halide crystals leads to dark radiographs
- *Improper safe light:* The light having more intensity than safe light will cause more ionization.

B. *Over exposure:* Lead to more ionization
- Excessive mA.
- Excessive KVP
- *Excessive time:* More the exposure time more will be ionization of metal halide crystals
- *Insufficient film:* Source distance. If the film source distance decreases the intensity of X-ray radiation increases leading to dark radiographs.

3. *Insufficient contrast*
Radiographic contrast is the difference in the intensity of densities between the various regions on a radiograph. Causes are:
A. Underdevelopment
B. Under exposure
C. Excessive tube voltage
D. *Excessive film fog:* When film is over developed then unionized crystals also get developed resulting in production of chemical film fog. Improper safe light causes film fog leading to insufficient contrast.

4. *Film fog*
Film fogging is fault caused by stray radiation or scattered radiation which are of low energy as compared to X-ray photons
A. Improper safe lighting conditions
- *Improper filter:* Filtration of higher energy radiation will be improper so the ionization occurs in dark room leading to film fog
- *Excessive bulb wattage:* This will produce more energy or higher energy radiation leading to film fogging
- *Inadequate distance between safe light and working surface:* As the distance decreases intensity increases in dark room leading to fogging of film

- Prolonged exposure of the film to safe light.

B. Light leaks
- Cracked safe light filter.
- Light from doors, vents, etc.

C. Use of expired films
D. Overdevelopment
E. Contaminated film solution
F. Deteriorated film which is stored at higher temperature, high humidity or exposed to irradiation.

5. *Dark spots*
Causes:
A. Finger print contamination
B. Black wrapping paper sticking to film surface which causes dark spot
C. Film in contact with tank or another film leads to non fixation of small area where the film is in contact with the tank
D. Film contaminated with developer before processing
E. Excessive bending of films.

6. *Light spots*
A. Film contaminated with fixer before processing-fixer contains clearing agent which washes off all the unexposed as well as exposed ionized metallic halide crystals.So during processing metallic halide crystals will not get converted to metallic halide ions which leads to light spots on radiographs
B. Film is in contact with tank.

7. *Yellow or brown stains*
A. *Depleted developer:* Oxidized product of developer is brown in color. These products interfere with developing reaction and stain the film
B. *Depleted fixer:* The clearing agent in fixer-Ammonium sulphate is unstable in acid environment causing stains on the film

C. Insufficient washing

D. Contaminated solution.

8. *Partial images*

   A. Part of film not immersed in developing solution

   B. Misalignment of X-ray tube head leading to 'Cone Cut'.

9. *Blurred radiographs*

   A. Movement of patient

   B. Movement of X-ray tube head

   C. Double exposure.

Q5 Describe in detail the procedure of taking periapical radiograph of maxillary central incisor.

Ans.

1. *Bisecting angle technique* (Fig. 1.1)

   • Position the film as close as possible to lingual surface of the teeth, resting in palate or floor of mouth

   • The plane of film and long axis of the teeth form an angle with its apex at the point where the film is in contact with the teeth

   • Construct an imaginary line that bisects this angle and direct the central ray of beam at right angles to this bisector. Consequently, the same length images are casted on the film as projected object.

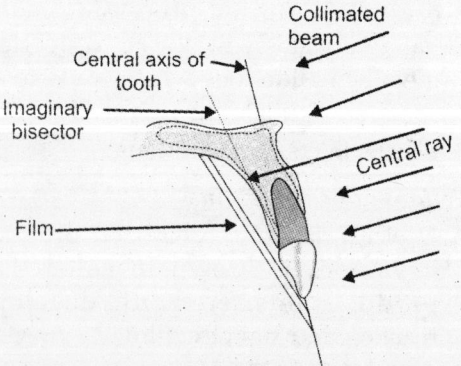

Fig. 1.1: Bisecting angle technique shows the central ray directed at a right angle to the plane that bisects the angle between the long axis of the tooth and the film

Image field: The field of view on radiographs (shaded area) should include both central incisors and their periapical region.

Bisecting angle technique

• *Film placement:* In Bisecting angle technique the film packet is held in place of palatal surface of central incisor in an angle similar to curvature of roots

• *Projection of central ray:* Direct the central ray at an angulation but perpendicular to plane of film

• Vertical angulation-45 degree

• *Point of entry:* Direct the point of entry form tip of nose.

2. *Paralleling technique (type A)* (Fig. 1.2)

   This is the technique in which X-ray film is supported parallel to long axis of the teeth and the central ray of X-ray beam is directed at right angles. This orientation of film, teeth and central ray minimized geometric distortion. Positioning of patient for maxillary arch patient's head should be upright with the sagittal plane vertical and the occlusal plane horizontal.

3. *Paralleling technique* (Fig. 1.3)

   • *Film placement:* Place a no. 1 film at level of second premolars to take advantage of maximal palatal height in the parallel cone technique. Position the X-ray film packet parallel to the long axis of central incisor

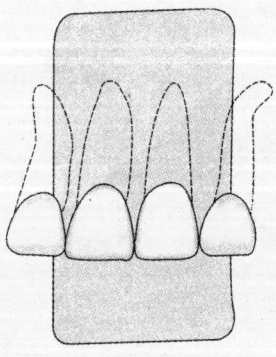

Fig. 1.2: Maxillary central incisor projection

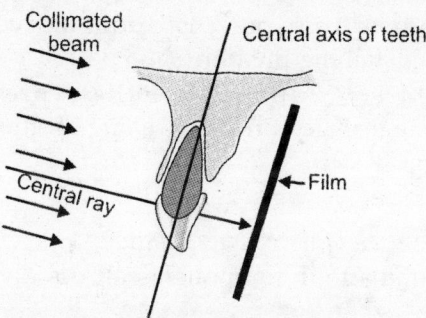

Fig. 1.3: Paralleling technique shows the parallelism between the long axis of the tooth and the film. The central ray is directed perpendicular to each

- *Projection of central ray:* Direct the central ray through contact point of central incisors and perpendicular to plane of films and roots of teeth. Vertical angulation of tube should be at 15–20 degree, horizontal angulation 0°
- *Point of entry:* Direct the point of entry of central ray high on lip, in the midline just below the septum of nostril.

Q6(i) Occlusal Film

Ans.

Occlusal Film

- Used to show larger areas of maxilla and mandible than may be seen on periapical film
- These films are used to obtain right angle views to the usual periapical view
- The patient holds the film by biting lightly on it to support it between occlusal surfaces of teeth.

Occlusal radiographs: Show an area of teeth and bone larger than periapical radiographs. An occlusal radiograph displays a relatively large segment of dental arch. It may include palate or floor of the mouth and a reasonable extent of contiguous lateral structures.

Occlusal radiographic projections for maxillary and mandible
- Anterior occlusal projections
- Lateral occlusal projections
- Cross sectional occlusal projections.

Uses

- They are useful when the patients are unable to open mouth wide enough for periapical radiographs or for other reasons cannot accept periapical radiography
- Location of objects in all 3 dimensions is displayed.

Indications

- To precisely locate roots and supernumerary un-erupted and impacted teeth (especially useful for impacted canines and third molars)
- To localize foreign bodies in the jaws and stones in the ducts of sublingual and submandibular glands
- To demonstrate and evaluate the integrity of the anterior, medial and lateral outline of maxillary sinus
- To aid in the examination of patients with trismus, who can open their mouths only a few mm
- To obtain information about the location, nature, extent and displacement of fractures of the mandible and maxilla
- To determine the medial and lateral extent of disease (Example: Cysts, osteomyelitis, malignancies) and to detect disease in palate or floor of mouth.

Cross Sectional Maxillary Occlusal Radiograph (Fig. 1.4)

- *Image field:* This projection shows the palate, zygomatic process of the maxilla, antero-inferior aspects of each antrum, nasolacrimal canals, teeth from second molar to second molar and nasal septum
- *Film placement:* Seat the patient upright with the sagittal plane perpendicular to the floor and occlusal plane horizontal. Place the film, with its long dimension perpendicular to the sagittal plane, crosswise in the mouth. Gently push the film in backward until it

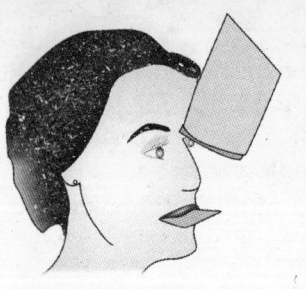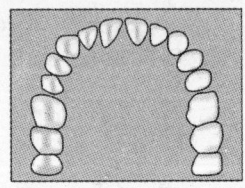

Fig. 1.4: Cross sectional maxillary occlusal projection

contacts the anterior border of the mandibular rami. The patient stabilizes the film by gently closing the mouth

- *Projection of the central ray:* Direct the central ray at a vertical angulation of +65° and a horizontal angulation of 0° to the bridge of nose just below the nasion, towards the middle of the film.

Q6(ii) Fixer and Developer

Ans.

Fixer

Function: The primary function of fixing solution is to dissolve and remove the undeveloped silver halide crystals from emulsion.

Composition

1. *Clearing agent:* After development the film emulsion must be cleared by dissolving and removing unexposed silver halide. An aqueous solution of ammonium thiosulfate dissolves silver halide grains and allow them to diffuse from emulsion
2. *Acidifier:* Acetic acid buffer system is present in fixing solution to keep the fixer pH constant which is required to promote good diffusion of thiosulfate into the emulsion. This also inactivates any carry over developing solution
3. *Preservative:* Ammonium sulfite prevents oxidation of thiosulfate clearing agent, which is unstable in acid environment of fixing solution. It also prevents oxidized developer from staining the film
4. *Hardener:* Aluminum Sulfate prevents damage of gelatin and swelling of emulsion.

Developer

Composition of developing solution:
It contains four components all dissolved in water.
A. Developer
B. Activator
C. Preservative
D. Restrainer.

A. *Developer*

- The primary function of developing solution is to convert the exposed silver halide crystals into metallic silver grains
- This process begins at the latent image sites where electrons from the developing agents are conducted into the silver halide crystals and reduce the constituent silver ions into solid grains of metallic silver
- Two developing agents are used:
  - Pyrazolidone type compound phenidone serves as a first electron donor that converts the silver ions into metallic silver at the latent image site. This electron transfer generates the oxidized form of phenidone
  - *Hydroquinone:* Hydroquinone provides an electron to reduce the oxidized phenidone back to its original active state so that it can continue to reduce silver halide grains to metallic silver.

B. *Activator*

- The developers are active only at alkaline ph values around 10. This is achieved by addition of alkali compounds/activators such as sodium or potassium hydrozide. Buffers are used to maintain this condition usually sodium bicarbonate

- The activator also cause the gelatin to swell so that the developing agents can diffuse more rapidly into the emulsion and reach the suspended silver bromide crystals.

C. *Preservative*

- The developing solution contains an antioxidant or preservative, usually sodium sulfite
- The preservative protects the developers from oxidation by atmospheric oxygen and thus extends their useful life
- The preservative also combines with the brown oxidized developer to produce a colorless soluble compound. If not removed, oxidation products interfere with the developing reaction and stain the film.

D. *Restrainer (anti-fog agents and increase contrast)*

- Bromide usually as potassium bromide, and benzotriazole are added to the developing solution to restrain development of unexposed silver halide crystals
- Bromide and benzotriazole depress the reduction of both exposed and unexposed crystals, they are much more effective in depressing the reduction of unexposed crystals.

2 *RGUHS March 1999*

QUESTION PAPER

PART A

1. Discuss the causes of pigmentation of oral mucosa
2. Define and classify anemia. Discuss in detail iron deficiency anemia.
3. Write short notes on
   a. Chronic atrophic candidiasis
   b. Angioneurotic edema.
   c. Erythrocyte sedimentation rate

PART B

4. What are common causes of faulty radiographs?
5. What are the intraoral radiographic techniques? Discuss any one in detail.
6. Write short notes on
   a. Ionization
   b. Developing solution
   c. Radiographic appearance of chronic focal sclerosing osteomyelitis

SOLUTIONS

PART A

Q1 Discuss the causes of pigmentation of oral mucosa

Ans.

Pigmentation in Oral Structure

The specific coloration, tint, location, multiplicity, size and configuration of pigmented lesions are of diagnostic importance. Blue, brown and black discolorations, constitute the pigmented lesions of the oral mucosa, and such color changes can be attributed to the deposition of either endogenous or exogenous pigments.

Causes

Pigmentation of oral mucosa can be due to following reasons:

1. Endogenous pigmentation
   • Hemoglobin

- Hemosiderin
- Melanin

2. Exogenous pigmentation
   - Silver amalgam
   - Graphite
   - Lead, mercury, bismuth
   - Chromogenic bacteria
3. Due to systemic disease.

Endogenous Pigmentation Explanation

1. *Hemoglobin:* This imparts red, blue or purple color to the mucosa and represents pigmentation associated with vascular lesions; coloration is rendered by circulating erythrocytes coursing through patent vessels
2. *Hemosiderin:* This appear brown and is deposited as a consequence of blood extravasation, which may occur due to trauma or defect in hemostatic mechanisms
3. *Melanin:* This is the pigment synthesized by melanocytes. Overproduction of melanocytes may be caused by a variety of mechanisms, including increased sun exposure, drugs, the pituitary adrenocortico tropic hormone (ACTH), and genetic factors (in association with certain syndromes), Benign nevi and malignant melanomas
4. Bilirubin.

Due to Intrinsic Processes

Peutz-Jeghers syndrome is an autosomal dominant disorder characterized by intestinal hamartomatous polyps in association with mucocutaneous melanocytic macules. Pigmented macules, often confluent and varying in size and shades of brown, appear in almost all cases periorally and on the lips and buccal mucosae. Any oral site may be involved, and the degree of pigmentation and oral involvement vary among affected individuals. Pigmented macules on the cutaneous surfaces covering the extremities and face are less frequently observed. The relative risk of developing cancer in this syndrome is increased 15-fold compared with that of the general population. The cancer primarily involves the GI tract (including the pancreas and the luminal organs), the female and male reproductive tracts, and the lungs.

Exogenous Pigmentation Explanation

These are usually traumatically deposited directly into the submucosa. However some may be ingested, absorbed, and distributed hematogenously to be precipitated in connective tissues, particularly areas subjected to chronic inflammation, such as gingiva

1. Silver amalgam–gray, black
2. Graphite–gray, black
3. Lead, mercury, bismuth-gray
4. Chromogenic bacteria–black, brown, green.

Oral Pigmentation due to Extrinsic Processes

The amalgam tattoo appears as a soft, painless, nonulcerated, blue/gray/black macule with no surrounding erythematous reaction. It is most frequently found on the gingival or alveolar mucosa, but many cases are also seen on the buccal mucosa. The tattoo is found more frequently in females than in males, probably because females are more likely to seek dental care. It is also seen more frequently with advancing patient age, presumably because of increased exposure to dental procedures over time. The tattoo is only moderately demarcated from the surrounding mucosa and is usually less than 0.5 cm in greatest diameter. Lesions with larger particles might be visible on dental radiographs.

Some patients demonstrate a long-term inflammatory response, with small, discolored papules produced, and in those who exhibit a strong macrophage response, the discolored patch can enlarge over time as the macrophages engulf the foreign material and attempt to move it out of the area.

Occasionally, deposits of amalgam are found in bone, usually as a result of the material being inadvertently dislodged from an adjacent restoration during tooth extraction or other surgical procedure, including the deliberate placement of amalgam into the apical canal of a root during endodontic surgery. These quickly become blackened and may impart a black discoloration to the adjacent bone.

Oral Pigmentation due to Hyperplastic or Neoplastic Processes

Melanotic macules may be solitary or multiple and can involve the gingiva, lip, as shown below, palate, buccal mucosa, and alveolar ridge, as shown below. Microscopically, this melanin deposit is mainly in the basal cell layers. Melanin may also be seen in the connective tissue near the basal cell layer.

Oral nevi are uncommon in the oral cavity. When they are present, they appear most commonly on the palate or gingiva. They can be intramucosal, junctional, compound, or blue nevi.

Junctional nevi are uncommon and are thought to arise primarily from melanocytes in the basal layer of the squamous mucosa. Junctional nevi reportedly can undergo malignant transformation to melanoma.

Oral melanomas are uncommon, and, similar to their cutaneous counterparts, they are thought to arise primarily from melanocytes in the basal layer of the squamous mucosa. The melanocytic density has a regional variation. In the oral mucosa, melanocytes are observed in a ratio of approximately 1 melanocyte to 10 basal cells. In contrast to cutaneous melanomas, which are etiologically linked to sun exposure, risk factors for oral melanomas are unknown. These melanomas have no apparent relationship to chemical, thermal, or physical events (e.g., smoking; alcohol intake; poor oral hygiene; irritation from teeth, dentures, or other oral appliances) to which the oral mucosa is constantly exposed. Although benign, intraoral melanocytic proliferations (junctional nevi) occur and are potential sources of some oral melanomas; the sequence of events is poorly understood in the oral cavity.

Currently, most oral melanomas are thought to arise de novo. Although rare, tumor transformation of nevi to melanoma involves the clonal expansion of cells that acquire a selective growth advantage. This transformation of melanocytes in an existing nevus, or of single melanocytes in the basal cell layer, must occur before the altered cells proliferate in any dimension. The oral mucosa has an underlying lamina propria, not a papillary and reticular dermis with easily discernible boundaries as is observed in skin. This architectural difference obviates the use of Clark levels for describing mucosal melanomas.

Iatrogenic Oral Pigmentation

Most iatrogenic pigmented lesions in the oral cavity are benign and their pigmentation is due to excessive production of melanin, which is produced by melanocytes. These cells are specialized dendritic cells present in the basal cell layer of the mucous membrane. The clinical visible pigmentation in the oral cavity depends on the number of melanocytes or the degree of melanin produced by these cells. The range of color pigmentation varies from gray to brown to black to dark blue. The closer the pigmentation to the surface, the darker the color (black); a melanin deposit before the basal cell layer will cause blue color.

Smoker's melanosis is due to long-term tobacco smoking. The pigmentation is usually distributed along the gingival layer in the upper and lower anterior teeth. It may also be seen in the soft palate, buccal mucosa, and floor of the mouth. Smoking cessation is the treatment of choice. The hyperpigmentation then disappears in a few months.

Actinic lentigo is also referred to as a solar lentigo. Lentigo presents as light-tan macules on the face, but it also may involve the upper (and especially) the lower lip as a result of sun exposure. It is common in elderly white persons. Microscopically, marked melanin pigments are present within the basal keratinocytes.

Melasma is a symmetric hyperpigmentation of the face and, at times, the lips. It is usually associated with pregnancy or oral contraceptive intake, along with exposure to sunlight. Microscopically, increased melanin is present in the keratinocytes and superficial connective tissue.

Q2 Define and classify anemia. Discuss in detail iron deficiency anemia.

Ans.

Definition and Classification

Refer to Q2 of September 1998

Iron Deficiency Anemia

Etiology

- Chronic blood loss
- Inadequate dietary intake
- Faulty iron absorption
- Increased requirement for iron, during infancy, childhood and adolescence and during pregnancy.

Clinical Features

Atrophic changes in oral mucosa, pharynx, esophagus and vulva leading to dry, inelastic and glazed appearance.

Symptoms

Easy fatigability, headache, dizziness, nausea, vomiting, diarrhea, loss of appetite, shortness of breath, loss of weight, pallor.

Signs

Signs: Thin narrow lips with a narrow orifice
  i. Pale, dry atrophic skin
  ii. Brittle and spoon shaped finger nails
  iii. Dryness of conjunctiva.

Cracks and fissures at corners of mouth
- A lemon tinted pallor of skin,
- A smooth, red, painful tongue with atrophy of fill form and later fungi form papillae
- Dysphagia resulting from an esophageal stricture or web
- The mucous membrane of oral cavity and esophagus are atrophic and show loss of normal keratinization which may predispose to carcinoma Koilonychia (spoon-shaped finger nails) or nails that are brittle and break easily
- Splenomegaly has been reported.

Plummer-Vinson Syndrome

Is in manifestation Iron Deficiency anemia (Also known as Paterson Kelly's syndrome). This syndrome occurs in women in fourth and fifth decades of life. The syndrome is seen in iron deficiency anemia and is associated with cracks or fissures at corners of mouth, a lemon tinged pallor of skin, a smooth red painful tongue with atrophy of filiform papillae and later fungi form papillae and dysphagia resulting from esophageal stricture or web.

This syndrome is predisposed to oropharyngeal carcinoma associated with general symptoms of anemia.

Laboratory Diagnosis

Blood examination reveals a hypochromic microcytic anemia of varying degree. RBC count is between 30–40 lakh units per cubic millimeter and the hemoglobin is invariably low. Iron deficiency anemia can be confirmed by lack of reticulocyte response following administration of vitamin B_{12}.

Serum iron is low and there is an absence of free hydrochloric acid in stomach. The achlorhydria is the cause of faulty absorption of iron.

Treatment

• Follow up of patients is to be done
• Iron therapy- ferrous sulphate 100 mg
• High protein diet.
  {Referred from Shafers, Burkitt and Davidson text}

Q3(a) Chronic Atrophic Candidiasis

Ans.

This condition has now become synonymous with Denture sore mouth.
Definition: This is a diffuse inflammation of maxillary denture bearing area with or without cracking and inflammation of oral commisures.

Etiology

• Inflammation due to denture wearing
• *Candida albicans* and *Staphylococcus aureus* infection
• Riboflavin deficiency
• Iron deficiency anemia
• Vit-B, folic acid deficiency.

Clinical Features

• This occurs mostly in denture wearers
• The palatal mucosa will be velvety or like an over ripe berry and bleeds on slight pressure when palatal papillary hyperplasia is also present
• Localized, simple inflammation or pin point hyperemia
• More diffuse erythema involving a part or entire denture covered mucosa
• Granular type involving the central hard palate and alveolar ridges. Denture sore mouth is most often found under maxillary denture as the negative pressure excludes

salivary antibodies from this region and yeast may reproduce, undisturbed in the space between denture and mucosa.

Management

• Rinsing of the appliance with dilute house hold bleach
• Disinfection of the appliance
• Leaving out the appliance, allowing the mouth to heal using antifungal creams or gels (e.g. Daktarin) or tablets (e.g. Nystan, Fungilin, Diflucan) regularly for up to 4 weeks
• The appliance may require adjustment or changing
• Soft liners provide a porous space and opportunity for additional mechanical locking of plaque and yeast to the appliance so it is considered to be an additional hazard and should be avoided.

Q3(b) Angioneurotic Edema

Ans.

Angioneurotic edema Is a rather common form of oedema occurring in both hereditary and non-hereditary forms. It appears to be closely related to general urticaria.

Etiotiogy

Some cases of non-hereditary form of angioneurotic oedema are due to food allergy drugs, endocrine disturbance or focal infections.

Pathogenesis

There is biochemical abnormality in patients with the disease is the absence of normally occurring inhibitor of C'1 esterase which is a specific alpha–2 globulin in complement system in the serum. This deficiency causes increased consumption of C'2 and C'4, with formation of kinin like substance that causes an increase in vascular permeability and edema, release of histamine with transudation of plasma.

Clinical Feature

1. Angioneurotic edema manifests itself as a smooth, diffuse edematous swelling particularly involving the face around the lips, chin and eyes, the tongue, and sometimes the hands and feet

2. The swelling may involve any area, including the parotid gland

3. The eyes may be swollen shut and the lips extremely puffy. The symptoms appear rapidly, sometimes being present when the patient is awake in the morning

4. A feeling of tenseness or an itching or prickly sensation sometimes precedes the urticarial swelling

5. The condition usually lasts for only 24–36 hours although some cases persists for several days

6. There may be visual involvement in some hereditary form

7. Vomiting and abdominal pain may occur, and especially dangerous, edema of glottis which can result in death through suffocation.

Treatment

- Etiologic agent has to be eliminated from diet
- Antihistamine drugs
- In cases of respiratory obstruction, emergency tracheostomy
- Aminocaproic acid and androgens antifibrinolytic agent which blocks the activation of plasmin.

Q3(c) Erythrocyte Sedimentation Rate

Ans.

Erythrocyte Sedimentation Rate is the rate at which the red blood cells sedimentate when allowed to stand.

- *Normal values:* The normal values are 0–20 mm/1st hour in females and 0–10 mm/1st hour in males

- *Technique of determining the values:* If blood is mixed suitably with an anticoagulant (sodium citrate in popular Westergren method) and allowed to stand vertically in a special tube (Example: Westergren tube) the erythrocytes, because they have a higher specific gravity than plasma begin to settle down, leaving a clear supernatant plasma above

- The length of the column of this clear supernatant plasma in mm after the end of 1st hour is ESR.

ESR Increases in

- Tissue destructive disorders such as trauma, infections and malignancies
- Infections where increase in plasma fibrinogen and gamma-globulin is seen as acute or chronic infections
- Collagenous diseases- Rheumatoid arthritis
- Tuberculosis
- Cancers.

Significance

- ESR does not help in specific diagnosis so the values are important for prognostication as well as assessment of progress in a person under treatment.

{Referred from Choudhary–Physiology Text}

PART-B

Q4 What are common causes of faulty radiographs?

Ans.

Refer Q4 of September 1998.

Q5 What are the intraoral radiographic techniques? Discuss any one in detail.

Ans.

Types of intraoral radiographs.

1. *Periapical radiographs:* This shows all of a tooth including the surrounding bone.

Periapical radiography: Two intraoral projection techniques (for details refer September 1998 Q5)
- Paralleling technique
- Bisecting angle technique
  Anterior periapical (no. 1 film)
  Posterior periapical (no. 2 film)
  Bite wing (no. 2 film)

Uses: Periapical radiographs are useful in diagnosis of various dental diseases

IOPAR is used
- To visualize periapical region
- In the diagnosis of periapical pathology
- To study the crown and root length
- To determine root morphology
- To study the integrity of lamina dura
- Selection of tooth for endodontic treatment in the evaluation of fracture of teeth
- As a part of routine radiographic examination
- To evaluate root apex foundation
- To study eruption pattern and stage of eruption
- To rule out impacted teeth, supernumerary teeth
- Post surgical evaluation of sockets
- To detect the cyst formation, abscess or any bone abnormality.

2. *Bitewing radiographs:* Show only the crowns of teeth and adjacent alveolar crests.

Bitewing radiography
This is also called as inter proximal radiograph:
- Horizontal bitewing films
- Vertical bitewing films residual alveolar crests in the maxilla and the mandible will be recorded on the radiograph

Uses/Indications
- In the diagnosis of interproximal caries
- To study the height of pulp chamber
- To study the occlusion of the teeth

- In the diagnosis of pulp stones
- To study height of alveolar bone or assessment of bone loss
- In diagnosis of secondary caries
- To detect interproximal calculus, foreign bodies and subgingival calculus

3. *Occlusal radiographs:* Show an area of teeth and bone larger than periapical radiographs. An occlusal radiograph displays a relatively large segment of dental arch. It may include palate or floor of the mouth and a reasonable extent of contiguous lateral structures. Occlusal radiographic projections for maxillary and mandible are:
- Anterior occlusal projections
- Lateral occlusal projections
- Cross sectional occlusal projections

Uses
- They are useful when the patients are unable to open mouth wide enough for periapical radiographs or for other reasons cannot accept periapical radiography
- Location of objects in all 3 dimensions is displayed.

Indications
- To precisely locate roots and supernumerary un-erupted and impactedteeth (especially useful for impacted canines and third molars)
- To localize foreign bodies in the jaws and stones in the ducts of sublingual and submandibular glands
- To demonstrate and evaluate the integrity of the anterior, medial and lateral outline of maxillary sinus
- To aid in the examination of patients with trismus, who can open their mouths only a few mm
- To obtain information about the location, nature, extent and displacement of fractures of the mandible and maxilla

- To determine the medial and lateral extent of disease (Example: Cysts, osteomyelitis, malignancies) and to detect disease in palate or floor of mouth.

Q6 Write short notes on

(a) Ionization

Ans.

When the number of orbiting electrons in an atom is equal to number of protons in its nucleus, the atom is electrically neutral.

- If an electrically neutral atom loses an electron, it becomes a positive ion and the free electron is a negative ion. This process of forming an ion pair is termed ionization
- Electrons can be lost by heating or by interaction (collision) with high energy X-ray or particles such as protons. Such ionization requires sufficient energy to overcome the electrostatic force binding the electrons to nucleus.

(b) Developing Solution

Ans.

Refer to Q6.2 of September 1998.

(c) Radiographic appearance of chronic focal sclerosing osteomyelitis

Ans.

Definition

Chronic focal sclerosing osteo-myelitis is an unusual reaction of bone to infection, occurring in instances of extremely high tissue resistance or in cases of a low-grade infection.

Clinical Features

This arises exclusively in young persons before the age of 20. The tooth most commonly involved is the mandibular first molar, which presents a large carious lesion. The symptoms of this disease are mild pain associated with an infected pulp.

Radiographic Features

Well-circumscribed radiopaque mass of sclerotic bone surrounding and extending below the apex of one cr both the roots. The entire root is always visible, an important feature in distinguishing it from the benign cementoblastoma that may closely resemble. The border of this lesion, abutting the normal bone, may be smooth and distinct or appear to blend into the surrounding bone.

Chronic focal sclerosing osteomyelitis is basically a reaction of bone to a mild bacterial infection entering the bone through a carious tooth in persons who have a high degree of tissue resistance and tissue reactivity. In such instances the tissues react to the infection by proliferation rather than destruction, since the infection acts as a stimulus rather than as an irritant.

Histologic Features

This reveals only a dense mass of bony trabeculae with little interstitial marrow tissue. If interstitial soft tissue is present, it is generally fibrotic and infiltrated only by small numbers of lymphocytes. Osteoblastic activity may have completely subsided at the time of microscopic study.

Treatment and Prognosis

The tooth may be treated endodontically or extracted, since the pulp is infected and the infection has spread past the immediate periapical area. The dense area of bone is sometimes not remodeled but in many cases may be recognized years later. Surgical removal of the sclerotic lesions should not be attempted before symptomatic relief.

RGUHS October 1999

QUESTION PAPER

PART A

1. Classify white lesions of oral mucosa and describe the etiology, clinical features diagnosis and management of oral lichen planus.
2. Describe the etiology clinical features of and management of trigeminal neuralgia.
3. Write short notes on
   a. Angular Stomatitis
   b. Fissured tongue
   c. Postprandial blood glucose technique.

PART B

4. Discuss in detail effect of radiation on oral mucosa.
5. Enumerate various radiographic techniques for TMJ. Describe in detail Tansorbital view technique.
6. Write short notes on
   a. Dental X-ray machine
   b. Intensifying screen
   c. Radiographic appearance of multiple myeloma.

SOLUTIONS

PART A

Q1 Classify white lesions of oral mucosa and describe the etiology, clinical features, diagnosis and management of oral lichen planus.

Ans.

Classification based on keratotic and non keratotic.

- Keratotic white lesions
  - Leukoedema
  - Linea alba
  - Leukoplakia
  - Benign migratory glossitis
  - Peripheral scar tissue
  - Lichen planus
  - Lichenoid drug reactions

- White hairy tongue
- Oral submucous fibrosis
- Papilloma
- Verrucous carcinoma
- White sponge nevus.
• Sloughing pseudomembranous necrotic white lesion
  - Plaque
  - Traumatic ulcer
  - Pyogenic granuloma
  - ANUG
  - Candidiasis
  - Necrotic ulcers
  - Cancrum oris - Noma
  - Erosive Lichen planus.

Clinical Features

1. Skin lesion appears as small, angular, flat topped papules few mm in diameter
2. These are discrete or gradually coalesce into larger plaques, each of which is covered by a fine, glistening scale
3. Papules are sharply demarcated from surrounded skin
4. Early lesion appears red then reddish purple/violaceous hue. Later dirty brownish in color
5. Centre of papule is slightly umbilicated
6. Its surface is covered by characteristic fine grayish white lines called Wickam's striae
7. Lesions occur anywhere on skin surface, distributed bilaterally in symmetric pattern.

Oral Manifestations

Characterized by lesions consisting of radiating white/gray velvety thread like papules in a linear, annular or reticular patches, rings and streaks over the buccal mucosa and to lesser extent on lips, tongue and palate.

• A tiny white elevated dots are seen at the intersection of Wickam's striae

• Vesicle and bullae formation is seen

Erosive	Non erosive
Bullous	Hypertrophic
Vesicular	Annular
Atrophic	Linear
Ulcerative	Reticular
Papular	

Management includes diagnosis and treatment.

Diagnosis

1. *Clinically:* Lichen Planus is suspected when erosive or bullous lesions are accompanied by typical lichenoid white lesions
2. Biopsy is necessary for definitive diagnosis Papanicolau staining is done. Hydropic degeneration of epithelium is seen histologically
3. Direct immuno fluorscence is done to differentiate from pemphigus, pemphigoid or discoid lupus erythematosis.

Treatment

Group I: Lichen planus of reticular, Atrophic
　　　　No symptoms on oral examination.
Group II: Lichen planus of reticular, Atrophic or any other variety except the

Erosive
a. With mild to moderate pain/burning
b. With moderate to severe pain/burning
Group III: Erosive lichen planus with or without symptoms.
Group IV: Patients who are on regular drugs continuously for more than six months may show sight of lichenoid reaction.

There is high percentage of anxiety prone and tense individuals having these lesions so psychological testing has to be done.

Q2 Trigemial Neuralgia

Ans.

Refer to Q1 September 1998.

SHORT NOTES

Q3(a) Angular Stomatitis

Ans.

Definition

A painful inflammation at corners of mouth is also known as angular chelitis/Perleche/stomatitis.

Etiology

- Inflammation due to denture wearing
- Candida albicans and staphylococcus aureus infection
- Riboflavin deficiency
- Iron deficiency anemia
- Vit-B, folic acid deficiency.

Clinical Features

- Occurs in both young children and adults
- Characterized symptomatically by a feeling of dryness and a burning sensation at the corners of mouth
- Epithelium at the commissures appeared wrinkled and macerated
- In time the wrinkling becomes more pronounced to form one or more deep fissures or cracks which appear ulcerated, but do not tend to bleed, although a superficial exudative crust may form
- If patient has lip sucking habit, the whole lip may be involved but terminate at the mucocutaneous junction
- Subsequent remissions are common and the lesions rarely disappear completely.

Treatment

- Antifungal therapy
- Nystatin
  - Amphotericin.
  - Topical Antifungal ointment topical applications at lesion's site.
- Antimicrobial treatment is also helpful.

For further treatment details refer Q3a chronic atrophic candidiasis in March 1999 paper.

Q3(b) Fissured Tongue

Ans.

Definition

Fissured tongue is a malformation manifested clinically by numerous small furrows or grooves on dorsal surface, often radiating out from the central groove along the midline of the tongue.

Types

- Cerebriform
- Transverse
- Foliaceous

Etiology

- Vitamin deficiency
- Trauma during development

Clinical Features

Generally Painless except in occasional cases in which food debris tends to collect in grooves and produce irritation.

Treatment

Cleaning of tongue with tooth brush followed by Antimicrobial mouthwash is advised. Local anesthetic gels can be used for relieving pain due to Referred from Shafer's - Text book of Oral Pathology}

Q3(c) Postprandial Blood Glucose Technique

Ans.

Clinical Correlation

The fasting blood glucose level, which is measured after a fast of 8 hours, is the most commonly used indication of overall glucose homeostasis, largely because disturbing events such as food intake are avoided. Abnormalities in these test results are due to problems in the multiple control mechanism of glucose regulation. The metabolic response to a carbohydrate challenge is conveniently assessed by a postprandial glucose level drawn 2 hours after a meal or a glucose load (Fig. 3.1) (Table 3.1).

Indications

- To assess long-term control of glycemia in known diabetic patients
- Prior to any surgical procedure in a patient to assess blood glucose level.

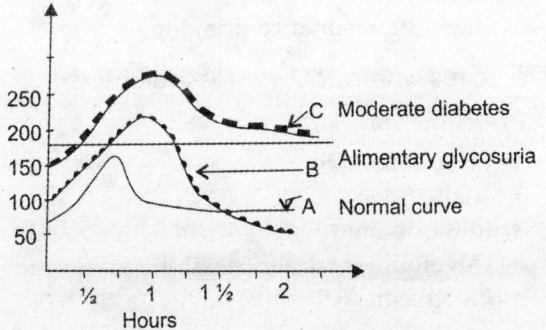

Fig. 3.1: Oral glucose tolerance test

Confirmatory test for
- Diabetes mellitus
- Cushing's disease

- Acromegaly.

Presence of diabetes symptoms plus casual (non-fasting) plasma glucose >= 200 mg/dl confirms diabetes.

Technique Procedure

1st a patient's blood sample is collected in the morning.

2nd 75 gms of glucose in 300 ml of water is given or heavy breakfast is advised.

3rd Blood samples are collected at half hourly interval for a minimum period of 2 hours.

Glucose concentration of every sample is estimated. Urinary samples are also collected for glucose concentration estimation.

Values

- Fasting plasma glucose 70–120 mg/dl
- Post prandial glucose level should not exceed a value twice that of fasting level and should return to normal within 2 hrs to rule out diabetes.

Q4 Radiation effects on oral mucosa

Ans.

Effects on Oral Mucous Membrane (OMM)

- The OMM contains basal layer composed of radiosensitive vegetative and differentiating intermitotic cells

Table 3.1: Causes of abnormal glucose levels

Persistent hyperglycemia	Transient hyperglycemia	Persistent hypoglycemia	Transient hypoglycemia
Reference Range, FBG: 70-110 mg/dl			
Diabetes Mellitus	Pheochromocytoma	Insulinoma	Acute Alcohol Ingestion
Adrenal cortical hyperactivity Cushing's Syndrome	Severe Liver Disease	Adrenal cortical insufficiency Addison's Disease	Drugs: salicylates, antituberculosis agents
Hyperthyroidism Acromegaly	Acute stress reaction Shock	Hypopituitarism Galactosemia	Severe Liver disease Several Glycogen storage diseases
Obesity	Convulsions	Ectopic Insulin production from tumors	Hereditary fructose intolerance

- End of 2nd week of therapy-cells die and mucous membrane begins to show areas of redness and inflammation (MUCOSITIS)
- The irradiated mucous membrane breaks down with the formation of a white to yellow pseudomembrane (desquamated epithelial layer)
- End of therapy-mucositis is severe, discomfort is at maximum, food intake is difficult. Secondary yeast infection by candida albicans is common
- After irradiation, mucosa heals but at later intervals mucous membrane tends to become atrophic, thin and relatively avascular
- Long term atrophy results from progressive obliteration of fine vasculature and fibrosis of underlying connective tissue
- Ulcers can result from denture sore, radiation necrosis, or tumor recurrence.

Effects on Taste Buds

- A loss of taste activity during the 2nd or 3rd week of radiotherapy.

Effects on Salivary Gland

- A marked progressive loss of salivary secretion in 1st few weeks of radiotherapy
- The extent of reduced flow is dose-dependant and reaches to zero at 60 Gy
- The mouth becomes dry (xerostomia) and tender, and swallowing is difficult and painful due to lack of lubrication.

Effects on Teeth

- There will be retardation of eruption of teeth if radiation exposure has occurred to teeth buds
- Radiation caries is a rampant form of dental decay that results from changes in salivary glands and saliva.

Effects on Bone

Degree of mineralization may be reduced, leading to brittleness and these changes are so severe that bone death results, the condition is called as osteoradionecrosis.

Q5 Enumerate various radiographic techniques for TMJ. Describe in detail transorbital view technique.

Ans.

Various TMJ Imaging Techniques

1. Panoramic radiography
2. Transcranial projection
3. Transpharyngeal projection
4. Transorbital projection
5. Submentovertex projection
6. Skull views
7. Conventional tomography
8. Computed tomography
9. Arthrography
10. Magnetic resonance imaging.

The cases where TMJ view is Indicated:

Hard Tissue Imaging

- Bony ankylosis
- Arthritides
- Remodeling
- Developmental abnormabilities
- Neoplasm
- Trauma
- Range of motion.

Soft Tissue Imaging

- Disk position
- Disk perforation
- Fibrous ankylosis
- Joint effusion
- Inflammatory conditions
- Joint space calcification localization.

Transorbital View Technique

Indications

The conventional frontal TMJ projection in delineating the joint with minimal superimpositions is transorbital projection.

- Transorbital view produces relatively true frontal projection of condyle and a major portion of condylar neck

- It demonstrates convex articulating surface of condyle and the slightly concave or flat, broad ridge of articular eminence
- Indicated when tomography is not available
- Indicated in TMJ disorders, trauma
- Significant dysfunction or alteration in range of motion, sensory or motor alterations, or significant changes in occlusion.

Transorbital Projection

This is similar to the transmaxiliary in that both provide an anterior view of the TMJ, perpendicular to the transcranial and transpharyngeal projections. In the transorbital view, the patient's head is tilted downward 10 degrees so that the cantho-meatal line is horizontal. The X-ray beam is projected from the front of the front of the patient through the ipsilateral orbit and TMJ of interest. The film cassette is placed behind the patient's head perpendicular to the X-ray beam. The patient opens maximally or, as an alternative, protrudes the mandible, there by positioning the condlye at the summit of the articular eminence and avoiding super-imposition of the articular eminence or skull base on the condyle.

1. The entire mediolateral dimension of the articular eminence, condylar head, and condylar neck is visible, which makes this view particularly useful for visualizing condylar neck fractures. The morphology of the convex surface of the condylar head can be evaluated, making this projection a useful a adjunct to transcranial and transpharyngeal projections in the diagnosis of gross degenerative changes or other anomalies. The usefulness of this projection is limited by the ability of the condyle to move to the summit of the articular eminence.

Q6(a) Dental X-ray Machine

Dental X-ray machines: The most commonly used X-ray machine is the wall-mounted dental X-ray unit (Fig. 3.2). Because thebasic components and operating techniques of alldental X-ray machines are similar, we will only discuss the wall-mounted unit. The component parts of the wall-mounted machine discussed here are the tube head, cylinder, extension arm, ready light, and aseparate control panel.

Tube head: The tube head (Fig. 3.3) contains the X-ray tube and other components necessary for generating X-rays. When an exposure is made, X-rays pass through an aluminum filter that screens out unnecessary radiation. Angulation scales are on both sides of the tube head for precise positioning technique.

Cylinder: The cylinder (or cone) is affixed to the tube headand is used to align the tube head with the patient andthe X-ray film. It is open-ended and composed of leadlaminated material that establishes the minimum distance from the X-ray source to the patient's skin.

Q6(b) Intensifying Screen (Figs 3.4 to 3.6)

- Intensifying screens are used in extraoral radiography. The rare earth elements like gadolinium and lanthanum, are used which emit green light on interaction with X-rays
- The intensifying screens are used in pairs, one on each side of the film and they are positioned inside a cassette. The cassette is used to hold each intensifying screen in contact with the X-ray film to maximize the

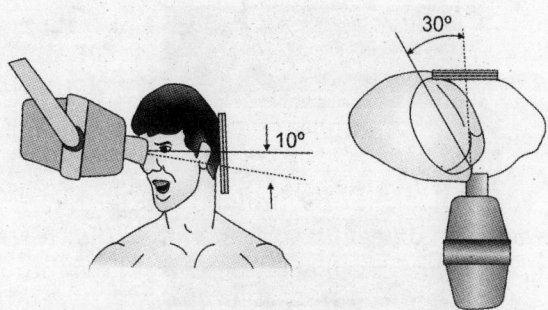

Fig. 3.2: Wall-mounted dental X-ray unit

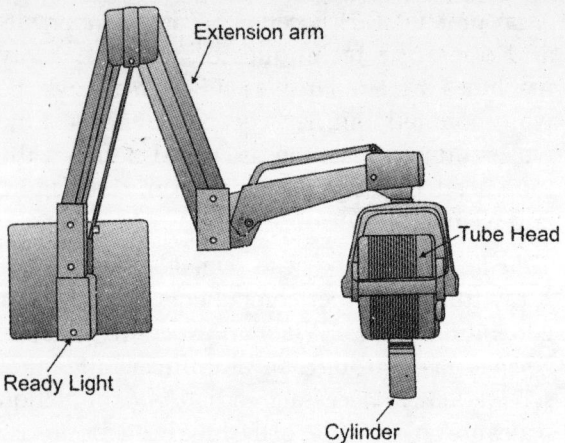

Extension arm

Tube Head

Ready Light

Cylinder

Fig. 3.3: tube head

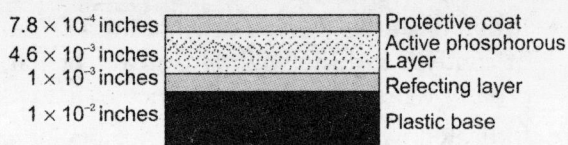

7.8×10^{-4} inches — Protective coat
4.6×10^{-3} inches — Active phosphorous Layer
1×10^{-3} inches — Refecting layer
1×10^{-2} inches — Plastic base

Fig. 3.5: Intensifying cross-screen section demonstrating the protective coat (which goes aginst the film), the active phosphor layer (which flouresces when exposed to X-ray photons), the reflecting layer (which reflects visible light back to the film), and the supporting plastic base.

sharpness of the image. Most cassettes are rigid but they may be flexible

- Intensifying screens are made up of a base supporting material, a phosphor and a protective polymeric coat.

1. *Base:* Some form of polyester plastic is used for base of radiographic film. About 0.25 mm thick base provides mechanical support for the phosphor. Function:
   - Base also is reflective and it reflects light emitted from the phosphor layer back toward the X-ray film. This increases the light emission of Intensifying Screens
   - Some Intensifying Screens omit the reflecting layer to improve image sharpness.

2. *Reflecting layer:*
   - In other Intensifying Screens, the base is not reflective, and a separate coating of titanium dioxide is applied to the base material to serve as a reflecting layer.

2. *Phosphor layer:*
   - This layer is composed of phosphorescent crystals suspended in a polymeric binder. When the crystals absorb X-ray photons, they fluoresce
   - The phosphor crystals contain rare earth elements, most commonly lanthanum and gadolinium
   - Their fluorescence can be increased by addition of thulinium, mobium, or terbium
   - The intensifying screens absorb 60% of photons that reach the cassette after passing through a patient
   - Different phosphor fluoresce in different portions of spectrum
   - Fast screen have large phosphor crystals and efficiently convert X-ray photons to

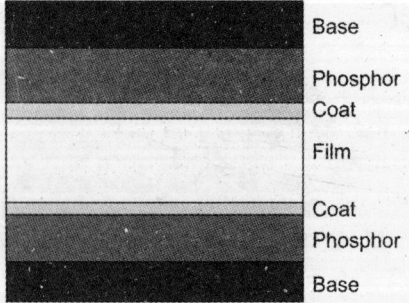

Base

Phosphor
Coat

Film

Coat
Phosphor

Base

Fig. 3.4: Two intesifying screens enclosing a film

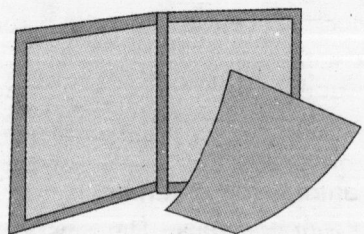

Fig. 3.6: Cassette for 8 × 10 inch film

visible light, but produce images with lower resolution.

3. *Protective coat:* A protective polymer coat (up to 15 mm thick) is placed over the phosphor layer to protect the phosphor and provide a surface that can be cleaned. When cassette is closed, the film is supported in close contact between two intensifying screens.

Uses of Intensifying Screen

1. For information in an X-ray beam to be translated into useful form, the intensities of radiation passing through the object must be recorded as a visual image
2. Used for extra oral radiography including panoramic, cephalometric, skull projections.
3. There will be substantial dose reduction to the patient.

Q6(c) Radiographic appearance of multiple myeloma
Ans.

Location

Multiple myeloma is seen more frequently in mandible than maxilla.

Periphery and Shape

- Periphery is well defined but not corticated and lack any sign of bone reaction
- The lesions are described as appearing "punched out". However many appear ragged and even infiltrate
- Some lesions have oval or cystic shape
- In periapical periodontal ligament region it appears as inflammatory periapical disease
- Soft tissue lesions appear as smooth bordered with underlying bone destruction.

Internal Structure

Islands of residual bone, yet unaffected by tumor gives the appearance of new trabecular bone.

Effects on Surrounding Structure

- If bone mineral is lost then teeth may appear to be "opaque" and stand out conspicuously from osteopenic background
- Neurovascular bundle loses its cortical boundary
- Mandibular lesions cause thinning of lower border of mandible or endosteal scalloping.

4 RGUHS March 2000

QUESTION PAPER

Long Essays

1. Classify the ulcerative and vesiculobullous lesions of oral cavity. Describe in detail recurrent aphthous stomatitis.
2. Enumerate the benign tumors of jaws and describe in detail ameloblastoma.

Short Essays

3. Describe the radiographic appearance of chronic osteomyelitis.
4. Describe radiographic appearance of periapical cemental dysplasia.
5. Describe radiographic appearance of dentigerous cyst.
6. Describe the clinical features of ANUG.
7. Describe clinical features of oral submucous fibrosis.
8. Mention predisposing factors of candidiasis.
9. Give the treatment plan of trigeminal neuralgia.
10. Give the treatment plan for erosive lichen planus.

Short Answers

11. Name the indications of bitewing X-rays.
12. Name the indications of PA Waters view.
13. Why salivary calculus is more common in Wharton's duct
14. Name the anatomical landmarks seen on upper anterior periapical film.
15. Name the causes of very light radiographs.
16. Why hydrogen peroxide mouth wash is given in ANUG.
17. Name the oral/systemic condition in which corticosteroids are contraindicated.
18. Name the drugs causing gingival enlargement.
19. Name the effects of X-ray radiation on oral cavity.
20. Name oral changes in AIDS patients.

SOLUTIONS

LONG ESSAYS

Q1 Classify the ulcerative and vesiculo-bullous lesions of oral cavity. Describe in detail recurrent aphthous stomatitis.

Ans.

Classification of ulcerative and vesiculo-bullous lesions of oral cavity.

CLASSIFICATION OF ORAL ULCERATION
Primary Ulcer
Traumatic Ulcer

- Physical–sharp tooth/denture
- Chemical–aspirin burn
- Psychological–cheek bite/emotional disturbance.

Infective Ulcer

- Actinomycosis
- ANUG
- Acute atrophic candidiasis
- Cancrum oris
- Infectious mononucleosis
- Syphilis.

Neoplastic Ulcer

- Squamous cell carcinoma
- Basal cell carcinoma.

Systemic Deficiency causing Ulcer

- Anemic ulcer
- Agranulocytosis
- Aphthous ulcer
  - Major ulcer
  - Minor ulcer
  - Behcet's syndrome
  - Reiter's syndrome.

Secondary Ulcer

Definition: Mucosal ulcerations caused secondarily to rupture of vesicle or bullae.

Intraepithelial Vesicular Formation

- Herpes zoster virus
- Herpangioma
- Herpes simplex virus
- Pemphigus vulgaris
- Pemphigus erythematosis.

Subepithelial Vesiculobullous Formation

- Erythema multiforme
- Epidermolysis bullosa
- Benign mucous membrane pemphigoid
- Bullous and erosive lichen planus.

BURKITT'S CLASIFICATION OF ORAL ULCERATION
Acute Multiple Ulcer
Herpes Simplex Virus

- Coxiella viral infection
- Varicella zoster
- Erythema multiforme
- Allergic stomatitis
- ANUG
- Oral ulcers secondary to cancer chemotherapy.

Chronic Multiple Ulcer

- Pemphigus vulgaris
- Bullous pemphigoid
- Erosive and bullous lichen planus
- Mucous membrane pemphigoid
- HSV in immunocompromised patient.

Recurrent Oral Ulcers

- Herpes labialis
- Recurrent aphthous stomatitis

- Behcet's syndrome
- Recurrent HSV infection
- Pscychic neutropenia including agranulocytosis.

Patient with Solitary Ulcer

- Histoplasmosis
- Blastomycosis
- Mucormycosis
- Traumatic ulcer
- Malignant ulcer.

RECURRENT APHTHOUS STOMATITIS

Definition

Characterized by painful, recurrent, solitary or multiple ulceration of oral mucosa.

Etiology

- Bacterial infection
- Immunologic abnormalities
- Iron, vitamin B_{12} and folic acid deficiency.
- Precipitation factors
- Trauma
- Endocrine condition
- Psychic disorder
- Allergic conditions.

Types of Recurrent Aphthous Stomatitis

1. Recurrent aphthous minor ulcer
2. Recurrent aphthous major ulcer
3. Recurrent herpetiform ulceration
4. Recurrent ulcers associated with Behcet's syndrome.

Clinical Features

1. *Recurrent aphthous minor ulcer*
   - Females are more prone than males
   - Age 10–30 years
   - Recurrent attacks of ulcers are seen every month or yearly
   - One or more small nodules occur with prodromal symptoms
   - Burning sensation followed by vesicle formation occurs within 24–48 hours
   - Oedema seen in the region
   - Paraesthesia in the region is noted
   - Malaise, low grade fever is also associated with the recurrent aphthous ulcer
   - Localized lymphadenopathy
   - The aphthous ulcer single or multiple will be covered by gray membrane with well circumscribed margin and surrounded by a halo
   - *Sites:* Buccal mucosa, labial mucosa, buccal and labial sulci, tongue, soft palate, pharynx, gingiva. This usually occurs in sites which are not bound to periosteum.

2. *Recurrent aphthous major ulcer*
   - Large, painful ulcers 1–10 in number
   - Lips, cheeks, tongue, soft palate are sites
   - They occur at frequent intervals
   - Ulcers persist for 6 weeks and heal with a scar
   - Recur in waves
   - Interfere with speech and eating.

3. *Recurrent herpetiform ulcer*
   - Crops of multiple, small, shallow ulcers 100 in number at one site (any intraoral site)
   - Small pinhead sized erosion that enlarge and coalesce. These are painful and present for 1–3 years with short remissions.

4. *Recurrent ulcers associated with Behcet's syndrome*
   Recurring oral ulcers, genital ulcers and eye lesions are seen.

Management of Recurrent Aphthous Ulcers (RAS)

The management includes diagnosis and treatment
- RAS is diagnosed by detailed case history and examination
- Laboratory investigation

- Biopsies are indicated to differentiate it from Crohn's disease
- The clinician should consider food allergy, malabsorption and HIV infection.

Treatment

Topical Therapy

Medication is prescribed according to severity of disease.

- In mild cases with two or three small lesions, emollient such as Orabase, Zilactin is necessary
- Pain relief of minor lesions can be obtained with use of topical anesthetic agent or topical Diclofenac (DOLO GEL)
- In more severe cases like in major ulcers with deep lesions that are larger than 1cm in diameter are extremely painful and interfere with speech and eating
- Topical Steroid preparation such as flucinomide, betamethasone or clobetasol are placed directly on the lesion shortens healing time and reduces the size of ulcers
- The gel can be carefully applied directly to the lesion after meals and at bedtime 2–3 times a day, or mixed with an adhesive such as orabase prior to application
- Larger lesions can be treated by placing a gauze sponge containing topical steroid on ulcer and leaving it in place for 15–30 min to allow for longer contact of medication
- Topical preparation like Amlexanox paste and topical 2% tetracycline which can be used as either mouth rinse or applied on gauze sponges
- Intralesional steroids are used to treat large indolent major RAS lesions.

Systemic Therapy

- Colchicine
- Pentoxifylline
- Dapsone
- Systemic steroids

- Thalidomide (side effects should be considered; used with extreme caution)

RAS associated with Behcet's syndrome is treated by Azathioprine with prednisone to reduce ocular disease as well as oral and genital involvement. Pentoxiphylline, Cyclosporine, Systemic Corticosteroids are also used. (Referred from Burkitt).

Q2 Enumerate the benign tumors of jaws and describe in detail ameloblastoma.

Ans.

Classification of Benign Tumors of Jaws

Ectodermal Origin

- Adenomatoid odontogenic tumor
- Ameloblastoma
- Calcifying epithelial odontogenic tumor
- Squamous odontogenic tumor
- Clear cell odontogenic tumor.

Mesodermal Origin

- Odontogenic myxoma
- Central odontogenic fibroma
- Cementomas
  - Periapical cemental dysplasia
  - Cementifying fibroma
  - Cementoblastoma.

Mixed Ectodermal and Mesodermal Origin

- Ameloblastic fibroma
- Ameloblastic fibro-odontoma
- Odontomas
  - Complex
  - Compound.

AMELOBLASTOMA

Definition

This is a slow growing benign neoplasm that has strong tendency to local invasion and that can grow to be quite large without metastasizing.

Clinical Features

- There is predilection for this lesion to occur in men and it develops more often in blacks
- Occurs at an age most commonly 3rd, 4th and 5th decade
- Both sexes are affected. 2/3rd of cases occur in posterior part of mandible followed by cuspid region
- Ameloblastoma grow slowly, and few, if any, symptoms occur in early stages
- Patient notices gradually increasing facial asymmetry. Swelling of cheek, gingival, hard palette is noted in untreated maxillary ameloblastoma
- Teeth in the involved region may be displaced and become mobile
- As the tumor enlarges, palpation may elicit a bony hard sensation or crepitus as the bone thins. If the lesion destroys overlying bone, the swelling may feel firm or fluctuant
- As it grows, this tumor can cause bony expansion and some times erosion through the adjacent cortical plate with subsequent invasion of the adjacent soft tissues
- An untreated tumor may grow to great size and is more of a concern in the maxilla, where it can extend to vital structures and reach into paranasal sinuses, orbit, nasopharynx, or vital structures at the base of the skull
- Recurrence rates are higher in older patients and in those with multilocular lesions.

Types

1. Follicular variant
2. Plexiform pattern
3. Acanthomatous
4. Granular variant
5. Cystic variant.

Radiographic Features

Location

- Molar ramus region of mandible. They may extend to symphyseal area

- Third molar area in maxilla and extend to maxillary sinus.

Periphery

- Ameloblastoma is well defined and frequently delineated by a cortical border which may be curved
- The periphery of lesion in maxilla is ill defined.

Internal Structure

- Varies from totally radiolucent to mixed radio opacity due to the presence of bony septa creating internal compartments
- These septa are usually coarse and curved and originate from normal bone that has trapped within tumor
- These septa are remodeled into curved shape providing honey comb, soap bubble appearance.

Effects on Surrounding Structure

- Ameloblastoma cause extensive root resorption, cyst like expansion with eggshell cracking of the bone
- Very advanced stage: Cortex gets eroded in one or more areas leading to perforated cortical plate giving ameloblastoma a multilocular appearance
- Bone perforation into surrounding soft tissues is seen in late stages.

Additional Imaging

- CT imaging is recommended
- MRI will provide superior images of the nature and extent of the invasion.

Differential Diagnosis

- Small unilocular ameloblastoma often cannot be differentiated from a dentigerous cyst

- Types of lesions that have internal septa are odontogenic keratocyst, giant cell granuloma, odontogenic myxoma and ossifying fibroma
- Giant cell granulomas generally occur anterior to the molars.

Management

- Complete eradication of lesion
- Reconstruction of resultant defect
- Curettage is contraindicated
- En bloc resection inraorally or extraorally can be done
- Segmental resection with continuity defect
- Radiation therapy may be used for inoperable tumors, especially those in the posterior maxilla.

SHORT ESSAY

Q3 Describe radiographic appearance of chronic osteomyelitis.

Ans.

Chronic suppurative osteomyelitis
1. Chronic focal sclerosing
2. Chronic diffuse sclerosing osteomyelitis
   - Sclerotic cemental
   - Florid osseous dysplasia.

CHRONIC FOCAL SCLEROSING OSTEOMYELITIS

Definition

Chronic focal sclerosing osteomyelitis is an unusual reaction of bone to infection, occurring in instances of extremely high tissue resistance or in cases of a low-grade infection. It is basically a reaction of bone to a mild bacterial infection entering the bone through a carious tooth in persons who have a high degree of tissue resistance and tissue reactivity. In such instances the tissues react to the infection by proliferation rather than destruction, since the infection acts as a stimulus rather than as an irritant.

Clinical Features

This arises exclusively in young persons before the age of 20 years. The tooth most commonly involved is the mandibular first molar, which presents a large carious lesion. The symptoms of this disease are mild pain associated with an infected pulp.

Radiographic Features

Well-circumscribed radiopaque mass of sclerotic bone surrounding and extending below the apex of one or both the roots. The entire root is always visible, an important feature in distinguishing it from the benign cementoblastoma that may closely resemble. The border of this lesion, abutting the normal bone, may be smooth and distinct or appear to blend into the surrounding bone.

Histologic Features

This reveals only a dense mass of bony trabeculae with little interstitial marrow tissue. If interstitial soft tissue is present, it is generally fibrotic and infiltrated only by small numbers of lymphocytes. Osteoblastic activity may have completely subsided at the time of microscopic study.

Treatment and Prognosis

The tooth may be treated endodontically or extracted, since the pulp is infected and the infection has spread past the immediate periapical area. The dense area of bone is sometimes not remodeled but in many cases may be recognized years later. Surgical removal of the sclerotic lesions should not be attempted before symptomatic relief.

Chronic diffuse sclerosing osteomyelitis it represents a proliferative reaction of the bone to a low-grade infection.

Clinical Features

- Occur at any age, but most commonly in elder patients with edentulous jaws.

- The disease is insidious in nature and presents no clinical indications of its presence
- On occasion there is an acute exacerbation of the dormant chronic infection,this results in suppuration and formation of fistula opening onto mucosal surface to establish drainage.in these casespatient may complains of vague pain and bad taste in the mouth.

Radiographic Features

Location

Site is posterior mandible often bilateral

Periphery

The periphery is well defined. There will be a gradual transition between the normal surrounding trabecular pattern and the dense granular pattern characteristic of this disease. The border between the sclerosis and the normal bone is often indistinct.

Internal Structure

This comprises regions of greater and lesser radiopacity compared with surrounding normal bone. Most of the lesion usually is composed of the more radiopaque or sclerotic bone pattern and radiolucency may be scattered through out the radiopaque bone.

Effects on Surrounding Structures

- Chronic osteomyelitis often stimulates the formation of periosteal new bone, which is seen radiographically as a single radiopaque line or a series of radiopaque lines (onion skin) parallel to the surface of cortical bone
- Over time the radiolucent strips that separates this new bone from outer cortical bone surface may be filled in with granular sclerotic bone
- The outer contour of mandible may be altered, assuming an abnormal shape, and

the girth of mandible may be much larger than on the unaffected side
- The roots of teeth may undergo external resorption and the lamina dura may become less apparent as it blends with the surrounding granular sclerotic bone
- If the tooth is non-vital periodontal ligament space usually is enlarged in apical region.

Q4 Describe the radiographic appearance of periapical cemental dysplasia.

Ans.

Periapical cemental dysplasia (PCD) is a localized change in normal bone metabolism that results in replacement of components of normal cancellous bone with fibrous tissue and cementum like material, abnormal bone, or a mixture of two.

Radiographic Features

Location

Epicenter of a PCD lesion lies at apex of tooth. The condition has predeliction for the periapical bone of mandibular anterior teeth.

In most cases lesion is multiple and bilateral, but occasionally a solitary lesion arises.

Periphery and Shape

Well defined periphery, often a radiolucent border of varying width is present, surrounded by a band of sclerotic bone that also can vary in width.
- The sclerotic bone represents a reaction of immediate surrounding bone
- The lesion may be irregularly shaped or may have an overall round or oval shape centered over the apex of tooth.

Internal Structure

- *Early stage:* Normal bone is resorbed and replaced with fibrous tissue that is usually continuous with the periodontal ligament which leads to radiolucency at the apex of involved tooth

- *Mixed stage:* Radiopaque structure appears in the radiolucent structure. This material usually is amorphous, has a round, oval or irregular shape and is composed of cementum or abnormal bone which is called as Cementicles
- *Mature stage:* Internal aspect may be totally radiopaque without any obvious pattern. Thin radiolucent margin can be seen at the periphery, because this lesion mature from the center to outward.

Effects on the Surrounding Structure

- The normal lamina dura of teeth is lost
- Periodontal ligament space either less apparent or gives a wider appearance
- Root resorption may occur
- Larger lesions may cause expansion of jaw
- The lesion may elevate the floor of antrum (For fig. Refer White and Phoroah page no. 492 for Fig. 23–9 and 23–10).

Q5 Radiographic appearance of dentigerous cyst.

Ans.

Definition

A dentigerous cyst is a cyst that forms around the crown of an unerupted tooth.

Radiographic Features

Location

The epicenter of a dentigerous cyst is found just above the crown of the involved tooth which usually is mandibular third molar or the maxillary canine.

- The cyst attaches at cemento-enamel junction
- Some dentigerous cyst are eccentric, developing from lateral aspect of follicle so that they occupy an area beside the crown instead of above the crown
- Cyst grow in to maxillary antrum and may become quite large before they are discovered

- Cyst attached to crown of mandibular molars may extend a considerable distance into ramus.

Periphery and Shape

Well defined cortex with a curved or circular outline. If infection is present, the cortex may be missing.

Internal Structure

Internal aspect is completely radiolucent except for the crown of involved tooth.

Effects on Surrounding Structure

- It displaces the associated tooth in an apical direction and resorbs the adjacent teeth
- The degree of displacement may be considerable; maxillary third molars or cuspids may be pushed to floor of the orbit, mandibular third molars may be moved to condylar regions or to inferior cortex of mandible
- The floor of the maxillary antrum may be displaced as the cyst invaginates the antrum
- The cyst may displace the inferior alveolar nerve canal in an inferior direction
- The slow growing cyst often expands the outer cortical boundary of involved jaw.

Q6 Describe the clinical features of ANUG (Acute Necrotizing Ulcerative Gingivostomatitis).

Ans.

Refer to Q 3.2 of September 1998.

Q7 Describe clinical features of oral submucous fibrosis (OSMF).

(Detail explanation of oral submucous fibrosis has been given here. The required part only has to be mentioned in the exam).

Ans.

Oral Submucous Fibrosis

A rare disorder involving inflammation and progressive fibrosis of tissues inside the mouth.

The condition starts with redness, blistering and ulceration inside the mouth that is eventually replaced with stiff fibrous tissue as it heals. The inside of the mouth can become stiff and hinder oral functions such as eating, speaking and even opening the mouth. Even the pharynx may occasionally be involved. The condition can become cancerous. The disorder is often associated with chewing betel nuts in Asian and Indian areas.

The condition is well recognized for its malignant potential and is particularly associated with areca nut, betel quid, tobacco chewing.

The mixture of this quid, or chew, is a combination of the areca nut (fruit of the *Areca catechu* palm tree, erroneously termed betel nut) and betel leaf (from the *Piper betel*, a pepper shrub), tobacco, slaked lime (calcium hydroxide), and catechu (extract of the *Acacia catechu* tree).

Lime acts to keep the active ingredient in its freebase or alkaline form, enabling it to enter the bloodstream via sublingual absorption. Arecoline, an alkaloid found in the areca nut, promotes salivation, stains saliva red, and is a stimulant.

Mortality/Morbidity

Oral submucous fibrosis has a high rate of morbidity because is causes a progressive inability to open the mouth, resulting in difficulty eating and consequent nutritional deficiencies. Oral submucous fibrosis also has a significant mortality rate because of it can transform into *oral cancer*, particularly squamous cell carcinoma, at a rate of 7.6%.

Race

Oral submucous fibrosis occurs on the Indian subcontinent, in Indian immigrants to other countries, and among Asians and Pacific Islanders as a result of the traditional use of betel quid endemic to these areas.

Sex

The male-to-female ratio of oral submucous fibrosis varies by region, but females tend to predominate

Clinical

Symptoms of oral submucous fibrosis include the following:
- Progressive inability to open the mouth (trismus) due to oral fibrosis and scarring
- Oral pain and a burning sensation upon consumption of spicy foodstuffs
- Increased salivation
- Change of gustatory sensation
- Hearing loss due to stenosis of the eustachian tubes
- Dryness of the mouth
- Nasal tonality to the voice
- Dysphagia to solids (if the esophagus is involved)
- Impaired mouth movements (e.g., eating, whistling, blowing, sucking)

Physical

Oral submucous fibrosis is clinically divided into 3 stages, and the physical findings vary accordingly, as follows:

Stage 1: Stomatitis includes erythematous mucosa, vesicles, mucosal ulcers, melanotic mucosal pigmentation, and mucosal petechia.

Stage 2: Fibrosis occurs in ruptured vesicles and ulcers when they heal, which is the hallmark of this stage.
- Early lesions demonstrate blanching of the oral mucosa
- Older lesions include vertical and circular palpable fibrous bands in the buccal mucosa and around the mouth opening or lips, resulting in a mottled, marblelike appearance of the mucosa because of the vertical, thick, fibrous bands running in a blanching mucosa. Specific findings include the following:
  – Reduction of the mouth opening (trismus)

- Stiff and small tongue
- Blanched and leathery floor of the mouth
- Fibrotic and depigmented gingiva
- Rubbery soft palate with decreased mobility
- Blanched and atrophic tonsils
- Shrunken budlike uvula
- Sinking of the cheeks, not commensurate with age or nutritional status

Stage 3: Sequelae of oral submucous fibrosis are as follows:

- *Leukoplakia* is precancerous and is found in more than 25% of individuals with oral submucous fibrosis
- Speech and hearing deficits may occur because of involvement of the tongue and the eustachian tubes.

Q8 Mention Predisposing factors of Candidiasis

Ans.

- Marked changes in the oral microbial flora following administration of antibiotics (especially broad spectrum), excessive use of antibacterial mouthrinses and xerostomia secondary to anticholinergic agents or secondary to salivary gland disease
- Chronic local irritants (dentures and orthodontic appliances: heavy smoking
- Administration of corticosteroids (topical, oral and aerosolized inhalant; systemic)
- Radiation to head and neck
- Age (infancy, preganancy, old age)
- Hospitalization age, debilitating disease, antibiotics
- Oral epithelial dysplasia (congenital or acquired keratotic oral lesions)
- Immunologic deficiency (congenital endocrine candidiasis syndrome, chronic familial mucocutaneous candidiasis, Digeorg's and Neolof's syndromes, thymoma, swiss and Bruton-type agammaglobulinemias), or acquired diabetes, leukemia and lymphomas, iatrogenic from cancer chemotherapy, bone marrow transplantation AIDS.

Q9 Give the Tratment Plan of Trigeminal Neuralgia.

Ans.

Refer to Q1 of September 1998

Q10 Give the treatment plan for Erosive Lichen Planus.

Ans.

Erosive lichen planus with or without symptoms are treated as follows:

- Immediate biopsy of lesion is indicated
- Local control of pain with Benzocaine 100% cream Xylocaine (Igmox) to relieve burning sensation. 2 mg diazepam for 2–3 weeks is recommended for this type for anxiety relief. Ointments, containing corticosteroid applied locally 3–4 times a day but considering the effect of the saliva and its washing out, its actual local effect could be questioned
- If the ulcer appears infected then a penicillin group of antibiotics like peptide or Oracyn K could be prescribed for 4 days
- If biopsy reports shows any evidence of premalignancy then immediate referral to a Oncology unit is mandatory.

Treatment

- Hydrogen peroxide mouthwash 2–3 times daily
- Ulcerated areas are dried with a sterile sponge and a corticosteroid ointment or cream rubbed gently into lesions several times daily
- Intralesional steroids are injected in severe cases
- Topical anesthetics are applied to relieve pain.

SHORT ANSWERS

Q11 Name the indications of Bitewing X-rays.

Ans.

Bitewing radiographs: show only the crowns of teeth and adjacent alveolar crests Bitewing

radiography. This is also called as interproximal radiograph
- Horizontal bitewing films
- Vertical bitewing films
  Residual alveolar crests in the maxilla and the mandible will be recorded on the radiograph.

Uses/Indications

Bitewing radiographs: show only the crowns of teeth and adjacent alveolar crests
- In the diagnosis of interproximal caries
- To study the height of pulp chamber
- To study the occlusion of the teeth
- In the diagnosis of pulp stones
- To study height of alveolar bone or assessment of bone loss
- In diagnosis of secondary caries
- To detect interproximal calculus, foreign bodies and subgingival calculus.

Q12 Name the indication of PA Waters view.

Ans.

1. Water's projection is useful for evaluation of the maxillary sinuses and is a variation of PA view
2. It demonstrates the frontal and ethmoid sinuses, the orbit, the zygomatico frontal suture, and nasal cavity
3. It demonstrates the position of coronoid process of mandible between the maxilla and zygomatic arch
   - *Image receptor and patient placement:* The Image receptor is placed in front of the patient and perpendicular to the midsaggital plane, the patients head is tilted upwards so that the canthomeatal line forms a 37-degree angle with the image receptor
   - *Position of the central X-ray beam:* The central beam is perpendicular to the image receptor and centered in the area of the maxillary sinuses

- Resultant image The midsagital plane should divide the skull images in two symmetric halves (Fig. 4.1).

Q13 Why salivary calculus is more common in Wharton's duct.

Ans.

Salivary calculus is more common in Wharton duct as
- Wharton's duct has sharp curves which is likely to trap mucin plugs or cellular debris
- Calcium levels are higher in saliva from submandibular gland
- The dependant position of submandibular gland increases the chance for stasis
- The viscosity of submandibular gland saliva is more
- Wharton's duct is more convoluted and has to travel against gravity.

Q14 Name anatomical landmarks seen on upper anterior periapical film.

Ans.

Radiographic anatomical landmark on anterior maxillary periapical film (Fig. 4.2).

Radiopaque Landmarks

1. Malar process
2. lower border of maxillary sinus

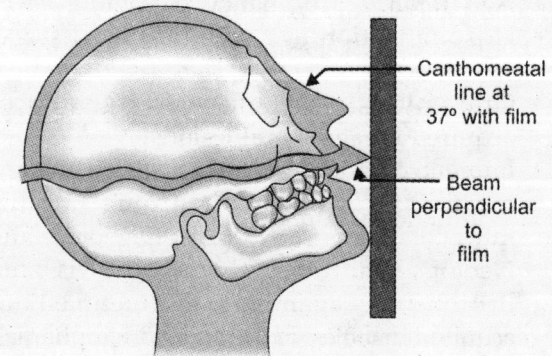

Fig. 4.1: Water's projection

3. Internasal septum
4. Anterior nasal spine
5. Lamina dura
6. Tip of coronoid
7. Pterygoid plate.

Radiolucent Landmarks

8. Nasopalatine canal
9. Maxillary sinus
10. Nasal fossae.

Q15 Name the causes of very light Radiographs.

Ans.

Causes of Light Radiographs

Processing Errors

1. Underdevelopment
   - Temperature too low
   - Time too short
   - Inaccurate thermometer
2. Depleted developer solution
3. Diluted or contaminated developer
4. Excessive fixation.

Underexposure

1. Insufficient mA
2. Insufficient KVP
3. Insufficient time
4. Excessive film-source distance
5. Film packet reversed in mouth.
   For details refer Q4 September 1998

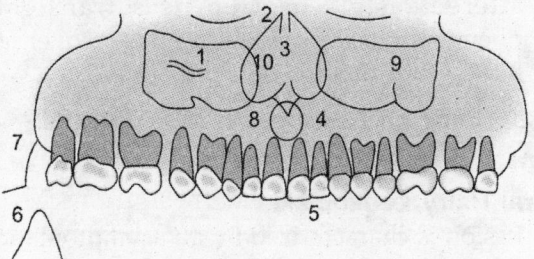

Fig. 4.2: Radiographic anatomical landmark

Q16 Why hydrogen peroxide mouth wash is given in ANUG.

Ans.

- Hydrogen peroxide is an oxygen liberating agent which is used as a mouth wash in dilute form
- Hydrogen peroxide reduces anaerobic atmosphere in punched out lesions of ANUG and reduces spirocheates, filamentous organism
- Because it kills nearly all types of harmful cells it touches it is widely regarded as one of the best things that you can use for cleaning cuts and wounds. It will also act as an anti-coagulant and help to slow any bleeding the wound might have. Some people also use solutions of **hydrogen peroxide** to help with fungal and ear infections as well, and it is even used as a mouthwash
- It prevents yeast infection.

Q17 Name the oral/systemic condition in which corticosteroids are contraindicated.

Ans.

Corticosteroids are contraindicated in
- Herpes simplex infection
- Peptic ulcer
- Bronchial asthma
- Hypertension or cardiovascular disease
- Peptic ulcer
- Osteoporosis
- Diabetes mellitus
- Tuberculosis or other infections
- Psychological difficulties
- Glaucoma
- Pregnancy
- Young patients.

Q18 Name the drugs causing Gingival Enlargement.

Ans.

Gingival overgrowth, also known as gingival hyperplasia occurs secondary to drugs

1. *Nifedipine:* Calcium channel blocker whereas nifedipine, which potentiates the effect of cyclosporine, reduces protein synthesis of fibroblasts. Nifedipine appears to have an additive effect when used together with cyclosporine in transplant recipients with hypertension

2. *Phenytion:* Antiepileptic drug. Phenytoin has been shown to induce gingival overgrowth by its interaction with a subpopulation of sensitive fibroblasts),

3. *Dilantin sodium:* Anticonvulsant drug.

4. *Cyclosporin:* Immunosuppressant. Cyclosporine has been suggested to affect the metabolic function of fibroblast (e.g., collagen synthesis)

Some of the risk factors known to contribute to gingival overgrowth include the presence of gingival inflammation (ie, gingivitis) resulting from poor oral hygiene. Furthermore, the presence of dental plaque may provide a reservoir for the accumulation of phenytoin or cyclosporine. In orthodontic patients, gingival overgrowth has been suggested to be due to nickel accumulation and epithelial cell proliferation.

Q19 Name the effects of X-ray radiation on oral cavity.

Ans.

Acute and Subacute Complications of Radiation Therapy

Acute reactions are those which arise during or shortly after radiation therapy and resolve within ninety days post-therapy.

1. Mucositis

- One of the first symptoms of radiation compli-cations is mucositis, which occurs 12–17 days after the initiation of therapy
- Mucosal inflammation varies with dosage, target size and duration of therapy. Oral mucositis can present as patchy mild erythema to frank confluent ulceration. Chemotherapeutic agents such as 5FU, procarbazine, methotrexate, etc. may increase the severity of these symptoms

- Currently, there are no drugs available to prevent mucositis, and it is imperative to distinguish these lesions from those caused by infections. Cultures may be needed to differentiate between fungal, bacterial and viral lesions versus those secondary to radiation effects

- This is accomplished by designing portals that limit the exposure to tissues not at risk for tumor reoccurrence. When interstitial implants are a part of a treatment protocol, soft tissues of the oropharynx are at greater risk for developing soft tissue ulcerations. Mucosa thickness, another important predictor of exaggerated tissue response, should be considered. The anterior commisures of the mouth and the medial surface of the angle of the mandible are sites which contain very thin mucosa and would benefit from field blocks if possible

2. Lack of saliva and damaged taste buds may alter the sensation of taste during radiotherapy. Often, patients complain that many foods taste excessively salty which may reduce the motivation for adequate oral intake. In response to their altered taste sensation, patients tend to compensate by increasing their intake of sugar

3. Increased risk of dental caries. However, altered taste sensorium is a transient phenomenon since the taste buds recover in two to four months post therapy.

Q20 Name oral changes in AIDS patients.

Ans.

Oral Hairy Leukoplakia

- Lesion is characterized by an asymptomatic poorly demarcated keratotic area ranging in size from few millimeters to centimeters

- Characteristic vertical striations imparting a corrugated appearance are present on the surface which may be shaggy or may appear hairy when dried
- The lesion cannot be rubbed off. Diagnosis of HL is an indication of both HIV infection and immunodeficiency; it is an indication for a work-up to evaluate and treat HIV disease. HL correlates with a statistical risk for more rapid progression of HIV disease.

Oral Candidiasis

- *Pseudomembranous candidiasis:* Present as painless or slightly sensitive white lesion that can be readily scraped off and separated from surface of oral mucosa, Site: soft and hard palate, buccal mucosa
- *Erythematous candidiasis:* Appear as red patches on buccal or palatal mucosa, there will be depapillation of tongue
- *Hyperplastic candidiasis:* Seen in buccal mucosa and tongue, it is more resistant to removal
- *Angular chelitis:* Commissures of lip appear erythematous with surface crusting and fissuring
  Fungal infection: Cryptococcus neoformans is also common in HIV.

Kaposi's Sarcoma (KS)

Oral cavity may be the first site of lesion. 71% develop lesions of the oral Mucosa palate and gingival and then the lesion develops in lower extremity.

- In early stages: oral lesions are painless, reddish purple macules on the mucosa. As the lesions progress, it becomes nodular and can be easily confused with other oral vascular entities such as hematoma, hemangioma, varicosity or pyogenic granuloma
- Lesions manifest as nodules, papules or non-elevated muscles that are usually blown, blue or purple in colour.

Bacillary (Epithelioid) Angiomatosis

- This is an infectious vascular proliferative disease with clinical and histologic features very similar to those of KS
- Gingival bacillary angiomatosis manifests as red pimple or blue edematous soft tissue lesions that may cause destruction of periodontal ligament and bone.

Oral Hyperpigmentation
Atypical Ulcers and Delayed Healing

Recurrent herpetic lesions and aphthous stomatitis. Herpes involve all mucosal surfaces and does not heal within 7–10 days but persists for months.

Periodontal Disease

HIV gingivitis: A persistent linear, easily bleeding erythematous gingivitis.

HIV Periodontitis: A necrotizing ulcerative, rapidly progressive form of periodontitis occurs more frequently among HIV patients

Oral Histoplasmosis
Non Hodgkin's lymphoma
Salivary Gland Enlargement

5 RGUHS September 2000

QUESTION PAPER

Long Essays

1. Enumerate "Sexually transmitted diseases". Describe in detail oral changes in AIDS. Add a note on cross-infection in dental clinic.
2. Enumerate periapical lesions and describe in detail periapical cyst and abscess.

Short Essays

3. Describe radiographic appearance of ameloblastoma.
4. Write briefly about radiation protection for patients.
5. Osteoradionecrosis
6. Describe clinical features of Plummer-Vinson syndrome.
7. Describe clinical feature and management of denture sore mouth
8. Describe clinical features of Steven Johnsons syndrome.
9. Give the treatment plan of pemphigus vulgaris
10. Give the treatment plan of ANUG

Short Answers

11. Name the indications of "True Occlusal View"
12. Name the indications of "Trans Orbital View"
13. Explain why sequestrum appears more radiopaque than adjacent bone.
14. Name the anatomical landmarks seen on upper posterior periapical film.
15. Name the causes of very dark radiographs.
16. Why corticosteroid is given in certain cases of herpes zoster.
17. Name systemic conditions which predispose the patients to inflammator gingival enlargements.
18. Name the types of recurrent aphthous stomatitis
19. State the purpose of toluidine blue test.
20. State the functions of lead/tin foil in dental X-ray film packet.

LONG ESSAYS

Q1 Enumerate "Sexually transmitted diseases". Describe in detail oral changes in AIDS. Add a note on cross-infection in dental clinic.

Ans.

Sexually Transmitted Diseases

The infections acquired exclusively through sexual intercourse and those for which sexual transmission is frequent enough to be considered a public health problem.

Bacterial and Chlamydial STD'S (potentially curable; rarely blood borne)

- Gonorrhea and related clinical syndromes (Urethirtis, Cervicitis, Salpingitis, Pelvic inflammatory disease Bacteremia, Disseminated Systemic infection, arthritis, proctitits, Pharyngitis)
- Non and post Gonococcal urethritis and related clinical syndromes
- Syphilis and other treponemal infections
- Chancroid
- Granuloma inguinale
- Limphogranuloma venereum
- "Gay Bowel Syndrome" associated with enteric pathogens.

Viral STDs

- Herpes simplex virus infection
- Infectious mononucleosis
- Cytomegalovirus infection
- Viral Hepatitis – Hepatitis A, B, C, D, E, F and G
- Human immunodeficiency virus infections and acquired immunodeficiency syndromes
- T-cell Lymphoma and Leukemia
- Warts condyloma acuminatum and papilloma virus infections
- Molluscum contagiosum.

Miscellaneous Bacterial, Fungal and Parasitic Infections which manifest as STD's

- Vulvovaginal candidiasis
- Trichomoniasis
- Vaginitis, Cervicitis, cystitis, pyelonephritis, peurperal and neonatal sepsis
- Bacterial Vaginosis
- Intestinal protozoal infections.
  {Refered from Shafers}

Oral changes in AIDS

Common Oral Conditions

Caries and dry mouth: Some medications used by people with HIV and even HIV itself may cause decreased salivary flow, or dry mouth, which is known to contribute to rampant caries.

Periodontal disease: Necrotizing ulcerative periodontitis (NUP) is a condition associated with rapid soft tissue and bone loss, including exposure of the bone; rapid deterioration of tooth attachment; and the premature loss of teeth.

Human papillomavirus: Human papillomavirus (HPV), the virus associated with genital and other warts, is one of the most common sexually transmitted infections. HPV-associated lesions frequently occur in the oral cavity, including the lip and sides of the tongue. They are usually raised, dull white and fleshy, smooth or rough, and may have a cauliflower-like appearance.

Conditions Found More Often in People with HIV

Oral candidiasis, Aphthous stomatitis, Herpes simplex.

Conditions Found Primarily in People with HIV

Oral Hairy Leukoplakia, Opportunistic Tumors

Oral lesions in HIV-infected patient's include oral candidiasis, oral hairy leukoplakia, atypical periodontal diseases, Kaposi's sarcoma and oral Hodgkin's lymphoma.

1. **Oral hairy leukoplakia**
   Clinical Feature
   Site-lateral borders of tongue, it has bilateral distribution and may extend to the ventrum.
   - Lesion is characterized by an asymptomatic poorly demarcated keratotic area ranging in size from few millimeters to centimeters
   - Characteristic vertical striations imparting a corrugated appearance are present on the surface which may be shaggy or may appear hairy when dried.
   - The lesion cannot be rubbed off.

2. *Oral candidiasis*
   Clinical feature:
   - *Pseudomembranous candidiasis:* Present as painless or slightly sensitive white lesion that can be readily scraped off and separated from surface of oral mucosa. Site: Soft and hard palate, buccal mucosa
   - *Erythematous candidiasis:* Appear as red patches on buccal or palatal mucosa, there will be depapillation of tongue.
   - Hyperplastic Candidiasis: Seen in buccal mucosa and tongue, it is more resistant to removal
   - *Angular chelitis:* Commissures of lip appear erythematous with surface crusting and fissuring.

3. *Kaposi's Sarcoma (KS)*
   - It is a rare multifocal vascular neoplasm occurring in the skin of lower extremities
   - It is a malignant tumor in its classical form and localized and slowly growing lesion. Oral cavity may be the first site of lesion. 71% develop lesions of the oral Mucosa palate and gingival
   - In early stages: Oral lesions are painless, reddish purple macules on the mucosa
   - As the lesions progress, it becomes nodular and can be easily confused with other oral vascular entities such as hematoma, hemangioma, varicosity or pyogenic granuloma
   - Lesions manifest as nodules, papules or non-elevated muscles that are usually blown, blue or purple in colour.

4. *Bacillary (Epithelioid) angiomatosis*
   - This is an infectious vascular proliferative disease with clinical and histologic features very similar to those of KS
   - Skin lesions are similar to those seen in KS or Cat scratch disease
   - Gingival bacillary angiomatosis manifests as red pimple or blue edematous soft tissue lesions that may cause destruction of periodontal ligament and bone.

5. *Oral hyperpigmentation*
   Oral pigmented areas often appear as spots or striations on the buccal mucosa, palate, gingiva or tongue

6. Atypical ulcers and delayed healing Recurrent herpetic lesions and aphthous stomatitis. Herpes involve all mucosal surfaces and does not heal within 7–10 days but persists for months

7. *Periodontal disease*
   HIV gingivitis: A persistent linear, easily bleeding erythematous gingivitis. The

gingival (gum) condition originally known as HIV-gingivitis, and now called linear gingival erythema (LGE), consists of a red band-like lesion along the gumline. LGE may be painful and bleed, and may progress to periodontal disease

- *HIV Periodontitis:* A necrotizing ulcerative, rapidly progressive form of periodontitis occurs more frequently among HIV patients, AIDS virus associated periodontitis. One particularly severe form (necrotizing ulcerative periodontitis) and a related condition (linear gingival erythema) appear to be unique to those with compromised immune systems

8. Oral histoplasmosis
9. Non Hodgkin's lymphoma
10. Salivary gland enlargement.

Cross Infection in Dental Clinic

Some sexually transmitted infections like all systemic infections are of professional concern to the dentist.

- Inadvertent contact between the dentist's finger and organisms present in the patients blood or saliva could conceivably lead to non-venereal infections in which organisms could enter the dentist's tissue by percutaneous or mucosal routes and lead to cross- infections

- *Among hospital-patient's and personnel:* cross infections and routes of transmission come directly under the scrutiny of physicians, nurses and surviellance of infection control personnel

- *Patient and personnel vulnerability:* When dental personnel get exposed to saliva, blood, and possible injury from sharp instrumentation while treating patients, they are more vulnerable to infections if they have not had the proper immunization or used the proper protective barriers.

Infection Control in Dental Clinic

- Develop clean habits-Wash hands before and after attending each patients
- Prevent cuts on your hands; if present use water occlusive dressing and use rubber gloves
- Health care workers with open skin lesions, wounds, weeping skin should refrain from looking after these patients.

Instrument Sterilization

- Only sterilized instruments should be used
- Needle stick and sharp injuries
- Only disposable needle and syringes should be used
- Infected waste should be discarded carefully
- Barriers; Use of gloves, masks, eye protection is strongly recommended
- Surfaces with potential for contamination as chairs, head rest, trays, switches, handles should be cleaned.
  {Refered from Studevent}

Q2 Enumerate periapical lesions and describe in detail periapical cyst and abscess.

Ans.

Classification of Periapical Lesions

Radiolucent Lesions

1. Acute apical periodontitis
2. Chronic apical periodontitis
3. Periapical abscess
4. Periapical granuloma.

Radiopaque Lesions

1. Rarefying osteitis
2. Sclerosing osteitis/focal sclerosing osteitis.

Classification of Periradicular Lesions

1. Acute periradicular diseases
   Acute alveolar abscess

Acute apical periodontitis
- Vital
- Non-vital.

2. Chronic periradicular diseases with areas of rarefaction
- Chronic alveolar abscess
- Granuloma
- Radicular Cyst
- Condensing osteitis
- External root resorption.

Classification of Periapical Cyst

(Apical periodontal cyst, root end cyst, Radicular Cyst)

- This is a sequelae of periapical granuloma. Originating as a result of bacterial infection and necrosis of the dental pulp, nearly always following carious involvement of the tooth
- It is true cyst as the lesion consists of pathologic cavity that is lined by epithelium and is often fluid filled
- *Pathogenesis:* This type of periodontal cyst exhibits a lumen that is lined by stratified squamous epithelium, while wall is made up of condensed connective tissue.

Clinical Features

1. Periapical cyst develops at the apex of the non-vital tooth
2. The tooth will often have a deep carious lesion, large restoration, or endodontic filling
3. Patient may not have any discomfort at the site of lesion
4. They tend to remain small but occasionally will cause a painless bony expansion. The expansion is labial or buccal in mandible or palatal in maxilla
5. It may be bony hard if cortex is intact, crepitant as the bone thins, or rubbery and fluctuant if the bone is destroyed
6. The cyst of long standing may undergo an acute exacerbation of inflammatory process

and develop rapidly into an abscess that may then proceed to cellulitis or from a draining fistula.

Radiographic Features

1. Radiolucent rounded or pear shaped unilocular lesion more than 1cm in diameter
2. The borders of the lesion are generally well defined and may or may not be eradicated
3. When a border is corticated, the radiopaque image will be continuous with the lamina dura around the associated root
4. The periapical cysts in posterior maxilla may extend into sinus and elevate its floor.

Management

1. Excision through extraction
2. Curettage
3. Endodontic therapy and Apical surgery
4. If the cyst is large, marsupilization is done.

Periapical Abscess

- It is an acute or chronic suppurative process of the dental periapical region. It usually arises as result of infection following carious involvement of tooth and pulp infection resulting in necrosis of pulp
- Abscess may develop directly as an acute apical periodontitis following an acute pulpitis.

Clinical Features

1. Acute periapical abscess presents the feature of an acute inflammation of apical peridontium
2. The tooth is extremely painful and is slightly extruded from its socket
3. As long as this abscess is confined to the immediate periapical region there is seldom severe systemic manifestation although regional lymphadentitis and fever may be present
4. Rapid extension to bone marrow spaces frequently occurs producing an actual osteomyelitis

5. Chronic periapical abscess presents no clinical feature since it is mild. Well circumscribed area of suppuration, that shows little tendency to spread from local area.

Radiographic Features

- Acute periapical abscess shows slight thickening of periodontal membrane
- In chronic cases, developing periapical granuloma presents radiolucent area at apex of tooth.

Treatment

Drainage must be established by either opening the pulp chamber or extracting the tooth. Root canal therapy can be carried out.

SHORT ESSAYS

Q3 Describe radiographic appearance of ameloblastoma.

Ans.

Refer to Q2 in March 2000

Q4 Write briefly about radiation protection for patients.

Ans.

Despite the low risks to the patient from dental radiography, it is best to keep exposure to ionizing radiation to a minimum. Therefore, the ALARA concept should be kept in mind when exposing dental films. This can be done by

1. *Film selection:* Fast film should be used. Only the type 'E' or the Ektaspeed is recommended in dental practice to-day, since it reduces the exposure by at least 40% as compared to type 'D'
2. *Intensifying screens:* For extra oral films, lateral cephalogram, OPG, lateral oblique, etc. use of rare earth screens has reduced the dosage definitively
3. *Grids:* Use of grids reduces the fogginess of film due to secondary radiation, thereby reducing the need for repeat films
4. *X-ray machines:* Only the units which are manufactured by reputed companies should be used
5. *Kilovoltage:* Using an X-ray beam with low kilovoltage results in higher patient doses, primarily to the skin. They do not reach the film and therefore do not contribute to the diagnostic image. Units should be operated using at least 60–90 kVp
6. *Filtration:* Units operating at 70 kVp or above should have filtration equivalent to 2.5 mm of aluminum. This removes the low energy X-rays from the beam and reduces radiation exposure
7. *X-ray collimation:* The beam should be collimated so that it is no more than 7 cm in diameter at patients face
8. *Position-indicating devices:* Open-ended, circular or rectangular lead lined cylinders are preferred for directing the X-ray beam. PID will reduce exposure to patient
9. *Film holding devices:* Leads to more stable positioning of the film
10. Proper processing is must, to avoid retakes.

Q5 Osteoradionecrosis

Ans.

Definition

Osteoradionecrosis refers to an inflammatory condition of bone (Osteomyelitis) that occurs often after the bone has been exposed to therapeutic doses of radiation usually given for the treatment of malignancy of head and neck region.

Clinical Features

- The mandible is much more commonly affected than the maxilla
- This is likely due to the microanatomy and reduced vasculature of this bone
- The posterior mandible is affected more often than the anterior portion

- Loss of mucosal covering and exposure of bone is the hallmark of osteoradionecrosis
- Pathologic fracture also may occur
- The exposed bone become necrotic as a result of loss of vascularity from the periosteum and subsequently sequestrates, often leading to exposure of more bone
- Intense pain may occur, with intermittent swelling and drainage extra orally.

Radiographic Features

Location

Mandible is more affected.

Periphery

It is ill defined and similar to that in osteo-myelitis. If the lesion reaches the inferior border of mandible, irregular resorbtion of this bony cortex often occurs.

Internal Structure

A bone formation to bone destruction occurs, with balance heavily towards more bone formation, giving the affected bone an overall sclerotic or radiopaque appearance.

Effects on surrounding Structures

Inflammatory periosteal new bone formation is uncommon, because of the deleterious effects of radiation on potential osteoblasts in the periosteum.

Management

Decortication with sequestrectomy and hyperbaric oxygen with antibiotics have shown limited success because of poor healing after surgery.

Conservative Treatment

Maintain the integrity of lower border of mandible and to keep the site free of infection and patient free of pain.

Q6 Describe clinical features of Plummer-Vinson syndrome.

Ans.

Refer to Q1 of September 1998.

Q7 Describe clinical feature and management of denture sore mouth.

Ans.

Refer Q3.1 of MAR 1999.

Q8 Describe clinical features of Steven's-Johnson syndrome.

Ans.

Stevens-Johnson syndrome is a severe vesiculobullous forms of the disease erythema multiforme (EM) Generalized vesicles and bullae involve the skin, mouth, eye and genitals in EM.

Etiology

Inflammatory conditions due to Autoimmune reactions
- Viral infections may trigger EM
- Drug intake (Barbiturates, phenylbutazone, digitalis, iodides, mercurials, birth control pills)
- Vaccination
- Radiation therapy
- Crohn's disease.

Clinical Features

- Erythema multiforme
- Stevens Johnson Syndrome
- Oral mucous membrane lesions
- Eye lesions
- Keratoconjunctivitis sicca
- Genital lesions.

Q9 Give the treatment plan of pemphigus vulgaris

Ans.

The pemphigus vulgaris is treated by early diagnosis and lower doses of medication can be used for shorter periods of time to control the diseases.

Treatment Plan of Pemphigus Vulgaris

a. High doses of systemic corticosteroids given in dosages of 1–2 mg/kg/day

b. When steroids are used for long period of time adjuvants such as azathioprine or cyclophosphamide are added to the regimen to reduce complications of long-term corticosteroids

c. Prednisone–used in low doses as maintainance therapy

d. Oral pemphigus is treated by combining topical with systemic steroid therapy, either by allowing the prednisone tablets to dissolve slowly in the mouth before swallowing or by using potent topical steroid creams

e. *Other therapies*
   1. Parenteral gold therapy
   2. Dapsone
   3. Tetracycline
   4. Plasmapheresis–used in patients, refractory to corticosteroids.

Q10 Give the treatment plan of ANUG

Ans.

Treatment Plan

i. Alleviation of acute inflammation plus treatment of chronic disease either underlying the acute involvement or elsewhere in the oral cavity

ii. Alleviation of generalized toxic symptoms such as fever and malaise

iii. Correction of systemic conditions that contribute to initiation or progress of gingival changes

1. The acutely involved areas are isolated with cotton rolls and dried.
   - A topical anesthetic is applied
   - Supragingival scaling is done
   - Patient is told to rinse mouth every 2 hours with a glassful of an equal mixture of warm water and 3% Hydrogen Peroxide
   - Twice daily with 0.12% Chlorhexidine are also effective
   - Patient is instructed to avoid tobacco, smoking, alcohol

2. Patient with moderate or severe ANUG and local lymphadenopathy or other systemic symptoms are placed on an antibiotic regimen. Systemic antibiotics
   a. Penicillin 250/500 mg orally every 6 hrs
   b. For penicillin–sensitive patients Erythromycin 250/500 mg every 6 hours
   c. Metronidazole–250/500 mg three times daily for 7 days

Contouring of gingiva as an adjunctive procedures in cases of severe gingival necrosis.

Topical drug therapy is only an adjunctive measure.

Escharotic drugs–phenol, silver nitrate and chronic acid should not be used as they may cause necrosis and destroy nerve endings.

3. *Oxygen liberating agents:* Hydrogen peroxide
4. *Mercurial derivatives:* Tincture nitromersol 1: 200
5. *Spirocheticides:* Sodium carbonate 10% aqueous solution
6. *Aniline dyes:* Gentian violet
7. Others: Vancomycin/surgical pack.

Supportive systemic treatment
- Copious fluid consumption
- Administration of analgesics for relief of pain
- Bed rest is necessary for patients with toxic systemic complications

Nutritional supplements
- Intake of water soluble vitamin B and C
- Patient is placed on a balanced diet.

SHORT ANSWERS

Q11 Name the indications of "True Occlusal View"

Ans.

Various radiographic techniques are employed in imaging the unerupted maxillary canine tooth (Figs 5.1 and 5.2).

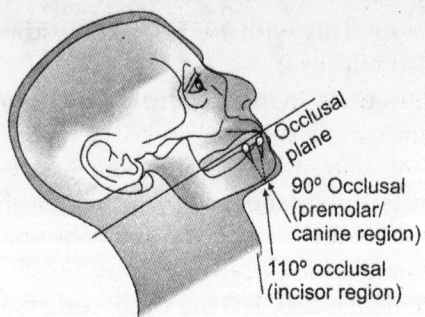

Fig. 5.1: Taking a true occlusal view of the lower jaw for the canine/premolar region and for the incisor region

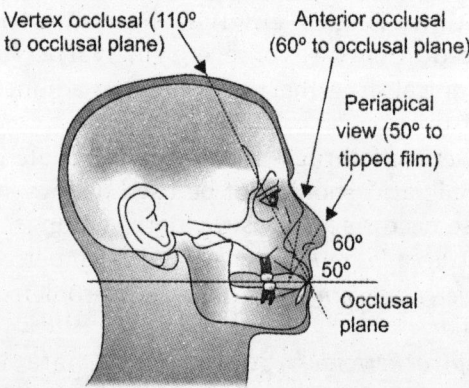

Fig. 5.2: incisor inclination, film position, and central X-ray beam, differentiating the periapical view, the anterior (oblique) occlusal view, and the true vertex occlusal view

This describes an extraoral technique in imaging the maxillary dentition in the superoinferior aspect. The radiograph obtained is very similar to the conventional vertex/true occlusal radiograph. A marked reduction in radiation dose is achieved with this new technique.

- It is useful in orthodontic treatment of impacted tooth
- To view the dentigerous cyst associated with impacted tooth
- True occlusal view acts as complement to the per apical film when tooth displacement is severe.

Technique of taking true occlusal view

True Occlusal View for mandibular arch

Lower canine or premolar region should depict all the posterior standing teeth in cross-section, and as such, and also provide bucco-lingual positional information of tooth and any associated structure in the plane at 90 degree to that seen on the peri apical film.

For anterior mandible: Head need to be tipped back further and the tube positioned at symphisis menti, at an angle of 110° to the horizontal, in line with long axis of the incisor teeth.

True occusal view of anterior maxilla is a view in which the central of the X-ray beam runs parallel to the long axis of the central incisors.

Q12 Name the indications of "Trans Orbital View"

Ans.

The conventional frontal TMJ projection in delineating the joint with minimal superimpositions is transorbital projection.

- Transorbital view produces relatively true frontal projection of condyle and a major portion of condylar neck
- It demonstrates convex articulating surface of condyle and the slightly concave or flat, broad ridge of articular eminence
- Indicated when tomography is not available
- Indicated in TMJ disorders, trauma
- Significant dysfunction or alteration in range of motion, sensory or motor alterations, or significant changes in occlusion

Also refer Q5 of OCT 1999.

Q13 Explain why sequestrum appears more radiopaque than adjacent bone.

Ans.

A sequestrum is a piece of dead bone that has become separated during the process of *necrosis* from normal/sound bone.

It is a complication (sequela) of *osteomyelitis*. The pathological process is as follows:

- Infection in the bone leads to an increase in *intramedullary* pressure due to inflammatory exudates
- The *periosteum* becomes stripped from the osteum, leading to vascular thrombosis bone necrosis follows due to lack of blood supply sequestra are formed.

An X-ray of a child's femur showing a bony sequestrum highlighted by the arrow (Fig. 5.3).

The sequestra are surrounded by sclerotic bone which is relatively avascular (without a blood supply). Within the bone itself, the *haversian canals* become blocked with scar tissue, and the bone becomes surrounded by thickened periosteum.

Due to the avascular nature of this bone, antibiotics which travel to sites of infection via the bloodstream poorly penetrate these tissues. Hence the difficulty in treating chronic osteomyelitis.

In cases of infections and inflammation of jaws of facial bone such as osteomyelitis sequestrum is formed by detachment of segments of necrotic bone. The sequestra is more radiopaque as there is irregular calcification of bone. The sequestra are usually more dense and better defined with a sharper outline than the surrounding vital bone.

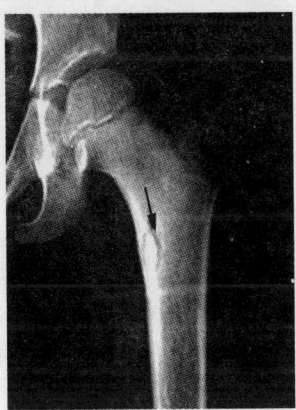

Fig. 5.3: Child's femur showing a bony sequestrum

a. Their increased density is the result of sclerosis
b. Also the inflammatory reaction probably stimulates the demineralization of vital bone surrounding the sequestra, there by enhancing the contrast.

Q14 Name the anatomical landmarks seen on upper posterior periapical film.

Ans.

Normal anatomic landmarks seen in upper periapical radiographs: Images of distal half of the second premolar, the three maxillary permanent molars, and some of the tuberosity, zygomatic arch

Radiolucencies seen in maxillary radiographs

1. *Intermaxillary suture:* Thin radiolucent line in the midline between two portions of premaxilla
2. *Nasal fossa:* It appears as a radiolucent image which lies above the oral cavity
3. *Incisive foramen:* It is oral terminus of nasopalatine canal. It may appear smoothly symmetric between the regions of roots
4. Superior foramina of nasopalatine canal-openings are on each side of nasal septum close to the antero inferior border of nasal cavity
5. *Lateral fossa:* Gentle depression in maxilla near apex of the lateral incisor appear as diffuse radiolucent
6. *Nasolacrimal canal:* It is found above apex of canine on the region of molars
7. *Maxillary sinus:* It is air containing cavity lined with mucous membrane. It is considered as a 3-sided pyramid with base, medial wall adjacent to nasal cavity and apex extending laterally to zygomatic process of maxilla

Radiopacities seen in maxillary radiographs

1. Anterior nasal spine is located in midline 1.5–2.0 cm above alveolar crest

2 Zygomatic process and zygomatic bone: This is an extension of lateral maxillary surface that arises in the region of apices of the first and second molars

3. *Nasolabial fold:* An oblique line demarcating a region that appears to be covered by a veil of slight radiopacity frequently transverses periapical radiographs of premolar region

4. *Pterygoid plates:* The mesial and lateral pterygoid plate lie posterior to tuberosity of maxilla.

Q15 Name the causes of very dark radiographs.

Ans.

Refer Q4 in March 1999.

Q16 Why corticosteroid is given in certain cases of herpes zoster.

Ans.

Herpes zoster is caused due to varicella zoster a DNA virus which becomes reactivated in some individuals causing lesions.

Combined antiviral and corticosteroid therapy for uncomplicated herpes zoster Steroids should not be given alone (without antiviral therapy) due to concern about promotion of viral replication. The effect of steroids on the incidence of secondary skin infection is unknown. Corticosteroids are given in cases of Herpes zoster to reduce the inflammation and thereby to decrease the rate of morbidity. The benefit of steroids included accelerated healing of lesions and more rapid resolution of acute pain.

In patient's over 60 years corticosteroids should be administered to prevent or minimize the occurence of post herpetic neuralgia.

Q17 Name systemic conditions which predispose the patients to inflammatory gingival enlargements.

Ans.

"Conditioned gingival enlargement" occurs when systemic conditions of the patient exaggerates or distorts the usual gingival response to dental plaque

- Hormonal–pregnancy, puberty
- Nutrition–associated with Vitamin C deficiency
- Allergic
- Systemic diseases causing gingival enlargement
- Leukemia
- Granulomatous diseases
- Sarcoidosis.

{Referred from Carranza Periodontia Text}

Q18 Name the types of recurrent aphthous stomatitis

Ans.

Classification

Aphthous ulcers are classified according to the diameter of the lesion.

1. *Minor ulceration*

   "Minor aphthous ulcers" indicate that the lesion size is between 3 mm (0.1 in)–10 mm (0.4 in). The appearance of the lesion is that of an erythematous halo with yellowish or grayish color. Extreme pain is the obvious characteristic of the lesion. When the ulcer is white or grayish, the ulcer will be extremely painful and the affected lip may swell. They may last about 1 week

2. *Major ulcerations*

   Major aphthous ulcers have the same appearance as minor ulcerations, but are greater than 10 mm in diameter and are extremely painful. They usually take more than a month to heal, and frequently leave a scar. These typically develop after puberty with frequent recurrences. They occur on movable non-keratinizing oral surfaces, but the ulcer borders may extend onto keratinized surfaces. They may last about 10 to 14 days

3. *Herpetiform ulcerations*

This is the most severe form. It occurs more frequently in females, and onset is often in adulthood. It is characterized by small, numerous, 1–3 mm lesions that form clusters. They typically heal in less than a month without scarring. Supportive treatment is almost always necessary

4. Recurrent ulcer associated with Behcet's syndrome.

Q19 State the purpose of Toluidine blue test.

Ans.

Indications

- To diagnose early carcinomatous or premalignant lesions such as leukoplakia, erythroplakia
- To differentiate between different inflammatory and dysplastic disorders
- Lesions, which are not indicated for biopsy. Composition of Toluidine Blue Solution
- Toluidine Blue 1 gm
- Acetic Acid 10 cc
- Absolute Alcohol 4.2 cc
- Distilled water 86 cc
- The pH is adjusted to 4.5.

Procedure

- Isolate and dry the area which has lesions
- Apply 1% acetic acid with camel hair brush
- Wait for 20 sec and rinse with water
- Apply Toluidine blue solution 1% with fresh brush
- Wait for 10–20 sec
- Decolorize with 2% acetic acid
- Apply Lugol's iodine solution
- Area is photographed and biopsy is planned.

Disadvantage

False negative and false positive results are common. So biopsy is necessary for confirmation.

Q20 State the functions of lead/tin foil in dental X-ray film packet.

Ans.

- The X-ray film packet has a thin lead foil backing between the wrappers
- The lead/tin foil layer is included in the film packet on the back side of the film away from tube to shield the film from back scattered (secondary) radiation, which would fog the film
- It may also effect slight reaction in patient exposure
- Additional Information

(If the film is placed back wards in patients mouth so the tube side of the film is not facing the tube, the lead foil will be positioned between the object and film. This will cause much of the radiation intended for the film to be absorbed by the lead foil, resulting in the light image).

RGUHS March 2001

QUESTION PAPER

Long Essays

1. How will you diagnose carcinoma of tongue? Mention the treatment planning for carcinoma of tongue?

2. Enumerate periapical radiolucencies and radiopacities. How would you diagnose systemic diseases with periapical changes in radiographs?

Short Essays

3. Moth-eaten appearance.
4. Pyogenic granuloma.
5. Potter bucky diaphragm.
6. Smear examination for candida albicans.
7. Liths in orotacial region.
8. Pain in migraine and periodic migranous neuralgia.
9. Drugs to relieve muscular spasm.
10. Myofacial pain dysfunction syndrome.

Short Answers

11. Café-au-lait spots.
12. Alkaline phosphatase.
13. Verruccous Carcinoma.
14. HIV.
15. Hairy tongue.
16. Age in examination.
17. Multilocular cyst.
18. PUS
19. Focal sepsis.
20. Target Lesion

LONG ESSAYS

Q1 How will you diagnose carcinoma of tongue? Mention the treatment planning for carcinoma of tongue.

Ans.

Diagnosis of Carcinoma of Tongue

1. Carcinoma of tongue is diagnosed by proper case and clinical examination.

   a. *Site:* Carcinoma of tongue is most common in the anterior 2/3rds of tongue at or near the edges.

   b. Growth itself

   - Carcinomatous ulcer of tongue looks irregular in shape with typical raised and everted edge, yellowish gray slough on the floor and thin serous discharge

   - Papilliferous or warty carcinoma looks like a papilloma which is usually pallor than surrounding epithelium. The base is broad and firm and invaded edge is indistinct

   - Carcinomatous lump is oval in shape with long axis parallel to long axis of tongue. Its surface is irregular; the edge is indistinct and consistency is hard.

   c. Examination of lymph nodes.

   Particularly the submandibular, submental and jugulodigastric groups are enlarged due to secondary infection of growth.

2. Radiography and lateral soft tissue films-Demonstrate extent of tumor infiltration in oropharynx.

3. *CT scan:* Define the degree of oropharyngeal adnexal tissue involvement with advanced lesions.

4. *MRI (Magnetic resonance imaging)*
   - Used preoperatively to define lingual tumor boundaries

   - Degree of vascularity to the tumor can be known and proximity of these tumors to large vessels and other anatomic structures.

5. Radionucleotide scanning

   Gallium 67 scanning has 89% specificity, but a tumor size threshold of at least 2 cm is required. It has limited resolution

6. Frozen section examination of margins of tissues prior to surgery.

TNM Staging

Carcinoma of tongue – Jacobson's malignancy grading system that asserts tumor cell population and tumor host relationship.

Site – Tumor – Node – Metastases – Pathology (STNMP)

Treatment Planning of Carcinoma Tongue

Treatment of carcinoma of tongue can be divided into

A. Treatment of primary growth.

B. Treatment of secondary lymph nodes.

1. T1 and small T2 categories: Early carcinoma of tongue respond equally well to treatment by surgical excision, partial glossectomy or radiation

   Prognosis 50–70% patients who are adequately treated survive and 25% of patients in this category die from the disease and extent of tumor spread may not be apparent without surgery

   Aggressive surgical treatment is recommended

2. Early lingual carcinoma/carcinoma in-situ

   - Occult regional metastasis to cervical nodes from T1 carcinomas of anterior tongue-elective surgical or radiation treatment of regional nodes

   - Small lesions of posterior tongue-Partial glossectomy is done

- Disadvantage is Speech impairment
- Irradiation
- Complications of irradiation are late effect of radiation, xerostomia, osteoradone-crosis, secondary radiation induced tumors, increased frequency of recurrences at primary site with radiation versus surgical treatment

3. Advanced T3 Stage Lingual Carcinoma
   Combined surgical and radiation therapy
   Prognosis-Poor
4. Carcinoma of anterior 2/3rd with evidence of node involvement may require–radical neck dissection
   - Partial mandibulectomy
   - Intraoral dissection (Commando operation)
5. Carcinoma of base of tongue
   Combined surgery and radiation.
   Two modes of treatment.

Surgery

a. If the growth is less than 1 cm in diameter the growth is removed along with a wide margin of mucosa of not less than 1 cm
   This excised growth should be sent for histopathological examination. Monthly follow–up should be continued
b. In case of larger growth preliminary treatment should be radiotherapy. In case where radiotherapy fails and growth is localized partial glossectomy or subtotal glossectomy is carried out
c. When growth reaches within 2 cm of the jaw, Hemimandibulectomy is required along with excision of growth.

Radiotherapy

a. When growth is more than 1 cm in diameter in anterior 2/3rd: Interstitial radiotherapy
b. Teletherapy-Cobalt 60 unit is used in posterior 1/3rd of the tongue
c. If large tumor with palpable nodes: Both primary lymphnodes and neck are irradiated to 4500 rads. Then 6–8 units later excision is carried out in continuity. (Commando operation).

Chemotherapy

Regional intra-arterial administration of a cytotoxic drug, e.g.
Treatment of Secondary lymph nodes –
a. If lymph nodes are palpable and secondarily involved by metastasis: Block dissection

Block Dissection

Sometimes Block dissection may be performed along with hemiglossectomy and this is called Commando operation
b. When enlarged lymph nodes are fixed and cannot be excised, deep radiation therapy is employed.

Q2 Enumerate periapical radiolucencies and radiopacities. How would you diagnose systemic diseases with periapical changes in radiographs?
Ans.

Periapical Lesions Showing Radiolucencies and Radiopacities

Radiolucent Lesions

- Dental granuloma
- Radicular cyst
- Residual cyst
- Periapical cyst
- Apical scar
- Cementoma (first stage).

Radiopaque Lesions

- Cementoma
- Compound odontoma
- Complex odontoma
- Ossifying fibroma
- Osteogenic sarcoma.

Diagnosis of systemic disease with periapical changes in radiographs.

Systemic disease and radiographic changes in Periapical region

1. *Hyperparathyroidism:* Endocrinal abnormality
   - Demineralization and thinning of cortical boundaries occur in jaws in cortical boundaries such as the inferior border, mandibular canal, and the the cortical outlines of maxillary sinus
   - A change in normal trabecular pattern result in ground–glass appearance of numerous, small, randomly oriented trabeculae Periapical radiographs reveal loss of lamina dura around one tooth or all the teeth
   - Brown tumors of hyperparathyrodism may appear in any bone. These lesions may be multiple with in a single bone.

2. *Hypoparathyroidism*
   Dental enamel hypoplasia, external root resorption, delayed eruption or root dilaceration.

3. *Hyperpituitarism*
   - Enlargement of jaws notably mandible
   - The increase in length of dental arches results in spacing of teeth
   - In Acromegaly, angle between ramus and body of mandible may increase. Thickness and height of alveolar processes may also increase
   - Roots of posterior teeth often enlarges as a result of hyper cementosis
   - Supra eruption of posterior teeth may occur.

4. *Hypopituitarism*
   - Jaws are small and result in crowding and malocclusion
   - Exfoliation of primary teeth is delayed by several years
   - Eruption of permanent teeth is delayed.

5. *Hyperthyroidism*
   - Early eruption and advanced rate of dental development
   - Premature loss of primary teeth
   - Generalized decrease in bone density.

6. *Hypothyroidism*
   - Delayed eruption, short roots, and thinning of the lamina dura
   - Maxilla and mandible are relatively small.

7. *Diabetes mellitus*
   Periodontal disease associated with diabetes leads to interdental bone loss and horizontal bone loss.

8. *Cushing's syndrome*
   Generalized osteoporosis which may have a granular bone pattern. The skull shows diffuse thinning
   - The teeth may erupt prematurely, and partial loss of lamina dura may occur.

9. *Osteoporosis*
   - Overall reduction in the density of bone
   - Periapically, lamina dura may appear thinner than normal.

10. *Rickets*
    - Within the cancellous portion of jaws, the trabeculae reduces in density, number and thickness
    - In severe cases, the jaws appear so radiolucent that the teeth appear to be bereft of bony support
    - Retarded root eruption in early rickets
    - Lamina dura and cortical boundary of tooth follicles may be thin or missing.

11. *Hypophosphatasia*
    - Inherited disorder that is caused by reduced production or defective function of alkaline phosphatase
    - Generalized radiolusceney of mandible and maxilla
    - The cortical bone and lamina dura are thin, alveolar bone is poorly calcified and may appear deficient

- Primary and permanent teeth have a thin enamel layer and large pulp chambers and root canals.

12. *Renal osteodystrophy (renal rickets)*
- Hypoplasia and hypocalcification of teeth are possible, resulting in loss of any radiographic evidence of enamel
- The lamina dura may be absent or less apparent in instances of bone sclerosis.

13. *Hypophosphatemia*
- Jaws are osteoporotic and radio lucent
- Teeth may be poorly formed, with thin enamel cusps and large pulp chambers and root canals
- Periapical rarefying osteitis
- If disease is severe, patient experiences premature loss of teeth
- The lamina dura may become sparse and cortical boundaries around tooth crypts may be thin or entirely absent.

14. *Osteopetrosis*
- Increased radiopacity of jaws
- Periapically even the roots of teeth may not be apparent
- The increased bone density and relatively poor vascularity results in susceptibility of mandible to osteomyelitis
- Delayed eruption, early tooth loss, missing teeth, malformed roots, crowns and poorly calcified teeth
- Lamina dura and cortical borders may appear thicker than normal.

15. *Progressive systemic sclerosis (scleroderma)*
- There will be an unusual pattern of mandibular erosions at regions of muscle attachment such as the angles, coronoid process, digastric region or condyles
- Periapical radiographs reveal an increase in the width of the periodontal ligament spaces around the teeth

- Periodontal ligament spaces are at least twice as thick as normal and both anterior and posterior teeth are affected
- The lamina dura remains normal.

16. *Sickle cell anemia:* It is an autosomal recessive, chronic hemolytic disorder. *Radiographic features:* General osteoporosis, decrease in volume of trabecular bone and thinning of cortical plates.
- Bone marrow hyperplasia a cause enlargement and protrusion of maxillary alveolar ridge.

17. *Thalassemia*
- Defect in hemoglobin synthesis
- Severe bone marrow hyperplasia prevents pneumatizations of paranasal sinuses, especially maxillary sinus and expansion of maxilla that results in malocclusion
- Jaws appear radiolucent, with thinning of cortical borders and enlargement of marrow spaces
- Lamina dura is thin, and the roots of teeth may be short.

SHORT ESSAYS

Q3 Moth-eaten appearance
Ans.

Moth-eaten appearance is seen in radiographic examination of malignant diseases of jaws. This is the diagnostic feature of some malignant tumors in radiographs in their advanced stages. Moth-eaten appearance or hair on end appearance or the ragged border in the surrounding structure is seen in the following diseases:

- Osteosarcoma
- Osteomyelitis
- Ewing's sarcoma
- Sickle cell anemia
- Thalassemia.

Pathogenesis

- Moth-eaten appearance is usually seen in Malignancy whose features are destructive, the effect on surrounding structures mirrors this behavior because malignant tumors tend to grow rapidly, they invade by means of easier routes, such as through maxillary antrum or through the periodontal ligament space around teeth, resulting in irregular widening with destruction of lamina dura
- They may also spread through inferior alveolar neurovascular canal, causing similar widening
- Usually there will be no periosteal reaction, some tumors stimulate unusual periosteal new bone formation
- Lesions such as osteosarcoma, as well as other tumors, can stimulate the formation of thin straight spicules of bone, giving a "hair on end" or "sun burst appearance" in their advanced stages.

Explanation of each condition

1. Osteogenic sarcoma

It is a malignant tumor consisting of cells and tissues in different stages of bone development. This may be osteoblastic/sclerosing type.

Clinical features: Pain and swelling of involved bone are early features. Mandibular area is more prone than maxilla.

Radiographic features: It has ill defined borders in most instances and it may be radiolucent, mixed radiolucent-radiopaque, or radiopaque. The internal osseous structure may take agranular or sclerotic –appearing bone, cotton balls.

If the lesion involves the periosteum directly or by extensions, typical 'sunray' or 'hair on end' appearance is seen.

2. Ewing's sarcoma

Clinical features: Pain is the chief complaint with the presence of swelling which fairly increases in size. It is inflammatory condition. Paraesthesia of lip and chin depends on the location. Metastasis may be through lymphatic or blood stream.

Radiographic features: It has a radiolucency that is poorly demarcated in early stages but in advancing stages, the bone is destroyed in an uneven fashion, resulting in ragged border.

Motheaten destructive radiolucency of medulla and erosion of cortex with expansion occurs with stimulation of periosteum resulting in gross disturbances of overlying periosteum and takes the form of Codman's triangle or hair-on-end appearance.

3. Osteomyelitis

Motheaten appearance is seen in chronic bone infections, or osteomyelitis, which tend to show channels of purulent material in bone. It often stimulates the periosteal new bone which is seen as radiopaque lines parallel to surface of cortical bone. Most lesions are composed of more radiopaque or sclerotic bone pattern.

In other cases small regions of radiolucency may be scattered through out the radiopaque bone.

4. Thalassemia

Radiographic Features:Hyperplasia of the ineffective bone marrow and its subsequent failure to produce normal red cells. The skull shows generalized granular appearance, and a hair-on-end effect may develop.

Q4 Pyogenic Granuloma
Ans.

Definition

Pyogenic granuloma is a distinctive clinical entity originating as a response of the tissue to a non-specific infection.

Etiology

1. Botryomycotic infection or staphylococci, streptococci infection

2. May arise from trauma to tissues, which provides a pathway for invasion of non-specific types of microorganisms into vascular endothelium.

Clinical Features

Site

- Gingiva, lips, tongue and buccal mucosa
- The lesion is usually elevated, pedunculated or sessile mass with a smooth, lobulated or even a warty surface which commonly is ulcerated and shows a tendency for hemorrhage, either spontaneously or upon slight trauma
- Some lesions have brown cast if hemorrhage has occurred into the tissue. Pyogenic granuloma may develop rapidly, reach full size and then remain static for indefinite period. The lesions may vary from few millimeters to centimeter or more in diameter.

Radiographic Features

A periapical granuloma also known as Pyogenic Granuloma is defined as a growth of granulomatous tissue continuous with the periodontal ligament resulting from death of pulp and diffusion of bacteria and bacterial toxins from root canal into the surrounding periradicular tissues through the apical and lateral foramina.

Radiographic Features

1. *Location:* Epicenter is at apex of involved tooth or at another region of tooth root
2. *Periphery:* The periphery of periapical granuloma is well defined, with a sharp transition zone. The area of rarefaction is well defined with lack of continuity of lamina dura
3. *Internal structure:* Radiolucency in the periapical region detectable of change in bone density, resulting in widening of periodontal ligament space
4. *Surrounding structure:* It is affected by resorption of bone and loss of lamina dura.

Histologic Features

- Pyogenic granuloma resembles granulation tissue except that it is exuberant and usually well localized
- The overlying epithelium is generally thin and atrophic
- There are vast numbers of endothelium lined vascular spaces and extreme proliferation of fibroblasts and budding endothelial cells
- There is infiltration of polymorphonuclear leukocytes lymphocytes and plasma cells.

Treatment and Prognosis

- Surgical excision
- The lesion occasionally recurs because it is not encapsulated
- When excising a pyogenic granuloma of the gingiva, extreme care should always be taken to scale the adjacent tooth and make certain that it is free of calculus, since calculus may act as the irritatant leading to recurrence of lesion.

Q5 Potter Bucky Diaphragm

Ans.

Potter Bucky Diaphragm (Fig. 6.1) reduces the white lead lines in the radiographic image. This is achieved by moving the grid sideways during exposure. Images of radiolucent grid lines on film can be deleted by moving the grid in direction of 90° to grid lines during exposure. This results in uniform exposure. It does not interfere with absorption of scattered photons. A moving grid is called as 'Bucky Grid'.

- It does not interfere with absorption of scattered photon
- This has effect of blurring out the radiolucent lines.

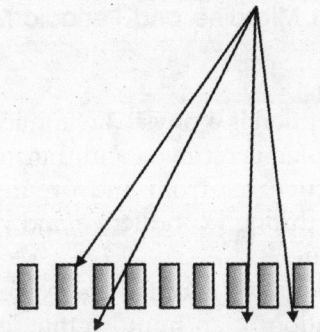

Fig. 6.1: Potter bucky diaphragm

Uses of Grids

- It reduces the amount of scattered radiations exciting a subject that reaches the film and results in more uniform exposure
- It removes scattered radiation
- It spares primary photons
- It reduces non-imaging exposure
- It increases subject contrast.

Q6 Smear examination for *Candida albicans*.

Ans.

Introduction

Candida albicans is a yeast like fungus which causes candidiasis. These organisms are common inhabitant of oral cavity, gastro-intestinal tract and vagina. There must be actual penetration of tissues with the organism and mere presence will not indicate the disease.

Candidiasis is an opportunistic infection. Oral candidiasis or thrush remains localized or may show extension to pharynx or even to lungs with fatal results.

Investigations

This include identification of predisposing factors, etiology and then laboratory diagnosis.
1. Collection of infected material from nail scrapings, mucous patches from mouth, etc.

2. Microscopic examination - Presence of mycelial forms indicate colonization and tissue invasion
3. Culture—Oval, budding cells, some pseudo-hyphae are seen.

Features

Rapid formation of hyphae, production of chlamydospores, fermentation and assimilation of sugars, nitrogen utilization, germ tube formation indicate candidial growth.

4. Smear examination
   - Fragments of the plaque material may be smeared on a microscopic slide, macerated with 20% potassium hydroxide and examined for typical hyphae
   - In addition the organism may be cultured in a variety of media, including blood agar, corn meal agar and sabouraud's broth, to aid in establishing the diagnosis
   - Histologic section of a biopsy from a lesion of oral candidiasis will show the presence of the yeast cells and hyphae or mycelia in superficial and deeper layers of involved epithelium.

These are more easily visualized if the sections are stained with periodic acid Schiff reagent (PAS) or methenamine silver, since the organism are positive in both instances.

Q7 Liths in Orofacial Region

Ans.

Sialolithiasis

This is the formation of a calcified structure within salivary duct leading to obstruction to salivary flow. The Liths can occur in:
- Submandibular gland - Warthon's duct (83% common)
- Sublingual gland - Bartholin's duct
- Parotid gland - Stenson's duct.

Clinical Features

1. Acute infections consequent to obstruction by a sialolith is similar to that of acute sialadenitis – Pain, pyrexia and tenderness of affected gland. Pus may be noticed at duct orifice

2. Salivary calculus may be palpable along the ducts intraorally

3. The gland involved may swell especially at meal times and may become tense and sore

4. Swelling reduces in size but swell again during the subsequent meal times when salivary flow is stimulated

5. Recurrent obstruction may lead to atrophy of the secretory cells and chronic sialdenitis and may lead to sialectasis

6. Calculi are radiopaque so radiographs demonstrate their presence.

Diagnosis

Salivary gland imaging is made by:

• Plain film radiography

• Panoramic and lateral oblique

• Antero posterior view used for parotid gland

• Sialography

• Radionucleotide salivary imaging

• CT scan and

• MRI (Magnetic Resonance Imaging).

Treatment

Analgesics, hydration, antibiotics, antipyretics.

a. *Conservative:* Salivary stimulants are used and the gland is massaged which will help to wash the fine debris and prevent stone formation and in drainage of pus

b. *Surgical:* Transoral sialolithotomy or if gland is severely involved then removal of gland through surgical intervention.

Q8 Pain in Migraine and Periodic Migranous Neuralgia.

Ans.

Pain perception is a physio anatomical process by which pain is received and transmission by neural structures from end organs or pain receptors, through conductive and perceptive mechanism.

Once the nerve endings are excited it leads to → Creation of an impulse that leads to → Self propagating wave of excitation along the nerve fibers.

Pain in Migraine

Clinical feature: This type of pain is characterized by unilateral frontal and temporal pain of throbbing variety, associated with irritability and nausea.

It is commonly seen in women in 20–30 age group and more so in educated women.

Premenstrual time aggravates this pain.

Treatment: Ergotamine tartarate dose.

• Migranil 7

• Amitryptyline–a tricyclic compound for prevention 100 mg per day Flunarin 7. Flunarizine 5 mg/10 mg tablets prophylaxis daily dose for adults is 10 mg in divided doses

• Inderal 7 Proranolol 10, 40, 80 mg tabs daily dose is 80–160 mg 2–4 times daily.

Periodic Migranous Neuralgia/ Sphenopalatine Neuralgia

Clinical feature: It is characterized by unilateral fits of pain in region of eyes. Mastoid, zygoma, upper face and nasal area.

No trigger zones are there and it comes at same time each day. Hence the term "Alarm clock headache". Spontaneous remissions reported.

Treatment: Alcohol injection in the sphenopalatine ganglion.

Drugs: Ergotamine is useful but side effects are present
- Propranalol 100 mg per day
- One of the most widely used method is cocainization of sphenopalatine ganglion or alcohol
- Injection of this structure, resection of ganglion as well as surgical correction of septal defect.

Q9 Drugs to relieve Muscle Spasm
Ans.

Muscle spasm is caused due to overstretching of muscles, sprain, tearing of ligaments and tendons, dislocation, fibrositis, bursitis, rheumatic disorders, etc.

Treatment

i. Centrally acting muscle relaxants

ii. Peripherally acting muscle relaxants

Centrally acting muscle relaxants reduce skeletal muscle tone by a selective action in cerebrospinal axis, without altering consciousness.

They selectively depress spinal and supraspinal polysynaptic reflexes involved in regulation of muscle tone without affecting monsosynaptically mediated stretch reflex.

1. Mephenesin group
   - Mephenesin
   - Carisoprodol
2. Benzodiazepine
   - Diazepam
3. GABA derivative
   - Baclofen

The centrally acting muscle relaxants decreases muscle tone without reducing voluntary power.
- Selectively inhibit polysynaptic reflexes in CNS
- Causes some CNS depression.
- Given orally sometimes parenterally
- Used in chronic spastic conditions like acute muscle spasm, tetanus.

Q10 Myofacial pain dysfunction syndrome
Ans.

Myofacial pain is the term used for the muscle pain that occurs with palpation

Clinical Features
Symptoms
- The pain may be intermittent/continuous in nature and usually do not progress to chronic pain and disability
- The pain aggravates with jaw functions such as chewing or opening wide

Signs
- Pain during palpation of TMJ and muscles of mastication
- A restricted range of mandibular movement or uncoordinated movements
- Irregularities of joint during movement
- Crating or grating sounds from TMJ.

Management

The treatment of MPDS cannot be designed to address a particular cause, multiple theories for controlling symptoms and restoring range of movement and jaw function are combined in a management plan

1. *Education and information*
   - Patient is educated on basis of self-care activities that he can perform to aid in control of symptoms
   - In developing strategies to avoid stress that aggravate symptoms or interfere with the ability to manage therapy
2. *Self-care and habit reversal*

Attention to jaw activities that are unrelated to function, as tooth clenching, jaw posturing habits, jaw muscle tensing and leaning on jaw, etc. is a critical beginning. So these behaviors need to be replaced with restful jaw postures. Home therapy like
   - Application of moist heat to the affected areas for 15–20 minutes twice daily

- Range of motion exercises that stay within the comfort zone
- As a part of initial therapy the patient is advised to be aware of habits
- Acquire correct position of jaw to avoid tooth contacts
- Modification of diet like soft food consumption is advised
- Certain postures are avoided,
- Other helping practices are adopted.

{Table-10.11 Page 290 Burkitt, New edition}

3. *Physiotherapy*
   - Education regarding biomechanics of jaw, neck and head posture
   - Passive modalities (heat and cold therapy, ultrasound, laser and TENS transcutaneous electrical nerve stimulation)
   - Range of motion exercises (active and passive)
   - Posture therapy
   - Passive stretching, general exercise, and conditioning program
   - *Ultrasound therapy:* Relies on high frequency oscillations that are produced and converted to heat as they are transmitted through tissue; it is a method of producing deep heat more effectively than the patient could achieve by using surface warming

4. *Intraoral appliances*
   - Cover all the teeth on the arch the appliance is seated on with splints, orthotics, appliances, orthopedic appliances, bite guards, night guards, or bruxing guards
   - Adjust the intraoral appliances to achieve simultaneous contact against opposing teeth
   - Adjust to a stable comfortable mandibular posture
   - Avoid changing mandibular position

Disadvantage: Avoid long term continuous use as this may risk for a permanent change in the occlusion

Advantages: Decreases masticatory muscle activity, relax the elevator muscles and decreases bruxism

Short term intermittent Repositioning therapy is helpful when transient episodes of jaw locking occur due to disk displacement

5. *Pharmacotherapy*
   - NSAIDS-non steroidal anti inflammatory drugs (Ibuprofin 400mg q.i.d.)
   - Antianxiety drugs
   - Tricyclic antidepressants (amitriptyline 10 mg)
   - Muscle relaxants–carisoprodol, methocarbamol
   - Clonazepam
   - Acetaminophen
   - In chronic pain disorders/acute injuries to TMJ opiods are used. Drug therapy should be used on fixed dose schedule rather than as needed for pain
   - COX-2 inhibitors-Rofecoxib and celecoxib are used for 2 weeks
   - Diclofenac Gel and Capsaicin Cream (0.025% to 0.075%) is applied externally on skin

6. *Behavioral therapy and relaxation techniques*
   - *Relaxation techniques:* Decrease sympathetic activity and arousal methods
     - Autogenic training
     - Meditation
     - Progressive muscle relaxation
     - Paced breathing and deep breathing

   This comforts body sensations, calms mind and reduces muscle tone
   - *Hypnosis:* It produces a state of selective or diffuse focus in order to induce relaxation. The technique includes pre and post suggestion to introduce specific goals
   - Cognitive behavioral therapy changes patterns of negative behavior and block pain from entering consciousness
   - Biofeed back is a treatment method that provides continuous feedback by moni-

toring the electrical activity of muscle with surface electrodes or by monitoring peripheral temperature

The monitoring instrumentation provides the training for the patient to achieve a more relaxed state.

7. *Trigger point therapy*
   - Cooling of the skin over the involved muscle by Fluromethane (a refrigerant spray) and the muscle is stretched
   - Intra muscular trigger point injections have been performed by injecting local anesthetic saline/sterile water or by dry needling Procaine dilute 0.5% with saline for 3–5 weeks.

8. *Oral health care delivery in MPDS patients*
   - Prior to dental treatment use hot compress with minor tranquilizer or skeletal muscle relaxant
   - Start the NSAID on the day of procedure
   - During the procedure
     a. Rubber mouth prop is used to support patient's comfortable opening position and it is removed periodically to reduce joint stiffness
     b. Give rest breaks and apply moist heat to muscles
   - After the procedure
     a. Extend muscle relaxants and NSAID use for 1–2 days
     b. Apply cold compress to TMJ and muscle areas

9. *Other treatment modalities*
   - Acupuncture-different forms of injection therapy using natural substances
   - Naturopathic
   - Homeopathic
   - Massage therapy, etc.

SHORT ANSWERS

Q11 Café-au-lait Spots

Ans.

Café-au-lait spots are pigmented black or brown lesions caused due to melanin pigmentation in orofacial region. This is seen in:

1. Hereditary intestinal polyposis syndrome (Peutz Jeghers Syndrome) Melanin pigmentation of lips and oral mucosa is present from birth and appears as small brown macules measuring 1–5 mm

2. *Neurofibroma:* Patients exhibit asymmetric areas of cutaneous melanin pigmentation. There will be loose overgrowths of thickened, pigmented skin which may hang in folds

3. *Polyostotic fibrous dysplasia:* Irregularly pigmented melanotic spots of light brown color are seen along with skeletal symptoms.

Q12 Alkaline phosphatase

Ans.

It is customary to order serum calcium, phosphorous and alkaline phosphatase level when diseases like fibrous dysplasia, primary or secondary hyperparathyroidism, osteoporosis, multiple myeloma, osteogenic sarcoma, or metastatic malignancies are suspected.

Alkaline phosphatase estimation is used as initial screening procedure.

Technique: Auto analyzer is used to determine abnormal values in the absence of signs and symptoms suggestive of bone disease.

- The normal values for serum alkaline phosphatase are 1 to 4 Bodansky units or 3-13 kind Armstrong units /dl and 30–110 per 100 ml

Inference: Alkaline phosphatase occurs mainly in osteoblast and in other tissues. Increases in serum concentration of this enzyme are seen in increased osteoblastic activity but also seen in association with obstructive liver disease and variety of miscellaneous conditions such as malignancy or absess of the liver, amyloid disease, leukemia and sarcoidosis

- The value decreases in Osteoporosis

- In the absence of evidence of liver disease, the rise is usually assumed to be the result of increased osteoblastic activity such as in Paget's disease.

Q13 Verrucous Carcinoma

Ans.

Verrucous carcinoma is a form of epidermoid carcinoma or oral cavity which occurs in the larynx, esophagus, nasal fossae and paranasal sinuses, external auditory meatus, lacrimal duct, skin and odontogenic cyst lining.

Clinical Features

Elderly patients with mean age of 60–70 years. Males have high predilection rate.

Site: Buccal mucosa, gingiva or alveolar ridge, palate and floor of mouth is occasionally involved.

Clinical manifestation: Neoplasm is chiefly exophytic and appears papillary in nature, with pebbly surface which is covered by a leukoplakic film. Regional lymph nodes are tender and enlarged.

Histologic Features

1. Epithelial proliferation with downgrowths of epithelium in connective tissue but without a pattern of true invasion
2. Cleft like spaces lined by thick layer of parakeratin
3. Parakeratin plugging also occur extending into epithelium.

Treatment

1. Surgical excision after accurate diagnosis
2. Radiation therapy
3. Combination of surgical and radiation therapy.

Q14 HIV

Ans.

The human immunodeficiency virus infection (HIV) is of major interest and concern to dentist and other oral health care workers because of pandemic nature of disease.

HIV is human immunodeficiency virus which is retro virus and leads to AIDS, i.e. Acquired immunodeficiency syndrome. Modes of transmission

A. Parenteral transmission
B. Perinatal transmission
C. Sexual transmission
D. Body fluids transmission.

Pathogenesis

HIV attacks the immune system specifically T-lymphocytes, B-lymphocytes, monocytes, promyelocytes, oligodendrocytes, capillary cell, epithelial cells, fibroblasts leading to cell death or irreversible immunosuppression.

Detection of HIV

AIDS detection is done by proper clinical analysis, history taking and HIV spot tests.

Confirmatory tests like ELISA, Western blot, Polymerase chain reaction are necessary.

Oral and dental management of HIV infected patients require the implementation of preventive protocol, aggressive treatment of established dental infection and use of antibiotic cover to prevent infection. A dentist should take

- Proper medical history of patient
- Barrier techniques like
  A. Eye protection (eye glasses)
  B. Mouth mask
  C. Disposable needles.
  D. Gloves

Proper sterilization of instruments and clothes HIV is sensitive to heat for 20 min. Autoclaving at 121°C for 15 min at 1 atm pressure kills this virus.

Q15 Hairy Tongue

Ans.

Definition

Hairy tongue is a non specific developmental disturbance or a condition where hypertrophy of filiform papillae occurs with the lack of normal desquamation which may be extensive and lead to thick matted layer on tongue.

Clinical Features

The papillae get stained due to food, tobacco smoke, candy and leads to yellowish white to brown color or even black.

Hypertrophied papillae at times touch the palate and cause gagging sensation.

If proper oral hygiene is not maintained, bacterial growth occurs on the papillae.

Treatment

Remove food debris and microbial flora by tongue cleaner. Tooth brush is used to clean the tongue.

Q16 Age in Examination

Ans.

The chronologic age of the patient has to be determined by the patient for the following reasons
1. Dental office record, hospital record
2. Some diseases are more common in particular age
3. During childhood, i.e. mixed dentition period, dental age has to be analyzed and interpreted for normal eruption of teeth with chronologic age
4. During puberty, females are more prone for gingivitis and oedematous gingiva
5. The immunity to fight against infections decreases as the patient grows old and other metabolic disorders like diabetes, hypertension is common
6. Mode of treatment can be analysed
7. Prognosis of treatment will be favorable in young individuals.

Q17 Multilocular Cyst

Ans.

Ameloblastoma is also known as multi-locular cyst which is a true neoplasm of enamel organ-type tissue which does not undergo differentiation to the point of enamel formation.

Clinical Features

a. Occurs at an age most commonly 3rd, 4th and 5th decade
b. Both sexes are affected. 2/3rd of cases occur in posterior part of mandible followed by cuspid region
c. Slow growing, painless growth unless secondarily infected. It can grow to huge dimensions.

Types

1. Follicular variant
2. Plexiform pattern
3. Acanthomatous
4. Granular variant
5. Cystic variant.

Sequelae: Ameloblastoma keeps on enlarging and it causes thinning of surrounding bone leading to fluctuation and egg shell cracking

Locally aggressive invasion in maxillofacial area may compress vital structure.

Management

1. Complete eradication of lesion
2. Reconstruction of resultant defect
3. Curettage is contraindicated
4. En bloc resection inraorally or extraorally can be done
5. Segmental resection with continuity defect.

Q18 PUS

Ans.

Pseudomembranous ulcerative stomatitis. It is a superficial infection of outer layers of the epithelium, and it results in the formation of patchy white plaques of flecks on the mucosal surface.

Removal of the plaques by gentle rubbing or scraping usually reveals an area of erythema or even shallow ulceration.

Clinical Features

- Bad taste
- Inflammation
- Erythema painful eroded areas
- Any mucosal surfaces may be involved.

Diagnosis

Smear demonstrating yeast or mycelia is seen.

Treatment

Antifungal agents are given.

Q19 Focal Sepsis
Ans.

Definition

Focal sepsis is the presence of microorganism in the blood. The metastasis from the focus of infection of organism or their toxins that are capable of injuring tissue.

Mechanism

1. Metastasis from infected focus by either hematogenous or lymphogenous spread
2. Toxins or toxic products may be carried, through blood stream or lymphatic channels from a focus to a distant site where they may incite a hypersensitive reaction in the tissues.
   Example: Scarlet fever in which erythrogenic toxin is liberated by infecting streptococci
3. *Rheumatic fever:* Develops as a result of an altered reactivity or hypersensitization of tissues to hemolytic streptococci
4. Subacute bacterial endocarditis.

Diagnosing Sepsis

- *Blood cultures:* Modular range of automated blood culture systems for real-time monitoring of blood samples. Bacterial growth is immediately detected and reported for earlier detection of causative pathogens
- *Identification and antibiotic susceptibility testing:*
  - Rapid identification of resistance phenotypes for relevant antibiotic choice
  - More refined prediction of therapeutic results
- *Procalcitonin (new marker of bacterial infection):* Is an automated test for early diagnosis and monitoring of sepsis and bacterial infection and is adapted to emergency situation.

Q20 Target Lesion
Ans.

These are characteristic features of Erythema Multiforme. The skin lesions contain petechiae in center of the lesion.

Bull's eye or target/Iris lesion: consists of central bulla or pale. Clearing area surrounded by edema and bands of erythema.

Site: Hands, feet, extensor surfaces of elbows and knees, (palms, soles).

Target tensions are symmetrically distributed whereas in other skin diseases gingiva is mostly involved and the lesions will be smaller.

- It take 2 weeks to heal.

Treatment

- Supportive treatment
- Topical anesthetics
- Systemic analgesics
- Mouth wash
- Prednisolone
- Patient is advised to have soft or liquid diet.

RGUHS September 2001

QUESTION PAPER

Long Essays

1. Pigmentation in Oral Structure Diagnostic clue to diagnose systemic disease–Discuss.
2. Radiographic changes of periapical region" in systemic disease. Discuss.

Short Essays

3. Myofacial pain dysfunction syndrome
4. Intensifying screen
5. Properties of radiation and X-rays
6. Tuberculous Ulcer in Tongue
7. Eagle's Syndrome
8. Subluxation of TMJ
9. Masseter Hypertrophy
10. Reticular Lichen Planus

Short Answers

11. Pink Spot
12. Tongue in AIDS
13. Multilocular
14. Definition of Leukoplakia
15. Elevation of Serum Calcium.
16. Acid Phosphatase
17. Biochemistry of Paget's disease
18. Cellulitis (Phlegmon)
19. Trotter's Syndrome
20. Soap Bubble Appearance

SOLUTIONS

LONG ESSAYS

Q1 Pigmentation in Oral Structure Diagnostic clue to diagnose systemic disease–Discuss.
Ans.

Introduction

Endogenous pigmentation
- Hemoglobin
- Hemosiderin
- Melanin.

Exogenous pigmentation
- Silver amalgam
- Graphite
- Lead, mercury, bismuth
- Chromogenie bacteria.

Oral mucosa pigmentation
- Systemic disease.

Pigmentation in Oral Structure

The specific coloration, tint, location, multiplicity, size and configuration of pigmented lesions are of diagnostic importance

- Blue, brown and black discolorations, constitute the pigmented lesions of the oral mucosa, and such color changes can be attributed to the deposition of either endogenous or exogenous pigments.

Causes of Pigmentation in Oral Mucosa

Endogenous pigmentation:

1. *Hemoglobin:* This imparts red, blue or purple color to the mucosa and represents pigmentation associated with vascular lesions; coloration is rendered by circulating erythrocytes coursing through Patent vessels

2. *Hemosiderin:* This appear brown and is deposited as a consequence of blood extravasation, which may occur due to trauma or defect in hemostatic mechanisms

3. *Melanin:* This is the pigment synthesized by melanocytes. Overproduction of melanocytes may be caused by a variety of mechanisms, including increased sun exposure, drugs, the pituitary adrenocortico tropic hormone (ACTH), and genetic factors (in association with certain syndromes), Benign nevi and malignant melanomas.

4. Bilirubin

Exogenous pigmentation

These are usually traumatically deposited directly into the submucosa. However some may be ingested, absorbed, and distributed hematogenously to be precipitated in connective tissues, particularly areas subjected to chronic inflammation, such as gingiva.

1. Silver amalgam–gray, black
2. Graphite–gray, black
3. Lead, mercury, bismuth–gray
4. Chromogenic bacteria–black, brown, green
   Table 7.1.

Q2 "Radiographic changes of periapical region" in systemic disease. Discuss.
Ans.

Radiographic changes of periapical region Systemic disorders affect the entire body, the radiogrophic changes manifested in the jaws are generalized. The general changes include the following:

1. A change in size and shape of bone
2. A change in the number, size and orientation of trabeculae
3. Altered thickness and density of cortical structure
4. An increase or decrease in overall bone density.

Systemic disease and radiographic changes in periapical region

1. Hyperparathyroidism Endocrinal abnormality

Table 7.1

Oral mucosal pigmentation giving diagnostic clue to systemic disease	Systemic disease
1. Blue, purple vascular lesions	
Present as tumor-like hamartoma, most are raised and nodular and some are flat, macular or diffuse. Tongue–multinodular and bluish red. Lip mucosa-localized, blue, raised.	Hemangioma • Port wine stain: Facial skin. • Concurrent history of seizures the condition represents encephalo trigeminal angiomatosis (Sturge-Weber's syndrome). • Hemodymanics in angiomas are perturbed and stasis with thrombosis occurs
Pathologic dilatations of veins or venules are varices or varicosities, at chief sites are: • Ventral surface of tongue • Lingual varicosities appear as tortuous, serpentine blue, red, and purple elevations that course over ventrolateral surface of tongue with extensions anteriorly • Lips and buccal mucosa have varices	Varix: A focal dilatations of a vein or a group of venules. • Occurs in older age group • Once formed, does not regress. • The traumatic event probably damages and weakens the vascular wall and culminates in dilation.
Red, blue or purple nodular tumors.	Angiosarcoma can arise from blood or lymph vessel endothelial cells, or from pericytic cells of vasculature.
Oral tumors of red, blue or purple, Site: hard palateIt is slowly progressive in growth. Oral lesions continue to show a predilection for the posterior hard palate, and they also being as flat red macules, of variable size and in irregular configuration.	Kaposi's sascoma: Skin tumors – localized in dorsal aspect of feet and great toe. Lymph node enlargement and may involve other node groups • Diagnostic sign of AIDS.
There are more than 100 purple papules on the vermilion and mucosal surfaces of the lips as well as on the tongue and buccal mucosa. • The lesions represent multiple microaneurysms, owing to weakening defect in adventitial coat of venules	Hereditary hemorrhagic telangiectasia • Facial skin and neck are also involved. The lesion is characterized by multiple round or oval purple papules measuring less than 0.5cm in diameter. • History of epistasis may be a complaint.
2. Brown melanotic lesions	
Ephelides can be encountered on the vermilion border of lips, with the lower lip being the favored site since it tends to receive more solar exposure. The lesion is macular and ranges from being quite small to over a centimeter in diameter.	Ephelis and oral melanotic macule Lesions are oval or irregular in outline, are brown or even black, and occur on gingiva, buccal mucosa and palate.
Nevocellular and blue nevi tend to be brown and may be macular or nodular in oral mucosaSite: Palate and gingiva or on buccal mucosa and on lips.	Nevocellur Nevus and Blue nevi

Contd...

Table 7.1 (Contd...)

Oral mucosal pigmentation giving diagnostic clue to systemic disease	Systemic disease
Melanomas in oral mucosa occur on anterior aspects of hard palate. Brown, black plaques with an irregular outline.	Malignant Melanoma Facial cutaneous melanomas may appear macular or nodular, coloration can be quite varied, ranging from brown to black, with zones of depigmentation
Pigmentations on oral mucosa can be large yet localized, to hard palate, or they can be multifocal, through out the mouth.	Drug induced Melanosis Quinolone, hydroxyquinoline and amodiaquine antimalarials, minocycline
Café-au-lait- spots on oral cavity and skin	Ephelis like macules to broad diffuse lesions. Café-au-lait Pigmentation.
Diffuse macular melanosis of buccal mucosa, lateral tongue, palate, and floor of the mouth.	Smoker's Melanosis occur due to cigarette smoking, tobacco smoke products
Bronzing of skin and patchy melanosis of the oral mucosa	Addison's disease and pituitary based Cushing's syndrome.
Hyperpigmentation of skin, nails, and mucous membrane • Diffuse multifocal macular brown pigmentation of buccal mucosa. • Gingiva, palate and tongue may be involved.	HIV oral Melanosis
Multiple focal melanotic brown macules are concentrated around the lips while the remaining facial skin is less involved. Macular appear as freckles or ephelides 0.5 cm in diameter	Peutz- Jeghers Syndrome Lesions on perioral areas are pathagnomonic ue Nevi

3. Brown Heme associated lesions

Bright red macule or as a swelling if a hematoma forms. Lesion will assume brown coloration but if multiple brown macular or swellings are observed.	Traumatic Ecchymosis– Hemorrhagic diathesis
Petechiae in soft palate	Viral or allergic pharyngitis.
Oral mucosal lesions are brown to gray diffuse macules that tend to occur in palate and gingiva	Hemochromatosis: Iron deposition in the submucosa,basilar melanosis is observed.

4. Gray / Black Pigmentation

Solitary or focal pigmentation lesions are mucular and bluish gray	Amalgam tattoo
Macular, focal gray or black traumatic implantation from lead.	Graphite tattoo
Hyperplastic papillae than pigmented by the colorization of chromogenic bacteria site: Dorsum of tongue	Hairy tongue
Pigmentation in free marginal gingiva–gray to black	Heavy metal ingestion

- Demineralization and thinning of cortical boundaries occur in jaws incortical boundaries such as the inferior border, mandibular canal, and the cortical outlines of maxillary sinus
- A change in normal trabecular pattern result in ground–glass appearance of numerous, small, randomly oriented trabeculae Periapical radiographs reveal loss of lamina dura around one tooth or all the teeth
- Brown tumors of hyperparathyrodism may appear in any bone. These lesions may be multiple with in a single bone.

2. Hypoparathyroidism: Dental enamel hypoplasia, external root resorption, delayed eruption or root dilaceration.

3. Hyperpituitarism
   - Enlargement of jaws notably mandible
   - The increase in length of dental arches results in spacing of teeth
   - In Acromegaly, angle between ramus and body of mandible may increase. Thickness and height of alveolar processes may also increase
   - Roots of posterior teeth often enlarges as a result of hyper cementosis
   - Supra eruption of posterior teeth may occur.

4. Hypopituitarism
   - Jaws are small and result in crowding and malocclusion
   - Exfoliation of primary teeth is delayed by several years
   - Eruption of permanent teeth is delayed.

5. Hyperthyroidism
   - Early eruption and advanced rate of dental development
   - Premature loss of primary teeth
   - Generalized decrease in bone density.

6. Hypothyroidism
   - Delayed eruption, short roots, and thinning of the lamina dura
   - Maxilla and mandible are relatively small.

7. Diabetes mellitus
   Periodontal disease associated with diabetes leads to interdental bone loss and horizontal bone loss.

8. Cushing's syndrome
   Generalized osteoporosis which may have a granular bone pattern. The skull shows diffuse thinning
   - The teeth may erupt prematurely, and partial loss of lamina dura may occur.

9. Osteoporosis
   - Overall reduction in the density of bone
   - Periapically, lamina dura may appear thinner than normal.

10. Rickets
    - Within the cancellous portion of jaws, the trabeculae reduces in density, number and thickness
    - In severe cases, the jaws appear so radiolucent that the teeth appear to be bereft of bony support
    - Retarded root eruption in early rickets
    - Lamina dura and cortical boundary of tooth follicles may be thin or missing.

11. Hypophosphatasia
    - Inherited disorder that is caused by reduced production or defective function of alkaline phosphatase
    - Generalized radiolusceney of mandible and maxilla
    - The cortical bone and lamina dura are thin, alveolar bone is poorly calcified and may appear deficient
    - Primary and permanent teeth have a thin enamel layer and large pulp chambers and root canals.

12. Renal Osteodystrophy (Renal Rickets)
    - Hypoplasia and hypocalcification of teeth are possible, resulting in loss of any radiographic evidence of enamel
    - The lamina dura may be absent or less apparent in instances of bone sclerosis.

13. Hypophosphatemia
   - Jaws are osteoporotic and radio lucent
   - Teeth may be poorly formed, with thin enamel cusps and large pulp chambers and root canals
   - Periapical rarefying osteitis
   - If disease is severe, patient experiences premature loss of teeth
   - The lamina dura may become sparse and cortical boundaries around tooth crypts may be thin or entirely absent.

14. Osteopetrosis
   - Increased radiopacity of jaws
   - Periapically even the roots of teeth may not be apparent
   - The increased bone density and relatively poor vascularity results in susceptibility of mandible to osteomyelitis
   - Delayed eruption, early tooth loss, missing teeth, malformed roots, crowns and poorly calcified teeth
   - Lamina dura and cortical borders may appear thicker than normal.

15. Progressive Systemic Sclerosis (Scleroderma)
   - There will be an unusual pattern of mandibular erosions at regions of muscle attachment such as the angles, coronoid process, digastric region or condyles
   - Periapical radiographs reveal an increase in the width of the periodontal ligament spaces around the teeth
   - Periodontal ligament spaces are at least twice as thick as normal and both anterior and posterior teeth are affected
   - The lamina dura remains normal.

16. Sickle cell anemia
   It is an autosomal recessive, chronic hemolytic disorder.
   Radiographic features: General osteoporosis, decrease in volume of trabecular bone and thinning of cortical plates
   - Bone marrow hyperplasia a cause enlargement and protrusion of maxillary alveolar ridge.

17. Thalassemia
   - Defect in hemoglobin synthesis
   - Severe bone marrow hyperplasia prevents pneumatizations of paranasal sinuses, especially maxillary sinus and expansion of maxilla that results in malocclusion
   - Jaws appear radiolucent, with thinning of cortical borders and enlargement of marrow spaces
   - Lamina dura is thin, and the roots of teeth may be short.

SHORT ESSAYS

Q3 Myofacial pain dysfunction syndrome
Ans.
Refer to March 2001 Q10.

Q4 Intensifying screen
Ans.
Refer October 1999 Q 6.2.

Q5 Properties of radiation and X-rays
Ans.
Properties of Radiation
Ionization

If an electrically neutral atom loses an electron, it becomes a positive ion and the free electron is a negative ion. This process of forming an ion pair is termed ionization.

Radiation is of two types:

1. Particulate radiation
   Consists of atomic, subatomic particles moving at high velocity. Example: Electrons, alpha particles, Beta-particles, protons, neutrons, cathode rays

2. Electromagnetic radiation
   It is the movement of energy through space and matter as a combination of electric and

magnetic field. It is generated when a velocity of an electrically charged particle is altered. Example Gamma-rays, X-rays, UV-rays, visible light, infra red rays, radar, TV, microwaves, radio waves.

Depending on the penetrating power
- Primary radiation
  - Short wavelength
  - High penetrating power
  - Directly coming from machine
  - Useful to produce image on screen.
- Secondary radiation / Scattered radiation
  - Long wavelength
  - Low penetrating
  - They may back scatter, degrading the image of object
  - They produce fogging effect on films.

Depending on nature of radiation
- Characteristic radiation
- Bremstrahlaung radiation.

Properties of X-rays

1. X-rays travel in straight line
2. Speed of X-rays is equal to that of natural light
3. X-rays cannot be reflected, refracted or deflected
4. X-rays do not have mass or weight
5. X-rays can produce fluorescence
6. X-rays penetrate matter
7. X-rays produce ionization
8. X-rays damage biologic tissues.

Q6 Tuberculous ulcer in tongue

Ans.

Tuberculosis is an infectious granulo-matous disease caused by the acidfast bacillus, *Mycobacterium tuberculae*. Pulmonary tuberculosis is the chief form of the disease. It may occur at any age and may either extend locally, become disseminated or, more commonly, become completely walled off and healed by fibrosis and calcification.

Clinical Features

- The signs and symptoms of tuberculosis is inconspicuous
- The patient may suffer from episodic fever and chills, fatigability and malaria
- There may be gradual loss of weight accompanied by persistent cough with or without associated hemoptysis.

Oral manifestations: The majority of tuberculosis lesions occur on the base of tongue, followed by the palate, lips, buccal mucosa, gingiva and frenulum.

The tuberculosis lesion is an irregular, superficial or deep, painful ulcer which tends to increase slowly in size. It is frequently found in areas of trauma and may be mistaken clinically for a simple traumatic ulcer or even carcinoma. {Refer Fig. 6. 1 P-343 Shafer 4th edition}

Tuberculosis gingivitis is an unusual form which may appear as a diffuse, hyperemic, nodular or papillary proliferation of gingival tissues. Tuberculosis may also involve the bone of maxilla or mandible.

Histological Features

- TB lesions exhibit foci of caseous necrosis surrounded by epithelioid cells, lymphocytes and occasional multinucleated giant cells
- Diagnosis of tuberculosis lesion can be confirmed only by microscopic examination of tissue with demonstration of the organisms in the lesions.

Treatment

The treatment of tuberculosis ulcer on tongue is secondary to treatment of the primary lesions combination therapy, usually 3–4 drugs to prevent resistance, chosen from the following isoniazid, rifampicin, ethambutol, rifabutin, streptomycin, pyrazinamide.

Prolonged therapy–6 months minimum indicated for slow growth rate of bacteria, increasing incidence of *Mycobacterium tuberculosis* drug resistance.

Oral Health Consideration

The risk of TB transmission from patients to dental care providers is considered to be minimal.

Administration of OSHA regulation gives the Detailed description of administrative procedures, infections control practices, engineering controls, and respiratory. Personal equipment appropriate for minimizing airborne microbial transmission.

Q7 Eagle's Syndrome
Ans.

Definition

The condition associated with ossification of stylohyoid ligament. Ossification of stylohyoid ligament usually extends downward from base of skull and commonly occurs bilaterally.

Clinical Features

1. The ossified ligament can be detected by palpation over the tonsil as a hard, pointed structure
2. There is vague, nagging to intense pain in the pharynx on swallowing, turning the head, or opening the mouth, especially on yawing
3. When this entity is associated with discomfort and the patient has a recent history of neck trauma (Example: Tonsillectomy), the condition is called Eagle's Syndrome. The elongated styloid process and local scar tissue probably causes symptoms by impinging on the glosso-pharyngeal neck.

Radiographic Features

- Ossification of sytlohyoid ligament
- The ligament may have at least some calcifications in individuals of any age.

Location

Region of mastoid process and crosses the postero-inferior aspect of ramus toward the hyoid bone.

Shape

Styloid process appears as long, tapering, thin, radiopaque, process that is thicker at its base and projects downward and forward.

- It normally varies from 0.5–2.5 cm in length
- The ossified ligament has roughly a straight outline but in some cases irregularity may be seen in outer surface.

Internal Structure

Small ossifications of stylohyoid ligament appear homogeneously radiopaque. As ossification increases radiopaque band is seen at periphery.

Management

- Steroid on lidocaine injections into the tonsillar fossa
- Amputation of stylohyoid process.

Q8 Subluxation of TMJ
Ans.

It is recurrent self reducible dislocation of the TMJ. In this condition, the capsule of the joint becomes so lax that the patient by virtue of habituation moves the mandible forward and backward (Fig. 7.1).

Clinical Features

It is seen in professional singers, musicians, speakers and aged people. It is a very embarrassing condition for the patient and is generally due to recurrent dislocation there by making the capsule and temporomandibular ligament sufficiently relaxed to allow such a free movement of the condyle.

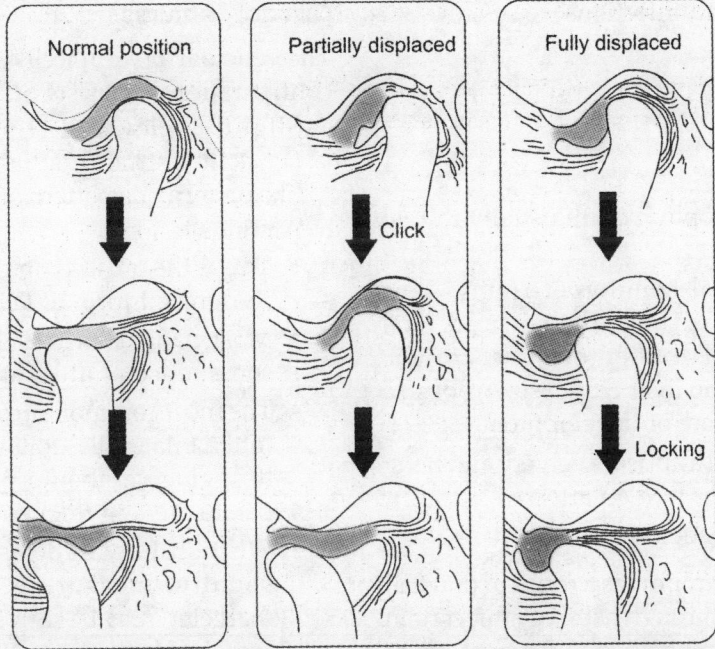

Fig. 7.1: Position and movement of disk during jaw opening

Diagnosis

TMJ Subluxation is diagnosed by soft tissue imaging of the joint magnetic resonance imaging and arthrography.

Arthrography with videofluorscopy provides a superior motion study of the joint. This gives information about disk position, function morphology and the integrity of diskal attachments, which is required for treatment plan.

Treatment

1. Immobilization of jaw by intermaxillary fixation gives good results in 3–4 weeks time but this is a crude method, as patient cannot eat anything during this period, so it rarely used
2. The Movement of mandible can be restricted by applying elastics on previously placed arch bar splints
3. Injection of sclerosing agents like sodium prylliate and sodium morrhuate in capsule help in fibrosis of capsule. The injections should preferably be given in space anterior and lateral to the joint to restrict the movements of mandible.

Surgical Treatment

The repair of capsule can be carried out through the conventional preauricular approach
1. The part of capsule is reduced by excising tissue
2. Shortening of temporalis tendon
3. Osteotomy of the zygomatic arch

Q9 Masseter Hypertrophy

Ans.

Hypertrophy of muscle refers to an increase in size of individual muscle fibers.

Etiology

Masseter hypertrophy is nonspecific and occurs in a variety of situations listed below
1. Developmental defects
2. Functional disturbances

3. Inflammation and infections
4. Metabolic changes
5. Neoplasms

Clinical Features

Masseteric hypertrophy occurs usually in two situations

1. Congenital facial hemihypertrophy. This exhibit enlargement of one half of head. Oral manifestations. Dentition of hyper-trophic side is abnormal in their crown size, root size and shape and rate of development.

   The buccal mucosa appears velvety and hang in soft, pendulous fold on affected side

   Treatment: Cosmetic repair.

2. Functional hypertrophy: as a result of unusual muscle function through habit or after certain surgical procedures involving the jaws where muscular function is inhibited

   Masticatory–Muscle hyperactivity progressing to a vicious cycle causes myo facial pain

   Treatment: Adequate rest to the muscle, stoppage of para functional habits, Relieve stress, physical therapy, Intraoral appliance therapy, pharmacotherapy and behavioral techniques.

Q10 Reticular Lichen Planus
Ans.

Definition

Lichen Planus is a common chronic inflammatory mucocutaneous disorder that varies in appearance from keratotic (reticular or plaque like) to erythematous and ulcerative.

Etiology

Nervous, high strung person malnutrition and inflection. Grinspan's syndrome–Diabetes millitus, Lichen planus and hypertension.

Clinical Features

The reticular form (lacelike keratotic mucosal configurations) consists of:

a. Slightly elevated fine whitish lines (Wickam's striae) that produce either a lace-like pattern or a pattern of fine radiating lines

b. Annular lesions.

   • This is the most common and most readily recognized form of lichen planus

   • Most patients with lichen planus exhibit some reticular areas at some time

   • The most common sites are Buccal mucosa (often bilaterally) followed by the tongue; lips, gingiva, the floor of mouth and the palate are less frequently involved

   • Whitish elevated lesions or papules, usually measuring 0.5–1.0 mm in diameter, may be seen on well keratinized areas of oral mucosa

   • However even large plaque like lesions may occur on cheek, tongue and gingiva, and these are difficult to distinguish from leukoplakia.

Histologic Features

1. Hyperparakeratosis with thickening of granular cell layer and saw toothed rete pegs
2. Liquefaction degeneration
3. Dense subepithelial band of lymphocytes
4. Isolated epitheial cells, shrunken with eosinophillic cytoplasm and pyknotic nuclear fragments (civiatte bodies) are scattered with in epithelium.

Diagnosis

Immunoflouroscent study of biopsy specimen.

Treatment

• Corticosteroids have been the most predictable and successful medications for controlling signs and symptoms

- Topical/systemic costicosteroids 0.05% flurocinonide and 0.005% clobestol in form of paste or gel
- *Prednisone:* 40–80 mg daily for less than 10 days with out tapering (systemically)
- Retinoids are also useful
- Topical application of cyclosporine.

SHORT ANSWERS

Q11 Pink Spot
Ans.

Pink Spot is an unusual form of tooth resorption that begins centrally within the tooth due to internal resorption. Which is called as Pink tooth of mummery.

Definition

It is an unusual form of tooth resorption that begins centrally within the tooth apparently initiated by a peculiar inflammatory hyperplasia of pulp.

Etiology

1. Caries exposure and accompanying pulp infection
2. nvasion of pulp by granulation tissue arising in the periodontium.

Clinical Features

1. Pink hued area on crown of tooth which represents hyperplastic vascular pulp tissue filling the resorbed area and showing through the remaining overlying tooth substance
2. Multiple tooth may be involved.

Radiographic Features

Round or ovoid radiolucent area in central portion of tooth associated with the pulp but not with external surface of tooth.

Treatment

- Root canal therapy
- Extraction of tooth.

Q12 Tongue in AIDS
Ans.

AIDS is acquired immunodeficiency syndrome in which a patient is prone to all kinds of infections.

HIV infected patients have higher incidence of recurrent herpetic lesions and aphthous stomatitis, Herpes may involve all mucosal surfaces.

Clinical Feature

The Tongue has lesions, which persist and present as large, nonspecific, painful ulcers;

Healing is delayed so their lesions develop secondary infections and described as typical ulcers.

A wide variety of bacterial and viral infections may produce persistent and severe oral ulcerations in HIV infected individual.

For details refer to Q1 of September 2000.

Q13 Multilocular
Ans.

The radiographic interpretation of the lesion involves analysing internal structure or appearance of any lesion, which can be classified into totally radiolucent, totally radiopaque and mixed radiolucent and radiopaque (Mixed Density).

The mixed density internal structure is seen as the presence of calcified structures against a radiolucent (black) backdrop.

- When septa represents residual bone that has been organized into long strands or walls. If these septa divide the internal structure into at least two compartments, the term "Multilocular" is used. The length, width, and orientation of the septa can be assessed
- Curved, coarse septa seen in ameloblastoma giving internal pattern a multilocular, soap bubble appearance

- Septa seen in giant cell granuloma are described as "Wispy or Granular"
- Straight, thin septa in small number is seen in odontogenic myxoma.
{Refer Fig. 15-20 P-291 White and Pharaoh}

Q14 Definition of Leukoplakia
Ans.

Leukoplakia is defined as a whitish patch or plaque which cannot be characterized clinically or pathologically as any other disease entity and whose occurrence is not associated with any physical or chemical causative agents except for the use of tobacco.

Q15 Elevation of Serum Calcium
Ans.

Normal serum calcium level is 8.5 –10.5 mg/dl. High level of serum. PTH leads to excess bone resorption and brings about an increase in serum calcium level. The important signs of hypocalcemia are

1. Neural sedation as manifested by drowsiness
2. Renal stones and osteoporosis leading to development of bony cysts and pathologic fractures

The main uses of calcitonin so far are in the treatment of Hypocalcaemia and Paget's disease.

Paget's disease: Osteoclastic activity predominates and may cause hypercalcemia and severe bone pain.

Treatment: Calcitonin reverses severe hypocalcemia Etidronate is given in repeated courses.

Q16 Acid Phosphatase
Ans.

- Acid phosphatase is localized mainly in specific membrane–bound organelles, the lysosomes
- Osteoclasts in bone and odontoclasts in resorbing dentin exhibit an intense acid phosphastase activity. The enzyme is localized in the part of the cytoplasm that lies apposed to resorbing surface of bone and dentin
- Acid phosphates is serum enzyme whose normal value is 0.6–3.1KA units/100 ml; Tartarate–labile–ACP–0 to 0.8 KA unit%.

Concentration is increased in:
- Metastasizing prostatic carcinoma
- Gaucher's disease is autosomal recessive defect of lipid metabolism
- Slight to moderate rise in Paget's disease
- Hyperparathyroidism
- Osteolytic lesions from breast carcinoma
- Thrombocytosis
- Slight increase after rectal examination (PR)
- Chronic granulocytic leukemia
- Myeloproliferative lesions.
{Refered from P-98 Chatterjee Biochemistry Text}

Q17 Biochemistry of Paget's Disease
Ans.

- The serum calcium and serum Phosphorous levels are usually within normal limits, even in cases of advanced osteitis deformans
- The serum alkaline phosphate level may be elevated, however, to extreme limits
- Values as high as over 250 Bodansky units have been reported, particularly in-patient's in the osteblastic phase of disease, when there is rapid formation of new bone and when there is polyostotic involvement
- In the monostotic form of the disease, alkaline Phosphatase level seldom exceeds 50 Bodenskys units. In the early stage Phosphatase level may not be significantly elevated
- The serum acid phosphate level is not increased.

Q18 Cellulitis (Phlegmon)
Ans.
Definition

Cellulites are a diffuse inflammation of soft tissues which is not circumscribed confined to one area, but which, in contradistinction to the abscess, tends to spread though tissue spaces and along facial planes.

Etiology

Cellulitis occurs as a result of infection by micro-organisms that produce significant amounts of hyaluronidase and fibrinolysins which act to break down are dissolve, respectively, hyaluronic acid, universal intercellular sement substance and fibrin.

Clinical Features

1. Moderately ill and has an elevated temperature and leukocytosis
2. Painful swelling of involved soft tissues, which is firm and brawny
3. Skin is inflamed, sometimes purplish.
4. Regional lymphadenitis
5. In maxilla, Infections perforate the outer cortical layer of bone above Buccinator attachment and causes swelling of upper half of face
6. Typical facial cellulitis tends to be localized and facial absces may form, which may become suppurative and discharge on free surface.

Treatment

Administration of antibiotics and removal of cause of infection.

Q19 Trotter's Syndrome
Ans.

- Tumors of nasopharynx can produce pain similar to trigeminal neuralgia, generally manifested in the lower Jaw, tongue and side of head with an associated middle ear deafness
- This symptom complex, caused by a nasopharyngeal tumor, has been called Trotter's Syndrome. These patients also exhibit asymmetry and defective mobility of soft palate and affected side
- As the tumor progresses, trismus of internal pterygoid muscle develops, and patient is unable to open his mouth
- There will be involvement of mandibular nerve in foremen ovale through which tumor invades the calvarium.

Q20 Soap Bubble Appearance
Ans.

- Soap bubble appearance is the diagnostic feature of ameloblastama, adenocystic carcinoma and aneurysmal bone cyst during radiographic interpretation
- The number and arrangement of septa may give the area soap bubble appearance (larger compartments of variable size) in the molar–ramus region in ameloblastoma which is a true neoplasm of odontogenic epithelium, it is persistent and locally invasive tumor
- Adenocarcinoma is a salivary gland malignancy this spreads along nerve sheath
- Aneurysmal bone cyst is considered to be a reactive lesion of bone rather than a cyst or true neoplasm. The internal structure show multilocular appearance in radiography.

8

RGUHS March 2002

QUESTION PAPER

Long Essays

1. Enumerate conditions which produce multiple ulcers in the oral cavity. Describe the clinical features, investigations and management of acute herpetic gingivostomatitis

2. Discuss the importance of lamina dura in dental radiography and describe in detail periapical radiolucent lesions.

Short Essays

3. Oral manifestations of AIDS
4. Toluidine blue staining
5. Agranulocytosis
6. Angioneurotic edema
7. Rickets
8. Collimation and filtration
9. Dosimetry
10. Serological tests for syphilis

Short Answers

11. Nikolsky's sign
12. Eagle's syndrome
13. Paul-Bunnell test
14. Carcinoma in-situ
15. Erosive Lichen planus
16. Koplik's spot
17. Radiographic appearance of periapical cementoma
18. Anodontia
19. Ramsay-Hunt syndrome
20. Radiographic appearance of hyperparathyroidism.

Q1 Enumerate conditions which produce multiple ulcers in the oral cavity. Describe the clinical features, investigations and management of acute herpetic gingivostomatitis.

Ans.

Introduction

Conditions which Produce Multiple Ulcers in the Oral Cavity

- Acute lesions
- Chronic lesions
- Recurrent lesions

Acute Multiple Ulcers

- Herpes virus infection
- Primary herpes simplex virus infection
- Coxsackie virus infection
- Varicella Zoster infection
- Erythema multiforme
- Contact allergic stomatitis
- Oral ulcer secondary to cancer chemotherapy
- Acute necrotizing ulcerative gingivo-stomatitis

Chronic Multiple Ulcers

- Pemphigus
- Subepithelial bullous dermatitis
- Herpes simplex infection in immuno-compromised patients.

Recurrent Multiple Ulcers

- Recurrent aphthous stomatitis minor
- Recurrent aphthous stomatitis major
- Recurrent aphthous stomatitis herpetiform
- Recurrent aphthous stomatitis associated with Behcet's syndrome.

Clinical Features

Extra oral signs and symptoms

1. Cervical adenitis, fever as high as 101°F to 105°F and generalized malaise 1–2 days before oral lesions.
2. Patients give history of recent acute infection or febrile diseases such as pneumonia, meningitis, influenza and typhoid.
3. It also occurs in periods of anxiety, strain, or exhaustion and during menstruation.

Oral Manifestations

Oral Signs

1. Acute herpetic gingivostomatitis appears as a diffuse, erythematous, shiny involvement of gingiva and adjacent oral mucosa with varying degrees of edema and gingival bleeding.
2. *Initial stage:* Presence of discrete, spherical gray vesicles on gingiva, labial mucosa and buccal mucosa, soft palate, pharynx, sublingual mucosa and tongue.
3. *After 24 hours:* Vesicles rupture and forms painful small ulcers with a red elevated, halo like margin and a depressed yellowish or grayish white central portion. Occasionally it may be without overt vesiculation.
4. Diffuse erythematous, shiny discoloration and edematous enlargement of gingivae with a tendency toward bleeding leading to generalized acute marginal gingivitis.
5. The course of disease is limited to 7–10 days.
6. Scarring does not occur in the areas of healed ulcerations.

Oral Symptoms

1. Patient complains of generalized "soreness" of the oral cavity that interferes with eating and drinking.

2. The ruptured vesicles are the site of pain and are particularly sensitive to touch, thermal changes, foods such as condiments, fruit juices, etc.

Investigations

The typical clinical picture of primary herpetic gingivostomatitis can be diagnosed according to case history, laboratory test:

1. *Cytology:* The fresh vesicle can be opened and a scraping made from the base of the lesion and placed on a microscope slide. The slide may be stained with giemsa, wright's or papanicolau's stain and searched for multinucleated giant cells, syncytium and ballooning degeneration of nucleus.

2. *HSV Isolation:* Isolation and neutralization of a virus in tissue culture is the most positive method of identification and has a specificity and sensitivity of 100%.

3. *Antibody titers:* Conclusive evidence of a primary HSV infection includes testing for complement fixing or neutralizing antibody in acute and convalescent sera. However, it is rarely necessary in routine clinical situation and is often not helpful since the results are not available until the infection is gone.

In immuno-compromised patients, an acute serum specimen should be obtained within 3–4 days of onset of symptoms.

Absence of detectable antibodies plus isolation of HSV from lesions is compatible with the presence of primary HSV infection.

Presence of antibody to HSV will begin to appear in a week and reach a peak in 3 weeks.

Convalescent serum can confirm diagnosis by demonstrating fourfold rise in anti-HSV antibody.

If the antibody titers are similar in acute and convalescent sera, then the lesions from which HSV was isolated were recurrent lesions.

Management

1. *Mild cases:* Supportive care is necessary.
2. *Moderate cases:* Analgesics are given to relieve pain–Aspirin and to control fever acetaminophen is given.
3. *Anaesthetics:* To relieve burning sensation on eating and drinking
   - Dyclonine hydrochloride 0. 5%
   - Lidocaine
   - Diphenhydramie hydrochloride 5mg/ml mixed with milk of magnesia.
4. Antiviral drugs:
   - Acyclovir
   - Famciclovir
   - Valacyclovir
5. Antibiotics are given for controlling other toxic systemic complication along with HSV infection.
6. Fluids and electrolyte balance has to be maintained for proper hydration.
7. Dental treatment
   Supragingival scaling has to be done to relieve gingival inflammation.

Q2 Discuss the importance of lamina dura in dental radiography and describe in detail periapical radiolucent lesions.
Ans.

LAMINA DURA

The radiograph of sound teeth in a normal dental arch demonstrate that the tooth socket are bound by a thin radiopaque layer of dense bone. Lamina dura (hard layer) is derived from its radiographic appearance.

Structural Integrity

- Lamina dura is continuous with the shadow of particle bone at the alveolar crest.
- It is slightly thicher than cancellous bone.
- Appearane of lamina dura depends on the direction of X-ray beam

Importance in dental radiography

1. *Uniform thickness and density:* Varies according to amount of occlusal stress to which tooth is subjected.
   - Wider and more dense lamina dura – heavy occlusion
   - Thinner and less dense lamina dura – teeth which are not subjected to occlusal forces.
2. Variations and disruptions in continuity of lamina dura
   - Super impositions of trabecular pattern and small nutrient canals passing from mandibular bone to periodontal ligament.
   - Discontinuity in periapical region suggestive of inflammatory lesion.
3. Presence of intact lamina dura
   - Vital pulp
   - Early cases of pulpitis
4. Absence of lamina dura
   - Due to periapical abscess or cyst
   - May be a normal condition so clinical evaluation is must.
5. Periodontal ligament space can be identified and analysed with the help of lamina dura.

Periapical Radiolucent Lesions

1. *Dental granuloma*

Site occurs in either jaw at any age; either sex

Clinical feature: Asymptomatic; non vital tooth.

Radiographic features: Circumscribed radiolucency at apex of nonvital tooth less than 5 mm in diameter. There will be loss of bone density and which results in widening of periodontal ligament space.

Treatment: Root canal treatment or extraction of involved tooth.

2. *Radicular cyst*

Location–either jaw

Age/sex at any age;either sex

Clinical feature: Non vital tooth; due to caries deep periodontal pocket; radicular cyst also causes resorbtion of roots of adjacent teeth

Radiographic features: Circumscribed radiolucency at apex of tooth measuring more than 1 to 2 cms surrounded by well defined radio opaque cortical border if secondary infection is there then there will be loss of this cortex.

Treatment: RCT with or without apicoectomy

3. *Residual cyst*

Site: Edentulous space; apical area of extraction sitemore in mandible. Occur at any age.

Clinical feature: Usually solitary, asymptomatic; circumscribed radiolucency located in edentulous space; history of extraction in area

Radiographic features: Periapical radiolucency circumscribed by a cortical margin unless it becomes secondarily infected.

4. *Periapical (dentoalveolar) abscess*

Site: either jaw

Age/sex: Occur at any age and either sex

Clinical feature: Swelling, redness, pain in the region of periapical abscess and one or more teeth in area will be non vital, associated tooth will be very sensitive to percussion and sinus opening may be seen in the buccal sulcus. Mild fever may be present.

Radiographic features: Usually solitary, diffuse or fairly well circumscribed area of radiolucency

Treatment: Drainage and extraction of the offending tooth.

5. *Apical scar*

Location: Apical area

Age/sex: Adulthood/either sex

Clinical feature: A non vital tooth with root canal filling and apical surgery. Associated tooth will be asymptomatic

Treatment: None

6. *Cementoma*

Location: Anterior mandibular teeth.

Age/sex: Occur over 30 years / females

Clinical feature: Associated tooth will be vital. Cementoma causes external resorption of roots. Cementoma has to be distinguished from periapical cysts and granuloma radio-graphically

Radiographic features: Well defined radiopacity with a cortical border and wheel spoke pattern internally. The tumour can cause expansion of outer cortex of mandible. Small, multiple periapical areas of radiolucency is seen in incisor region.

SHORT ESSAYS

Q3 Oral manifestations of AIDS
Ans.
Refer to Ques.1 of September 2000.

Q4 Toludine Blue Staining
Ans. Introduction
- Procedure
- Indication
- Advantages
- Disadvantages

Procedure
- Toludine blue staining uses a 1% aqueous solution of the dye that is decolorizedwith 1% acetic acid. The dye binds to dysplastic and malignant epithelial cells with a high degree of accuracy.
- The dye is topically applied on lesion with swab or as an oral rinse and staining is observed.

Indications
- Early carcinomatous or premalignant lesion is diagnosed
- Leukoplakia
- Erythroplakia
- To differentiate inflammation and dysplastic areas.

Interpretations
After removal of irritants the lesion is tested by toludine blue staining.

- If it stains: It indicates extensive dysplasia/early carcinoma.
- If it doesn't stain: Then also it is not indicative of absence of disease so biopsy has to be done.

Advantages
- Easy technique
- Done in cases where biopsy is contra-indicated in early stages.
- Saves time

Disadvantages
- False positive test is possible due to over diagnosis. In some cases the epithelial cells get stained even if allergic reactions are there.
- False negative test is possible due to underdignosis, thus biopsy is necessary for confirmation.

Q5 Agranulocytosis
Ans.

Definition
Agranulocytosis is a serious condition characterized by an extremely low leukocyte count and absence of neutrophiles; it most often is caused by a drug or medication that interferes with cell formation or enhances cell destruction.

Classification
1. Primary agranulocytosis-etiology is unknown
2. Secondary agranulocytosis-etiology is known

Etiology
Ingestion of any one of a considerable variety of drugs which causes idiosyncrasy in form of urticaria, cutaneous rashes and edema. For example: Amidopyrine, Barpiturates, Benzene, Bismuth, Chloramphenicol Cinchophen, DDT, Gold salts, Phenacetin Phenothiazines.

Clinical Features

- Occur at any age and in particularly women
- Disease commences with a high fever, accompanied by chills and sore throat.
- The patient suffers malaise, weakness and prostration.
- The skin appears pale and anemic or in some eases jaundiced
- Most characteristic feature of the disease is the presence of infection, particularly in oral cavity, but also throughout the gastro-intestinal tract, genitourinary tract, respiratory tract and skin
- Regional lymphadenitis accompanies the infection in any of these locations.
- The clinical signs and symptoms develop rapidly in the majority of cases, usually within a few days and death may occur within a week.
- Oral manifestations
- The oral lesions constitute an important phase of clinical aspects of agranulocytosis.
- These appear as necrotizing ulcerations of the oral mucosa, tonsils and pharynx.
- *Site:* Gingiva and palate
- The lesions appear as ragged necrotic ulcers covered by a gray or even black membrane.
- There is little or no inflammatory cell infiltration
- Patients manifests excessive salivation.

So all oral surgical procedures particularly tooth extraction are contraindicated in cases of agranulocytosis.

Lab Findings

WBC count in aguanulocytesis–below 2000 cells/mm^3 with complete absence of granulocytes or polymorphonuclear cells.

RBC count and platelet count are usually normal, occasionally anemia is present.

Treatment

Not specific but etiology should be recognized and withdrawal of causative agent is must.

Prognosis

Death usually occurs due to massive infection so antibiotics are prescribed.

Q6 Angioneurotic Oedema
Ans.

Is a rather common form of oedema occurring in both hereditary and non-hereditary forms. It appears to be closely related to general urticaria.

Etiotiogy

Some cases of non-hereditary form of angioneurotic oedema are due to food allergy drugs, endocrine disturbance or focal infections.

Pathogenesis

There is biochemical abnormality in patients with the disease in the absence of normally occurring inhibitor of C'1 esterase which is a specific alpha–2 globulin in complement system in the serum. This deficiency causes increased consumption of C'2 and C'4, with formation of kinin like substance that causes an increase in vascular permeability and edema, release of histamine with transudation of plasma.

Clinical Feature

1. Angioneurotic edema manifests itself as a smooth, diffuse edematous swelling parti-cularly involving the face around the lips, chin and eyes, the tongue, and sometimes the hands and feet.
2. The swelling may involve any area, including the parotid gland.
3. The eyes may be swollen shut and the lips extremely puffy. The symptoms appear rapidly, sometimes being present when the patient awake in the morning.

4. A feeling of tenseness or an itching or prickly sensation sometimes precedes the urticarial swelling.

5. The condition usually lasts for only 24-36 hrs although some cases persists for several days.

6. There may be visual involvement in some hereditary form.

7. Vomiting and abdominal pain may occur, and especially dangerous, edema of glottis which can result in death through suffocation.

Treatment

• Etiologic agent has to be eliminated from diet.
• Antihistamine drugs
• In cases of respiratory obstruction, emergency tracheostomy.
• Aminocaproic acid and androgens anti-fibrinolytic agent which blocks the activation of plasmin.

Q7 Rickets
Ans.

Rickets refers to any disorder in vitamin D–calcium phosphorous axis which results in hypomineralization of bone matrix i.e. a failure of endochondral calcification.

Types

• Adult rickets (Osteomalacia)
• Vitamin D resistant Rickets (Familial Hypophosphatemia)
• Renal rickets (Renal Osteodystrophy)

Clinical Feature
General

• Change in the bones are found in the epiphyseal plate, the metaphysis and the shaft.
• The changes in the lips and long bones of children. Oral manifestations
• Developmental abnormalities of dentin and enamel.

• Delayed eruption
• Mal-alignment of teeth in jaws
• Rachitic teeth is seen in which an abnormally wide predentition zone and much interglobular dentin is present

Treatment

Dietary enrichment of Vitamin D,
• Hormonal therapy
• Fluoride administration.

Q8 Collimation and Filtration
Ans.
Collimation

1. The tissue area (and volume) exposed to the primary X-ray beam should not exceed the minimum coverage consistent with meeting diagnostic requirement and clinical feasibility so collimation limit the size of X-ray beam and reduces patient exposure.

2. The field of radiation at the patient's skin surface is contained in a circle having a diameter of no more than 7 cm (2¾ inches) when the X-ray tube is operated above 50 kVp and the dimensions of no. 2 intraoral film (3.2 × 4.1 cm).

So limiting the size of the X-ray beam is necessary to significantly reduce the X-ray beam.

Types of Collimation

1. *Rectangular position indicating device (PID)* May be attached to the radiographic tube having exit opening of 3.5 × 4.4 cm reduces area of patient's skin surface exposed by 60% over that of a round (7 cm)

2. Film holders with rectangular collimators may be used with round PIDS.

3. Precision instrument XCP instrument film holders are clipped to aiming ring.

(Fig. 8.1) 'A'-A larger volume of irradiated tissue results from 'A' (with shorter FSFD) than from 'B'(in which the longer FSFD produces a less divergent beam).

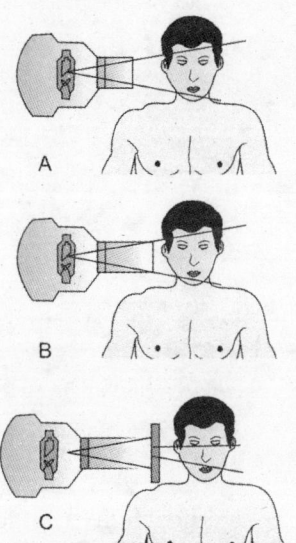

Fig. 8.1: Effect of FSFD (Focal spot-to-film distances) and collimation on the volume of tissue irradiated

In 'C' the Collimator between round PID and the patient produces the effect of a rectangular PID on tube housing or a rectangular collimating face shield on film holding instrument.

This rectangular collimator (close to patient in 'C') results in a smaller, less divergent beam and a smaller volume of tissue irradiated than in 'A' and 'B'.

Filtration

Types of Filtration

1. Inherent filtration

   Consists of the materials that the X-ray photons encounter as they travel from the focal spot on the target to form the usable beam outside the tube enclosure. These materials include:

   - Glass wall of the X-ray tube
   - Insulating oil that surrounds many dental tubes.
   - Barrier material that prevents the oil from escaping through X-ray port.

Inherent filtration ranges from the equivalent of 0.5–2 mm of aluminum.

2. External filtration

This is supplied in the form of aluminium disks placed over the port in the head of the X-ray machine.

When an X-ray beam is filtered with 3 mm of aluminium, the surface exposure is reduced to about 20% of that with no filtration. 1.5 mm to 70 kVp and 2.5 mm of aluminum for all higher voltages.

Uses of Filtration

1. Selective filtration of excessively high energy as well as excessively low energy radiation.
2. Filtering an X-ray beam with aluminium preferentially remove low energy photons, thereby reducing the beam intensity and increasing its mean energy.
3. Total filtration is the sum of inherent filtration plus any added external filtration. When total filtration is reduced, the surface exposure is reduced.
4. There will be no loss of radiological information.
5. Image quality will be good because of an increase in contact, sharpness and resolution.

Q9 Dosimetry
Ans.

Definition

Determining the quantity of radiation exposure or dose is termed as dosimetry.

The term dose is used to describe the amount of energy absorbed per unit mass at a site of interest, exposure is a measure of radiation based on its ability to produce ionization in air under standard conditions of temperature and pressure (STP) Quantity

Quantity	SI unit	Traditional unit	Conversion
Exposure	Air kerma	Roentgen (R)	1Gy = 100 rad 1 rad = 0.01Gy
Absorbed dose	Gray	Rad	1Gy = 100 rad 1 rad = 0.01Gy
Equivalent dose	Sievert (Sv)	Rem	1 Sv = 100 rem 1 rem = 0.01Sv
Effective dose	Sievert (Sv)	–	–
Radio activity	Becquerel (Bq)	Curie	1Bq = 2.7×10–11Ci 1 Ci = 3.7 × 10–10

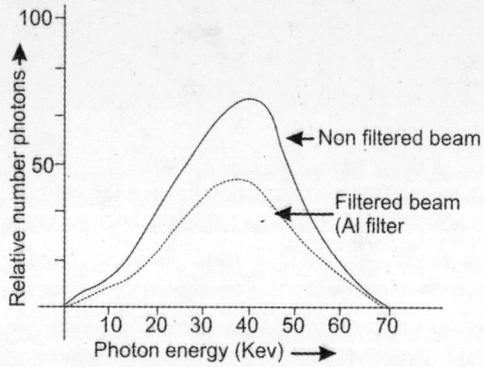

Fig. 8.2: Relative number of photons vs photon energy (KeV)

Units of Measurement

Exposure

It is a measure of radiation quantity, the capacity of radiation to ionize air.

Absorbed Dose

It is a measure of energy absorbed by any type of ionizing radiation per unit mass of any type of matter.

Equivalent Dose (H_T)

This is used to compare the biologic effects of different types of radiation to a tissue or organ. It is sum of products of absorbed dose (D_T) averaged over a tissue or organ and radiation weighing factor (W_R)

$$HT = \Sigma W_R \times D_T$$

Equivalent dose is expressed as a sum to allow for the possibility that the tissue or organ is exposed to more than one type of radiation (Fig. 8.2).

Effective Dose (E)

This is used to estimate the risk in humans. It is sum of products of equivalent dose to each organ or tissue (H_T) and tissue weighing factor

$$E = \Sigma W_T \times H_T$$

Radioactivity

The measure of radioactivity (A) describes the decay rate of a sample of radioactive material.

Q10 Serological tests for syphilis
Ans.

STANDARD TEST FOR SYPHILIS

Lipoidal or cardiolipin Antigen(Ag) is used.

Wasserman Test

Complement fixation test in which patient's serum is incubated with cardiolipin Ag and guinea pig Complement.
a. If serum contains antibody to Cardiolipin-complement is used up in Ag- Ab reaction
b. If antibody is absent in serum –complement will be left behind

The presence of complement is detected by adding indicator (hemolytic system consisting of sheep RBC'S and antisheep RBC antiserum prepared by immunization of rabbits)

Interpretation: Antibody is absent: Test is Negative for syphilis

Antibody is present: Test is Positive for syphilis.

Kahn's Test

It is tube flocculation test. 0.15 ml serum is taken in 3 tubes and mixed with antigen in different quantities, i.e. 0.05 ml; 0.025 ml and 0.0125 ml Antigen at 37°C.

Tubes are shaken in Kahn shakes at 280 oscillations per minute and examined after adding saline.

Interpretations: Floccules appear-positive test. Uniform opalesence: Negative Test.

VRDL

Venereal Disease Research Laboratory Test is a slide flocculation test in which 0.05 ml of inactivated serum is taken in special VDRL slides and 1drop of freshly prepared antigen is added. Then slide is rotated in VDRL rotator at 120 oscillations for 4 min.

Interpretations

i. Uniform distribution of crystals in the drop–Antibody absent-negative test
ii. Formation of clumps-Antibody present-positive test.

TREPONEMAL TESTS
Reiter Treponemal Test
Treponema Pallidum Test

A. *Using live T. pallidum: serum +Cl : Antibody present*

Examined under dark ground illumination— If 50% immobilized Positive test. If 20% immobilized negative test.

B. *Using killed T. pallidum: TPA- Treponema pallidum agglutination test*

TPIA-Treponema pallidum immune adherence; T. pallidum will be adhered to erythrocytes in presence of antibody
FTA-Fluorescent Treponemal antibody in which indirect immunofluorescent test using smear prepared with Nichol's stain is examined under UV microscope and interpreted by the presence of Fluorescent Treponemas

C. *Test using Treponema pallidum extract - it has high degree of sensitivity.*

ELISA (ENZYME LINKED IMMUNOSORBENT ASSAY)

Antigen coated + Antihuman gamma globulin, i.e. labeled with enzyme. Substance is acted upon by bound enzymes.

SHORT ANSWERS
Q11 Nikolsky's sign
Ans.

Definition
The loss of epithelium occasioned by rubbing apparently unaffected skin is termed Nikolsky's sign.

Clinical Manifestation

• Nikolsky's sign is characteristic feature of pemphigus, caused by prevesicular edema which disrupts the dermal-epidermal junction.
• The non-ulcerated gingivae are massaged under lateral pressure. The epithelium readily strips or slides from the connective tissue to leave the raw sensitive surface which bleeds readily.
• This feature is seen in chronic desquamative gingivitis.
• Oral lesions are similar to those occurring on skin although intact bullae are rare since they tend to rupture as soon as they form.

Q12 Eagle's syndrome
Ans.
Refer Sept 2001 Q.7.

Q13 Paul-Bunnell test
Ans.
This is a laboratory test for infectious mononucleosis. This test is both characteristic and pathognomonic of the disease.

This is a laboratory test for infectious mononucleosis. This test is both characteristic and pathognomonic of the disease.

1. Patient exhibits typical lymphocytes in the circulating blood as well as antibodies to the Ebstein Barr virus and increased heterophil antibody titer
2. Increased heterophil is present only in small minority of children with the disease. The normal titer of agglutinins and hemolysins in human blood against sheep's red blood cells does not exceed 1:8,
3. The titer may rise to 1:4096 in infectious mononucleosis and is referred to as positive Paul Bunnel test
4. Patients have more than 50% lymphocytosis of which 10% is of atypical form.

Q14 Carcinoma in-situ
Ans.

Severe dysplastic changes in a red or white lesion indicate considerable risk for the development of cancer.

- The more severe grades of dysplasia merge with the condition referred to as carcinoma in situ, which implies that intra epithelial changes are the same as those seen in invasive cancers, even though there is no histologic evidence in the specimen submitted, that malignant cells have left the confines of epithelium.
- WHO has used the term carcinoma in situ only when the dysplastic change affects the whole or almost the whole thickness of epithelium involved.

Clinical Features

Shiny atrophic patches to leukoplakia to erythroplakia.

Treatment

Local excision with a wide border of normal tissue.

Example: Bowen's disease is an intra epidermal squamous cell carcinoma that may progress to invasive carcinoma over time.

Q15 Erosive Lichen planus
Ans.

Lichen planus is the dermatologic disease which manifests in the oral cavity. It is the common chronic immunologic inflammatory disorder which varies in appearance from Keratotic to erythematous and ulcerative.

Clinical Features

Thin epithelium gets abraded or ulcerated from inflamed areas of oral mucosa. These areas may be present as a patchy distribution among keratotic lesions or as extensive involvement.

Symptoms–burning to severe pain, sensitive to hot, acidic, spicy food and extensive areas of ulceration may be painful. They may be hemorrhagic with slight trauma caused due to brushing.

Histopathology

Hyperkeratosis, hydropic degeneration of basal layer, dense infiltration of lymphocytes

Treatment

- Hydrogen peroxide mouthwash 2–3 times daily.
- Ulcerated areas are dried with a sterile sponge and a corticosteroid ointment or cream rubbed gently into lesions several times daily.
- Intralesional steroids are injected in severe cases.
- Topical anesthetics are applied to relieve pain.

Q16 Koplik's spot
Ans.

- These are small white lesions with erythematous bases on buccal mucosa and inner aspect of lower lip.

- These lesions are pathagnomonic of early measles infections as this occurs 2–3 days before cutaneous rashes.
- Measles is a disease with prodromal phase that is characterized by symptoms of upper respiratory tract infection, tonsillo-pharyngitis and Koplik's spot.

Treatment

- Symptomatic treatment
- Antipyretics, analgesics.

Q17 Radiographic appearance of periapical cementoma
Ans.
(Also known as periapical cemental dysplasia/ cementoma)

Location
Periapically near apex of tooth root occasionally lesions localized near mental foramen

Internal Structure

- *Earliest stage:* Formation of circumscribed area of periapical fibrosis accompanied by localized destruction of bone: Osteolytic stage
- *Second stage:* Development of lesion is beginning of calcification in the radiolucent area of fibrosis : Cementoblastic stage
- *Third stage:* Excessive amount of calcified material is deposited in the focal area and appear as a well defined radiopacity that is usually bordered by a thin radiolucent line or band: Mature stage.

Q18 Anodontia
Ans.

Definition

The expression of develop-mentally missing teeth may range from the absence of one or a few teeth (Hypodontia) to failure of all teeth to develop (Anodontia).

Clinical Features
1. Hypodontia is in permanent dentition excluding third molars
2. Missing primary teeth,
3. Absence of teeth may be unilateral or bilateral,

Diagnosis

- Missing teeth are identified clinically and by counting the existing teeth.
- Eruption of some teeth are developmentally delayed which can be identified in radiograph
- Tooth may be considered missing when it can not be discerned clinically or radio-graphically and if no history exists about its extraction.
- Patients with ectodermal dysplasia have Anodontia as the common feature.

Q19 Ramsay-Hunt syndrome
Ans.
This syndrome consists of special form of herpes zoster infection of geniculate ganglion, with the involvement of external ear and oral mucosa.

Clinical Manifestations
Facial paralysis, Pain of external auditory meatus and pinna of ear, vesicular eruptions in oral cavity and oropharynx, Tinnitis, Vertigo and other disturbances.

Diagnosis
- Cytologic examination
- Tzank test to detect multinucleated giant cells

Q20 Radiographic appearance of hyperparathyroidism

Ans.

General Radiographic Features in Hyperparathyroidism

- Subtle erosions of bone from subperiosteal surfaces of phalanges of hands
- Demineralization of skeleton
- Osteitis fibrosa cystica are localized regions of bone loss produced by osteoclastic activity, resulting in a loss of all apparent bone structure
- Brown tumors occur late in life
- Pathologic calcifications

Radiographic Features of Jaws in Hyperparathyroidism

- Demineralization and thinning of cortical boundaries such as the inferior border, mandibular canal, and the cortical outlines of maxillary sinuses.
- Density of jaws is decreased resulting in radiolucent appearance that contrast with the density of teeth.
- Teeth stand out in contrast to radiolucent jaws
- Ground glass appearance of numerous small randomly oriented trabeculae.
- Brown tumors may be multiple within single bone.
- They have variably defined margins and may produce cortical expansion.

Radiographic Features of Teeth and associated Structures

- Loss of lamina dura around one tooth may occur.

9

RGUHS September 2002

QUESTION PAPER

Long Essays

1. Classify oral ulceration with a suitable example of each condition. Describe the clinical feature and management of recurrent aphthous ulcers.

2. Describe in detail sialography and its significance in various diseases of the salivary glands.

Short Essays

3. Investigations and management of oral candidiasis.

4. Clinical features and radiographic features of osteosarcoma.

5. Clinical features and management of osteoradionecrosis.

6. Uses and types of Grids.

7. Clinical and laboratory diagnosis of Anemias.

8. Indication and radiographic technique for maxillary standard occlusal view.

Short Answers

9. Paul bunnel test.

10. Turner's tooth

11. Lipshutz bodies

12. Exfoliative cytology

13. Radiographic view to detect fractured zygomatic arch

14. Enumerate two differences between periapical abcess and periodontal abcess.

15. Café-au-lait spots.

16. Composition of X-ray film.

17. Four conditions associated with cervicofacial lymphadenopathy.

18. Clinical features of Bell's palsy.

SOLUTIONS

LONG ESSAYS

Q1 Classify oral ulceration with a suitable example of each condition. Describe the clinical feature and management of recurrent aphthous ulcers.

Ans.

Refer to March 2000 Q1 solution.

Q2 Describe in detail Sialography and its significance in various diseases of the salivary glands.

Ans.

Description of Sialography

1. Sialography is a radiographic technique wherein a radiopaque contrast agent is infused into the ductal system of salivary gland before imaging with plain films, fluoroscopy, panoramic radiography, conventional tomography, or CT scan.

2. Sialography remains the most detailed way to image the ductal system. The parotid and submandibular glands are more readily studied with this technique. Although the sublingual gland is difficult to infuse intentionally, it may be fortuitously opacified while infusing Warthon's duct to image the submandibular gland.

3. With this technique, a lacrimal or periodontal probe is used to dilate the sphincter at the ductal orifice before the passage of a cannula (blunt needle or catheter) connected by extension tubing to a syringe containing contrast agent.

4. Lipid soluble (Example: Ethiodol) or non lipid-soluble (Example: Sinografin) contrast solution is then slowly infused until the patient feels discomfort (usually between 0.2 and 1.5 ml, depending on gland being studied). These iodine containing agents render the ductal system radiopaque.

5. The filling phase can be monitored by fluoroscopy or with static films The intend is to opacify the ductal system all the way to the acini the image appears as "tree limbs" with no area of the glands devoid of ducts.

6. With acinar fillings the "tree" comes into bloom which is the typical appearance of the parenchymal opacification phase.

7. The gland is allowed to empty for 5 minutes without stimulation. If postevacuation images suggest contrast retention, a sialogogue such as lemon juice or 2% citric acid may be administered to augment evacuation by stimulating secretion.

Non lipid-soluble contrast agents are preferred because of reports of inflammatory reactions subsequent to inadvertent extravasation of lipid soluble agents.

Significance or Indication of Sialography

1. To study normal anatomy, physiologic function of the gland.

2. To detect any shrinkage or obstruction of the duct.

3. To study pathologic condition like inflammation, stones/sialolithiasis, space occupying lesions (benign tumors and malignancies).

4. Detection of calculi/foreign bodies and determination of extent of destruction of salivary gland tissue.

5. Detection of fistulae, deverticuli and strinctures

6. Detection and diagnosis of recurrent swelling and inflammatory process

7. Selection of site of biopsy.

8. Detection of residual stone, residual tumor, fistulae prior to lithotomy/surgical procedure is done after sialography.

Significance in Salivary Gland Diseases

Obstructive and Inflammatory Disorders

- Sialolithiasis-cigar/ oval shaped radiopacity is seen in sialogram. Sialography is contraindicated if stone is distally placed in radiograph as it may get displaced in the duct.
- Bacterial sialadenitis
  - In acute infections sialography is contraindicated as it results in foreign body reaction and severe pain.
  - In chronic infections it is a useful procedure, the sac like acini and mildly dilated terminal ducts are demonstrable.
  - An even distribution through out the gland is seen in recurrent parotitis and autoimmune disorders.
- Sialodochitis-Dilation of ductal system is a prominent sialographic presentation – Interstitial fibrosis is apparent
- Autoimmune sialadenitis- Sialography is helpful in diagnosis and staging.
  - *Early stage:* Initiation of punctuate (less than 1 mm)and globular 1–2 mm spherical collections of contrast agent is evenly distributed.
  - *Disease progression:* Collections of contrast agent greater than 2 mm and irregular in shape is seen.
  - *End point:* Complete destruction of the gland occurs.

Non Inflammatory Disorders

- *Sialadenosis:* Enlargement of glands are seen.
- *Cystic lesions:* On sialographic examination, cystic masses are visualized.

Benign Tumors

- Sialography may suggest a space occupying mass when the ducts are compressed or smoothly displaced around the lesion (ball in hand appearance).

SHORT ESSAYS

Q3 Investigations and management of oral candidiasis

Ans.

Investigations

This includes identification of predisposing factors, etiology and then laboratory diagnosis.

1. Collection of infected material from nail scrapings, mucous patches from mouth, etc.
2. *Microscopic examination:* Presence of mycelial forms indicate colonization and tissue invasion
3. *Culture:* Oval, budding cells, some pseudo-hyphae are seen.

Features

Rapid formation of hyphae, production of chlamydospores, fermentation and assimilation of sugars, nitrogen utilization, germ tube formation indicate candidial growth.

4. *Smear Examination*
   - Fragments of the plaque material may be smeared on a microscopic slide, macerated with 20% potassium hydroxide and examined for typical hyphae.
   - In addition the organism may be cultured in a variety of media, including blood agar, corn meal agar and sabouraud's broth, to aid in establishing the diagnosis.
   - Histologic section of a biopsy from a lesion of oral candidiasis will show the presence of the yeast cells and hyphae or mycelia in superficial and deeper layers of involved epithelium
   - These are more easily visualized if the sections are stained with periodic acid Schiff reagent (PAS) or methenamine silver, since the organism are positive in both instances.

Management

a. Control the underlying predisposition

b. Cutaneous candidiasis is treated with topical Azole ointment.

c. Topical application–Nystatin
   - Clotrimazole
   - Econazole
   - Amphotericin

5. Oral administration–Miconazole 250 mg 6 hrly
   - Ketoconazole 200 mg daily
   - Fluconazole 50–200 mg daily

6. For intravenous infusion–Amphotericin 1 mg/kg/day
   - Miconazole 600 mg 8 hourly

7. Mucosal infections responds well to lozenges or suspensions of Nystatin or Amphotericin.

8. Persistent infections and nail infection s require oral Ketoconazole 100 mg daily which may need to be maintained for some months.

9. Systemic infections should be treated with IV Infusion.

Q4 Clinical features and radiographic features of osteosarcoma

Ans.

Osteosarcoma is a malignant mesen-chymal tumor in which tumor cells produce bone matrix. It is a most common primary malignant tumor of bone which accounts for 20% of bone cancers.

Approximately 5% of osteosarcoma occurs in the jaws.

Clinical Features

Osteosarcoma arise in several clinical settings include pre-existing bone abnormality as Paget's disease, Fibrous dysplasia, giant cell tumor, bone infarct and prior to irradiation.

Site: Any bone may be involved

Age: It has bimodal age distribution so it is seen in patients younger than 20 years of age and elderly patients.

Classification of Osteosarcoma

1. Conventional type—arising with in the medullary cavity
2. Juxtacortical type—arising from periosteal tumor
3. Extra skeletal type—arising rarely in soft tissue.

Symptoms or sign is swelling, which may be present as long as 6months before diagnosis; swelling is usually rapid.

Other indications are pain, tenderness, erythema, of overlying mucosa, ulceration, loose teeth, epistaxis, hemorrhage, nasal obstruction, exophthalmos, trismus and blindness. Hypoesthesia is also reported in cases involving neurovascular canals.

Radiographic Features

- *Location:* The mandible is more affected than maxilla. The posterior areas are also more commonly affected in the maxilla, with the most frequent site being the alveolar ridge, antrum, and palate. The lesion may cross the midline.

- Periphery and shape It has ill defined borders. When viewed against normal bone, the lesion is usually radiolucent with no peripheral sclerosis or by extension, typical sunray spicules or "hair on end trabeculae". This occurs when periosteum is displaced, partially destroyed, and disorganized. If the periosteum is elevated and maintains its osteogenic potential but is breached in the center, a Codman's triangle at the edges is formed. Rarely laminar periosteal new bone may be present.

- *Internal structure:* Osteosarcoma may be entirely radiolucent, mixed radiolucent-radiopaque, or quite radiopaque. The internal osseous structure may take the appearance of granular or sclerotic – appearing bone, cotton balls, wisps, honeycombed internal structure in areas with adjacent destruction of pre-existing osseous architecture.

- *Effects on surrounding structure:* Widening of the periodontal membrane is associated. The antral or nasal wall cortices may be lost in maxillary lesions. Mandibular lesions may destroy the cortex of neurovascular canal or it may be widened or enlarged.

Q5 Clinical features and management of Osteoradionecrosis.

Ans.

Clinical Features

- The mandible is much more commonly affected than the maxilla.
- This is likely due to the microanatomy and reduced vasculature of this bone.
- The posterior mandible is affected more often than the anterior portion
- Loss of mucosal covering and exposure of bone is the hallmark of osteoradionecrosis.
- Pathologic fracture also may occur
- The exposed bone become necrotic as a result of loss of vascularity from the periosteum and subsequently sequestrates, often lead in to exposure of more bone.
- Intense pain may occur, with intermittent swelling and drainage extra orally.

Management

Prevention of PRON

1. The irradiation should be done after proper healing of surgical site.
2. The irradiation should not be done in close proximity to bone.
3. A high dose of irradiation with/without proper fractionization should not be given.
4. Intraoral implants should not be used in combination with external radiation.
5. Good oral hygiene should be maintained and irritants are eliminated.
6. Proper home care programs are advised.

7. Prosthetic appliances should not be used after radiation therapy.
8. Physical and nutritional status should be improved.
9. Teeth in high dose fraction with questionable prognosis should be extracted prior to radiotherapy and radiotherapy is planned after 21 days suggested as healing time.

Classification of PRON has been described to identify stages and to select the therapy.

Stage 1: Resolved Healed
- No pathologic fracture
- Past pathologic fracture

Treatment: Prevention of recurrence

Stage 2: Chronic non-progressive
- No pathologic fracture
- Pathologic fracture

Treatment
- Local wound care: Topical antibiotic tetracycline or antiseptic chlorhexidine rinses or gels may reduce the potential local irritation of microbial flora. For chronic cases, regular follow up should be done.
- HBO if indicated: Hyperbaric oxygen therapy (HBO) increases oxygenation of tissue, increases angiogenesis, and promotes osteoblast and fibroblast function.
- HBO is prescribed as 20–30 dives at 100% oxygen and 2 to 2.5 atmosphere of pressure.

Stage 3: Active, progressive
- No pathologic Fracture
- Pathologic fracture

Treatment

Local wound care
- HBO therapy is an important part of therapy. Prophylactic HBO may be considered when surgery is required following radiation therapy, when the patient is felt to be at extreme risk due to high-dose radiation to the bone with a high biologic effect (TDF>109)
- Surgery if indicated

- Sequestra may be managed with limited resection or may require mandibulectomy. If surgery is required, postsurgical HBO of 10 dives is recommended.

{Referred from Burkitt 9th edition and Neelima Malik Oral surgery text}

Q6 Uses and types of Grids

Ans.

The scattered radiation originating within the patient's tissues travel in different directions than the primary beam and causes deleterious effects in the film.

In a prallel grid the absorber plates are parallel to the anode.

- A grid or scatter grid is used to prevent the scattered radiation from reaching the film (Fig. 9.1).
- The grid is positioned between object and the film.
- Grid consists of a large number of long number of long parallel strips of radio-opaque material (Example: Lead) inter-spersed with radiolucent interspace material.

Types of Grids

1. *Linear Grid* (Fig. 9.2)

The strips of lead are placed parallel to each other, while using the linear grid, cut off of the beam can occur as some of primary beam may get absorbed by the lead in the peripheral region.

2. *Focused Grid* (Fig. 9.3)

The lead strips are angled from the center to the edge so that the interspaces are directed at the focal spot.

3. *Pseudo-focused Grid* (Fig. 9.4)

The extra reduction of primary radiation away from the center of the beam can be minimized by using a pseudo-focused grid, in which, the height of the lead strips are progressively reduced from the center to the periphery.

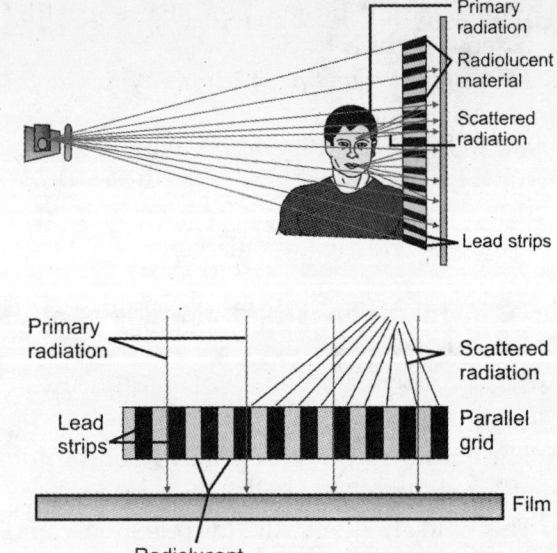

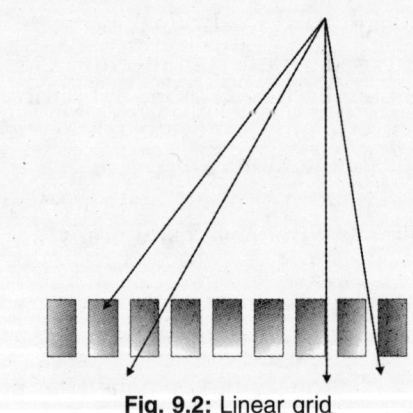

Fig . 9.1: An X-ray grid absorbs scattered X-ray photons from the primary beam and prevents them from fogging the film.

Fig. 9.2: Linear grid

4. *Crossed Grid*

Two grids are placed on top of each other and at right angles. This minimises the scattered radiation traversing in same line as primary beam.

5. *Moving Grid/Potter Bucky Diaphragm*

This reduces the white lead lines in the radiographic image. This is achieved by moving

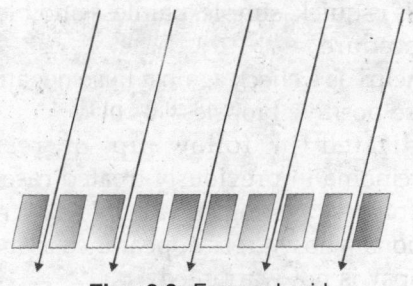

Fig . 9.3: Focused grid

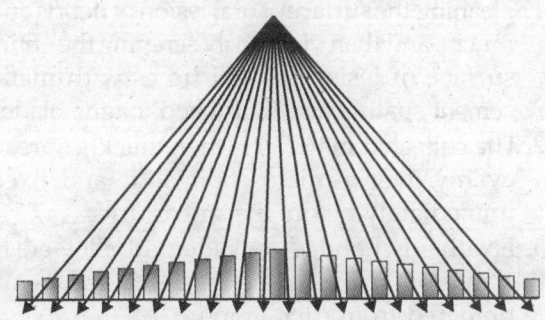

Fig . 9.4: Pseudo-focused grid

the grid sideways during exposure. Images of radiolucent grid lines on film can be deleted by moving the grid in direction of 90° to grid lines during exposure. This results in uniform exposure. It does not interfere with absorption of scattered photons. A moving grid is called as 'Bucky Grid'.

- It does not interfere with absorption of scattered photon.
- This has effect of blurring out the radiolucent lines.

Uses of Grids

- It reduces the amount of scattered radiations exciting a subject that reaches the film and resuts in more uniform exposure.
- It removes scattered radiation.
- It spares primary photons
- It reduces non-imaging exposure
- It increases subject contrast.

Q7 Clinical and laboratory diagnosis of anemias.
Ans.
Clinical Diagnosis of Anemia
Symptoms

Lassitude, fatigue, breathlessness on exertion, palpitations, throbbing in head and ears, dizziness, tinnitus, head ache, dimness of vision, insomnia, paraesthesia of fingers and toes, angina.

Signs

Pallor of skin, mucous membranes, palms of hands, conjunctivae, tachycardia, cardiac dilatation, systolic flow murmurs, oedema.

Laboratory Diagnosis of anemia

- Red blood cell count–decreases than 1 lakh per cubic millimeter.
- Blood smear-BT, CT, hemoglobin level
- Serum iron level
- Hemoglobin level decreases
- Mean corpuscular volume
- Mean corpuscular hemoglobin
- ESR is determined
- Leukocyte count
- Bone marrow analysis.

Q8 Indication and radiographic technique for maxillary standard occlusal view
Ans.
Refer to Q6.1 of September 1998.

SHORT ANSWERS
Q9 Paul-Bunnel Test.
Ans.
Refer to Q13 March 2002 Solution.

Q10 Turner's Tooth
Ans.
Turner's tooth is a type of hypoplasia involving a single tooth most commonly maxillary permanent incisor, maxillary or mandibular premolar.

Clinical Features

The hypoplasia may be of any degree ranging from mild brownish discoloration of the enamel to severe pitting and irregularity of the tooth crown.

Etiology

1. Bacterial infection involving periapical tissue of deciduous tooth may disturb the ameloblastic layer of permanent tooth and result in a hypoplastic crown.
2. Trauma to deciduous teeth when it has been driven into alveolus and has disturbed the permanent tooth bud.

Treatment

- Veneering, composite restoration
- Pulpally involved tooth is RCT treated and restored with crown.
- Bleaching can be done for mild cases of discoloration.
  (Referred from White and Phoroah-Radiology text)

Q11 Lipshutz Bodies

Ans.

These are intranuclear inclusions which are eosinophilic, ovoid, homogeneous structures, with in the nucleus these inclusions tend to displace the nucleolus and nuclear chromatin peripherally.

- Lipshutz bodies are seen in primary herpes labialis and recurrent herpetic stomatitis.
- The displacement of chromatin often produces a peri-inclusion halo.

Clinical Significance

Lipshutz bodies are diagnostic feature of HSV infections.

Q12 Exfoliative Cytology

Ans.

- Exfoliative cytology is an adjunct to the surgical biopsy

- This is quick, simple, painless and bloodless procedure
- It helps as a check against false negative and false positive biopsies
- Indicated in follow up of recurrent carcinoma in previously treated cases
- Exfoliative cytology is valuable for screening lesions whose gross appearance is such that biopsy is not warranted.

Technique

1. Cleaning the surface of oral lesion of debris and mucin, and then vigorously scraping the entire surface of lesion several times with metal cement spatula or a moistened tongue blade.
2. The collected material is then quickly spread evenly over a microscopic slide and fixed immediately before the smear dries.
3. Fixative is flooded on slide and allowed to stand for 30 min. to air dry. Two smears are prepared from each lesion.

The cytologic smear when examined fall into 5 classes:

- Normal
- Atypical
- Intermediate
- Suggestive of cancer
- Positive for cancer.

Uses

Diagnosis of lesions of herpes zoster, Pemphigus vulgaris, Benign familial pemphigus, Keratosis follicularis, Hereditary benign intraepithelial dyskeratosis, White sponge nevus and pernicious and Sickle cell anemia is done by Exfoliative cytology.

Q13 Radiographic view to Detect Fractured Zygomatic Arch

Ans.

The radiographic examination may provides the only means of determining the presence and extent of the injury.

- The submentovertex projection provides a good view of the Zygomatic arch.
- CT images can provide valuable three dimensional information.
- The Occipitomental (Water's) projection provides an image of whole zygoma and maxillary sinus.
- *Inference:* The zygomatic arch may fracture at its weaker point, about 1cm posterior to the zygomaticotemporal suture. Separation or fracture of the frontozygomatic suture may occur medially within the thin bone comprising the lateral wall of antrum.

Panoramic views of the zygomatic arch reveal the zygomaticotemporal suture as a radiolucent line, which may even have the appearance of discontinuity in the inferior border.

Q14 Enumerate two differences between periapical abscess and periodontal abscess
Ans.

Periapical abscess	Periodontal abscess
1-Occur due to caries	Occur due to periodontitis
2-The tooth will be tender on vertical	The tooth tender percussion associated will be be tender on horizontal percussion
3-Radiolucency seen at apex of the tooth	Radiolucency is seen lateral to apex of the tooth
4-Vitality of the tooth is affected	Tooth may be vital as periodontium is involved

Q15 Café-au-lait Spots
Ans.

Café-au-lait spots are pigmented black or brown lesions caused due to melanin pigmentation in orofacial region. This is seen in

1. Hereditary intestinal polyposis syndrome (Peutz-Jeghers syndrome) Melanin pigmentation of lips and oral mucosa is present from birth and appears as small brown macules measuring 1–5 mm.
2. *Neurofibroma:* Patients exhibit asymmetric areas of cutaneous melanin pigmentation. There will be loose overgrowths of thickened, pigmented skin which may hang in folds.
3. *Polyostotic fibrous dysplasia:* Irregularly pigmented melanotic spots of light brown color are seen along with skeletal symptoms.

Q16 Composition of X-ray Film
Ans.
Composition of X-ray Film (Fig. 9.5)
X-ray film has two principal components
- Emulsion
- Base

Emulsion

Silver halide grains. These are sensitive to X radiation and visible light, and a vehicle matrix in which the crystals are suspended. The silver halide grains are composed of crystals of silver bromide.

Base

The function of the film base is to support the emulsion.

The base must have the proper degree of flexibility to allow easy handling of the film. The base is 0.18 mm thick and is made of polyester polyethylene terephthalate. The film base is uniformly translucent and casts no pattern on the resultant radiograph.

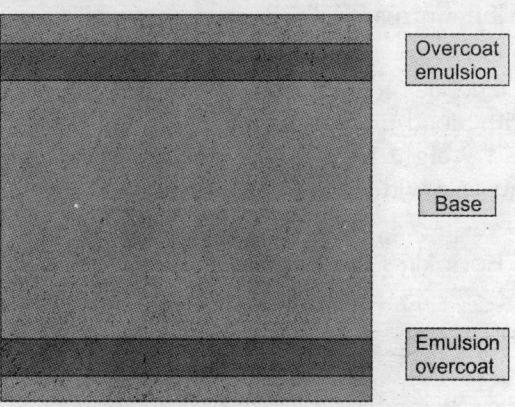

Overcoat emulsion

Base

Emulsion overcoat

Fig . 9.5: X-ray film

Q17 Four conditions associated with cervico-facial lymphadenopathy.

Ans.

1. Actinomycosis

The disease is characterized by the formation of painful abscesses in the mouth, lungs, or gastrointestinal tract. Actinomycosis abscesses grow larger as the disease progresses, often over months. In severe cases, they may penetrate the surrounding bone and muscle to the skin, where they break open and leak large amounts of pus. The purulent leakage via the sinus cavities contains "sulfur granules," not actually sulfur-containing but resembling such particles. These granules contain progeny bacteria.

2. Tuberculosis

Tuberculosis or TB (short for tubercles bacillus) is a common and often deadly infectious disease caused by various strains of mycobacteria, usually *Mycobacterium tuberculosis* in humans. Tuberculosis usually attacks the lungs but can also affect other parts of the body. It is spread through the air, when people who have the disease cough, sneeze, or spit. Most infections in humans result in anasymptomatic, latent infection, and about one in ten latent infections eventually progresses to active disease, which, if left untreated, kills more than 50% of its victims.

The classic symptoms are a chronic cough with blood-tinged sputum, fever, night sweats, and weight loss. Infection of other organs causes a wide range of symptoms.

3. Hodgkin's Lymphoma

It is a type of lymphoma, which is a cancer originating from white blood cells called lymphocytes Hodgkin's lymphoma is characterized by the orderly spread of disease from one lymph node group to another and by the development of systemic symptoms with advanced disease. When Hodgkin's cells are examined microscopically, multinucleated Reed-Sternberg cells (RS cells) are the characteristic histopathologic finding. Hodgkin's lymphoma may be treated withradiation therapy or chemotherapy.

Signs and Symptoms

- Night Sweats
- Unexplained weight loss
- Lymph nodes: the most common symptom of Hodgkin's is the painless enlargement of one or more lymph nodes. The nodes may also feel rubbery and swollen when examined. The nodes of the neck and shoulders (cervical and supraclavicular) are most frequently involved (80–90% of the time, on average). The lymph nodes of the chest are often affected, and these may be noticed on a chest radiograph.
- Splenomegaly
- Hepatomegaly: enlargement of the liver,
- Hepatosplenomegaly
- Pain
- Pain following alcohol consumption
- *Back pain:* Nonspecific back pain (pain that cannot be localized or its cause determined by examination or scanning techniques)
- Red-coloured patches on the skin, easy bleeding and petechiae due to low platelet count
- *Cyclical fever:* Patients may also present with a cyclical high-grade fever known as the Pel-Ebstein fever

4. AIDS

Acquired immune deficiency syndrome or acquired immunodeficiency syndrome (AIDS) is a disease of the human immune system caused by the human immunodeficiency virus (HIV). This condition progressively reduces the effectiveness of the immune system and leaves individuals susceptible to opportu-nistic infections and tumors. HIV is transmitted through direct contact of a mucous membrane or the bloodstream with abodily fluid containing HIV, such as blood, semen, vaginal fluid, preseminal fluid, andbreast milk. This transmission can involve anal, vaginal or oral sex, blood transfusion, contaminated hypodermic needles, exchange between mother and baby duringpregnancy, childbirth, breastfeeding or other exposure to one of the above bodily fluids. AIDS is now a pandemic.

Q18 Clinical features of Bell's Palsy.

Ans.

Bell's palsy or **idiopathic facial paralysis** is a dysfunction of cranial nerve VII (thefacial nerve) that results in inability to control facial muscles on the affected side. Several conditions can cause a facial paralysis, e.g. brain tumor, stroke, and Lyme disease Bell's palsy is defined as an idiopathic unilateral facial nerve paralysis, usually self-limiting. The trademark is rapid onset of partial or complete palsy, usually in a single day. It can occur bilaterally resulting in total facial paralysis in around 1% of cases.

Clinical Features

Bell's palsy is characterized by facial drooping on the affected half, due to malfunction of the facial nerve (VII cranial nerve), which controls the muscles of the face.

Facial palsy is typified by inability to control movement in the facial muscles. The paralysis is of the infranuclear/lower motor neuron type.

The facial nerves control a number of functions, such as blinking and closing the eyes, smiling, frowning, lacrimation, and salivation. They also innervate the stapedial (stapes) muscles of the middle ear and carry taste sensations from the anterior two thirds of the tongue.

Clinicians should determine whether the forehead muscles are spared. Due to an anatomical peculiarity, forehead muscles receive innervation from both sides of the brain. The forehead can therefore still be wrinkled by a patient whose facial palsy is caused by a problem in one of the hemispheres of the brain (central facial palsy). If the problem resides in the facial nerve itself (peripheral palsy) all nerve signals are lost on the ipsilateral (same side of the lesion) half side of the face, including to the forehead (contralateral forehead still wrinkles).

Differential Diagnosis

(Herpes zoster virus, Lyme disease)

The degree of nerve damage can be assessed using the House-Brackmann score.

Although defined as a mononeuritis (involving only one nerve), patients diagnosed with Bell's palsy may have "myriad neurological symptoms" including "facial tingling, moderate or severe headache/neck pain, memory problems, balance problems, ipsilateral limb paresthesias, ipsilateral limb weakness, and a sense of clumsiness" that are "unexplained by facial nerve dysfunction". This is yet an enigmatic facet of this condition.

Signs

- Paralysis of muscles on the side of the face
- Eye on affected side stays open
- *Bell's sign:* The eyeball moves upward when the patient tries to close his eyes
- Exposure keratitis occurs due to inability to close the eye leading to corneal ulceration
- Buccinator muscle weakness
- Creases of forehead are flattened
- Nasolabial fold is lost.

Symptoms

- Pain around the ear
- Drooling of saliva
- Mouth turns to opposite side
- Food is retained in upper and lower buccal and labial folds
- Impaired blinking
- Loss of taste on anterior two thirds of tongue
- Reduced salivary secretion.

10

RGUHS March 2003

QUESTION PAPER

Long Essays

1. Enumerate oral precancerous lesions and conditions. Describe clinical features and management of oral submucous fibrosis
2. Discuss the adverse effects of therapeutic radiation on oral tissues

Short Essays

3. Composition and uses of intensifying screens
4. Uses and side effects of oral penicillins
5. General and oral manifestations of Bismuthism
6. Investigations and management of primary herpetic gingivostomatitis
7. Collimation and filtration
8. Indication and radiographic technique for paranasal view

Short Answers

9. Eagle's syndrome
10. Clinical features of erosive lichen planus
11. Radiographic appearance of Ameloblastoma
12. Hutchinson's triad
13. Sturge-Weber syndrome
14. Indications for bitewing radiographs
15. Enumerate four differences between pemphigus vulgaris and Benign mucous membrane pemphgoid
16. Anodontia
17. Name four drugs causing gingival enlargement
18. Schimmer's test

SOLUTIONS

LONG ESSAYS

Q1 Enumerate oral precancerous lesions and conditions. Describe clinical features and management of oral submucous fibrosis.

Ans.

Precancerous lesion is defined as morphologically altered tissue in which cancer is more likely to occur than its apparent normal part.

- Leukoplakia
- Erythroplakia
- Smoker's palate (Stomatitis nicotina palatine)
- Chronic hyperplastic candidiasis
- Dyskeratosis congenita
- Dyskeratosis follicularis

Premalignant condition is defined as generalized state of body which is associated with significantly increased risk of cancer.

- Oral submucous fibrosis
- Siderogenic dysplasia
- Plummer-Vinson syndrome
- Lichen planus
- Syphilis

Clinical Features

Diagnosis is based on clinically discernable blanching and pallor, palpable bands and restricted mouth opening severe burning sensation of mouth, aggravated by the use of even moderately spicy food.

Histopathologically Atrophic oral epithelium+ loss of rete pegs + epithelial dysplasia + hyalinization of collagen bundles + Fibroblasts decreased and blood vessels obliterated.

Stage I: Early OSMF
- Mild blanching
- No restriction in mouth opening

- No restriction in tongue protrusion (mesioincisal angle of upper central incisor to tip of tongue when maximally extended with mouth wide open will be 6.07 cm in females and 6.73 cm in males.
- Third criteria cheek flexibility (Cf)
  $Cf = V1 - V2$
- Two points measured between at one third the distance from the angle of of mouth on a line joining the tragus of the ear and angle of mouth, (V2) the subject is then asked to blow his cheeks fully and the distance measured between two points marked on the cheek (V1)
- Burning sensation only on taking spicy food or hot liquids.

Stage II: Moderate OSMF
- Moderate to severe blanching
- Mouth opening reduced by 33% flexibility also demonstrably decreased.
- Burning sensation even in absence of stimuli
- Palpable bands felt
- Lymphadenopathy either unilateral or bilaterally.

Stage III: Severe OSMF
- Burning sensation very severe
- More than 66% reduction in mouth opening, Cheek flexibility and tongue protrusion. The tongue may appear fixed.
- Ulcerative lesions may appear on cheek Thick palpable bands Lymphadenopathy bilaterally evident.

Management

Grade I: Only blanching of oral mucosa and no other symptoms
Treatment:Stoppage of habits
- Less spicy food consumption
- Good oral hygiene
- Vitamin A, B synthetic administration

Grade II: Burning, dryness, vesicles and ulcers. This can be alleviated but OSMF is resistant to treatment.

In addition to Grade I Treatment, Palliative therapy is given

- Topical vitamin A and systemic vitamin A, vitamin B complex and beta carotene.
- Oral iron preparations
- Intralesional hydrocortisone- 75 mg/wk
- Topical anesthetics, beta carotene (systemic and topical)

Grade III: Burning, dryness, vesicles and ulcers with restricted mouth opening.

Treatment: Submucosal injected steroids

- Collaginase-2 mg 1ml of hyalurinidase
- Placentrix injection and hyalurinadase in 2% lidocaine placental extract 2cc weekly

Grade IV: Grade III + palpable bands all over the oral cavity except tongue.

- Systemic steroids- Dexamethasone
- Bethnazole – mouth wash/ rinse
- Intra lesional hydrocortisone-75mg/week
- Hyaluronidase injection
- Intralesional 1000/500 IU in 1% cc of lidocaine

Grade V: Grade IV + involvement of tongue.

Treatment:

- Surgical intervention of fibrous bands to relieve trismus is treatment of choice.
- Oral stent is used as an adjunct to surgery to prevent relapse.
- Surgical graft/excision can be done.

Grade VI: OSMF + history of proven oral cancer

Treatment:

- Anti cancer drugs
- Radiotherapy
- Surgical therapy
  Refer to Q3 Sept 2001

Q2 Discuss the adverse effects of therapeutic radiation on oral tissues.

Ans.

Introduction

- Effect of Radiation on oral tissues
- Measures of radiation protection

Effect of Radiation on Oral Tissues

The deterministic effects of a course of radiotherapy in normal tissues of oral cavity occurs when 2 Gy is delivered daily, bilaterally through 8×10 cm fields over the oropharynx, for a weekly exposure of 10 Gy which continues till 50 Gy is administered. The effects are as follows:

1. *Oral Mucous Membrane (OMM)*
   - The OMM contains basal layer composed of radio-sensitive vegetative and differentiating intermitotic cells
   - End of 2nd week of therapy—cells die and mucous membrane begins to show areas of redness and inflammation (MUCOSITIS)
   - The irradiated mucous membrane breaks down with the formation of a white to yellow pseudomembrane (desquamated epithelial layer)
   - End of therapy—mucositis is severe, discomfort is at maximum, food intake is difficult. Secondary yeast infection by candida albicans is common
   - After irradiation, mucosa heals but at later intervals mucous membrane tends to become atrophic, thin and relatively avascular
   - Long-term atrophy results from progressive obliteration of fine vasculature and fibrosis of underlying connective tissue. Ulcers can result from denture sore, radiation necrosis, or tumor recurrence

2. *Taste Buds*
   - Doses in therapeutic range cause extensive degeneration of the normal histologic architecture of taste buds

- Patients notice a loss of taste activity during the 2nd or 3rd week of radiotherapy
  - Bitter and acid flavors are severely affected when posterior 2/3rd of tongue is irradiated
  - Salt and sweet flavors are affected when anterior third of the tongue is irradiated

3. *Salivary Glands*
   - The parenchymal component of the salivary gland is radiosensitive. (Parotid gland is more sensitive than sub-mandibular or sublingual gland)
   - A marked progressive loss of salivary secretion in 1st few weeks of radiotherapy
   - The extent of reduced flow is dose-dependant and reaches to zero at 60 Gy
   - The mouth becomes dry (xerostomia) and tender, and swallowing is difficult and painful due to lack of lubrication
   - Saliva will be viscous and has a pH value 1 unit below normal (i.e. an average of 5.5 in irradiated patients compared with 6.5 in unexposed individuals)
   - Buffering capacity of saliva falls after irradiation the inflammatory response becomes more chronic and glands demonstrate progressive fibrosis and adiposis.
   - Changes in salivary condition leads to radiation caries.
   - There is increase in *Streptococcus mutans*, *Lactobacillus* and *Candida* organisms

4. *Teeth*
   - Irradiation of the teeth with therapeutic doses
     a. During their development retards growth
     b. If precedes calcification may destroy tooth bud
     c. After calcification has begun irradiation of teeth may inhibit cellular differentiation, causing malformation and arresting growth

- Children receiving radiation therapy to the jaw may show defect in permanent dentition such as
  - Retarded root development
  - Dwarf teeth
  - Failure to form one or more teeth
- The teeth may complete calcification and erupt prematurely
- Adult teeth is usually resistant to radiation exposure but pulpal tissue may demonstrate long term fibroatrophy
- Radiation caries is a rampant form of dental decay that results from changes in salivary glands and saliva.

Types of Radiation Caries

1. Widespread superficial lesions attacking buccal, occlusal, incisal and palatal surfaces
2. Involves primarily the cementum and dentin in the cervical region
3. Lesions progress around the tooth circumferentially and result in loss of crown
4. Final type–appears as a dark pigmentation of the entire crown

5. *Bone*
   - Mature bone is damaged due to irradiation of mandible during treatment of oral cancer as there is radiation induced damage to vasculature of periosteum and cortical bone.
   - Osteoblasts are destroyed. Normal marrow may be replaced with fatty marrow and fibrous connective tissue.
   - Marrow tissue becomes hypovascular, hypoxic and hypocellular
   - Endosteum becomes atrophic leading to necrosis
   - Degree of mineralization may be reduced, leading to brittleness and these changes are so severe that bone death results, the condition is called as osteoradionecrosis.
   - This renders the bone to get easily infected.

Measures of Radiation Protection

Position and distance rule: If no barrier is available, the operator should stand at least 6 feet from the patient, at an angle of 900–1350 to central ray of the X-ray beam when the exposure is made.

1. The operator can leave the room or take a position behind a suitable barrier or wall during exposure of film.
2. Operators should never hold the films in place.
3. Neither the operator nor patient should hold the radiographic tube housing during exposure.

To ensure that personnel–monitoring devices are used which are referred to as "Film Badges" these devices provide a useful record of occupational exposure.

SHORT ESSAYS

Q3 Composition and uses of intensifying screens.
Ans.
Refer to Q4 of September 2001 solution

Q4 Uses and side effects of oral penicillins
Ans.
Dental uses of oral penicillins:
1. Periodontal abscess
2. Periapical abscess
3. Acute suppurative pulpitis
4. Ludwig's angina
5. Vincent's angina-supportive infection of salivary gland
6. Postoperative and post traumatic infections, injury.

Medical uses of oral penicillin:
1. Sinusitis
2. Meningitis
3. Syphilis
4. Tonsillitis
5. Pharyngitis
6 Gonorrhea
7. Diphtheria
8. Tetanus
9. Anthrax
10. Actinomycosis
11. Skin, bone, soft tissue infections.

Side effects of penicillins
1. Anaphylactic shock
2. Skin rash, serum sickness like syndrome
3. Bone marrow depression
4. GI upset-Diarrhea is common with Ampicillin
5. Angioedema
6. J-H Reaction in syphilis when pencillin is given.

Q5 General and oral manifestations of Bismuthism.
Ans.
Bismuth was formerly used widely in the treatment of syphilis and its use is still common in treating certain dermatologic disorders. Ingestion of heavy metals or Metal salts can be an occupational hazard, since many metals are used in industry and paints. These ingested pigments tend to extravasate from vessels in foci of increased capillary permeability such as inflamed tissues.

General symptoms of toxicity includes:
• Behavioural changes
• Neurologic disorders
• Intestinal pain

Oral Manifestations

• Bismuth pigmentation of oral mucosa, particularly of gingival and buccal mucosa is most common oral feature of bismuth therapy.
• The pigmentation appears as a "bismuth line" a thin blue black line in the marginal gingiva which is sometimes confined to the gingival papilla.

- There may also be the same type of pigmentation of buccal mucosa, the lips the ventral surface of tongue, or in any localized area of inflammation such as around partially erupted third molar or around the periphery of the ulcer as an anachoretic phenomenon.
- This pigment represents precipitated granules of bismuth sulfide produced by the action of hydrogen sulfide on the bismuth compound in the tissues.
- The hydrogen sulfide is formed through bacterial degradation of organic material or food debris and is most common in sites of food retention.
- The bismuth line occur in patients receiving prolonged bismuth therapy and more frequent in unclean mouths.
- Patient complains of burning sensation of oral mucosa and a metallic taste in the mouth.

Q6 Investigations and management of primary herpetic gingivostomatitis.
Ans.

Investigations

The typical clinical picture of primary herpetic gingivostomatitis can be diagnosed according to case history, laboratory test:

1. *Cytology:* The fresh vesicle can be opened and a scraping made from the base of the lesion and placed on a microscope slide. The slide may be stained with giemsa, wright's or Papanicolau's stain and searched for multinucleated giant cells, syncytium and ballooning degeneration of nucleus.
2. *HSV Isolation:* Isolation and neutralization of a virus in tissue culture is the most positive method of identification and has a specificity and sensitivity of 100%.
3. *Antibody titers:* Conclusive evidence of a primary HSV infection includes testing for complement fixing or neutralizing antibody

in acute and convalescent sera. However, it is rarely necessary in routine clinical situation and is often not helpful since the results are not available until the infection is gone.

In immuno-compromised patients, an acute serum specimen should be obtained within 3-4 days of onset of symptoms. Absence of detectable antibodies plus isolation of HSV from lesions is compatible with the presence of primary HSV infection.

Presence of antibody to HSV will begin to appear in a week and reach a peak in 3 weeks.

Convalescent serum can confirm diagnosis by demonstrating fourfold rise in anti-HSV antibody.

If the antibody titers are similar in acute and convalescent sera, then the lesions from which HSV was isolated were recurrent lesions.

Management

1. Mild cases: supportive care is necessary.
2. *Moderate cases:* Analgesics are given to relieve pain–Aspirin and to control fever Aceta-minophen is given.
3. *Anaesthetics:* To relieve burning sensation on eating and drinking
   - Dyclonine hydrochloride 0.5%
   - Lidocaine
   - Diphenhydramie hydrochloride 5 mg/ml mixed with milk of magnesia.
4. *Antiviral drugs:*
   - Acyclovir
   - Famciclovir
   - Valacyclovir
5. Antibiotics are given for controlling other toxic systemic complication along with HSV infection.
6. Fluids and electrolyte balance has to be maintained for proper hydration.
7. *Dental treatment:* Supragingival scaling has to be done to relieve gingival inflammation.

Q7 Collimation and filtration.

Ans.

Refer to March 2002 Q8.

Q8 Indication and radiographic technique for paranasal view.

Ans.

The paranasal sinuses are air filled cavities of the craniofacial complex, comprising of maxillary frontal and sphenoid sinuses and ethmoid air cells The maxillary sinus is of particular importance to dentist because of their proximity to dental structures

Indications for Paranasal Sinus View

- Diseases associated with maxillary sinus
A. Intrinsic
  - Mucositis
  - Sinusitis
  - Empyema
  - Retention Pseudocyst
  - Polyps
  - Antroliths
  - Mucocele
  - Neoplasms-benign:
    - Epithelial papilloma
    - Osteoma
    - *Malignant:* Squamous cell carcinoma
  Pseudo tumor

B. Extrinsic
  - Periostitis
  - Odontogenic cysts and tumors
  - Fibrous dysplasia

- Traumatic injuries to paranasal sinuses can be detected

Radiographic Technique for Paranasal Sinus View

Various radiographic techniques are used to view paranasal sinuses

1. Maxillary lateral occlusal projection for maxillary sinus view

2. Panoramic radiograph depicts greater internal structure of maxillary sinus and parts of inferior, posterior and anteromedial walls

3. Standard series of playing film views of the sinuses include Occipitomental (Waters), Lateral submentovertex Caldwell 150 degree. PA view is used to evaluate frontal sinus and ethmoid air cells

4. Lateral skull views: 4 pairs of paranasal sinuses

5. Computed tomography and MRI (Magnetic Resonance Imaging) is important for evaluation of sinus disease

6. High resolution axial and coronal CT and MRI examinations are the most useful and non-invasive technique for paranasal sinuses and adjacent structures

Submentovertex Projection (Fig. 10.1)

- Image receptor and patient placement
  Image receptor is placed parallel to patient's transverse plane and perpendicular to the mid sagital and coronal planes. To achieve this, the patient's neck is extended as far backwards as possible, with the cantho-meatal line forming a 10 degree angle with the image receptor
- Position of the central X-ray beam
  The central beam is perpendicular to the image receptor, directed from below the mandible towards the vertex of the skull

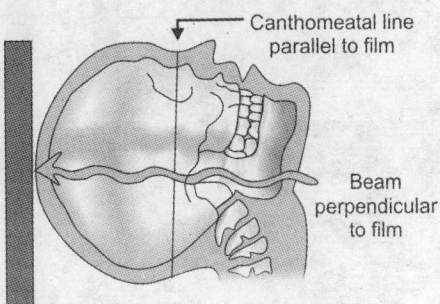

Canthomeatal line parallel to film

Beam perpendicular to film

Fig. 10.1: Submentovertex projection

(hence the name submentovertex, or SMV), and centered about 2 cm anterior to a line connecting the right and left condyles
• Resultant image

The mid sagital plane (represented by an imaginary line extending from the interproximal space of the maxillary central incisors through the nasal septum, to the middle of the anterior arch of atlas, and to the dens) should divide the skull in two symmetric halves

Water's Projection (Figs 10.2 and 10.3)

• Image receptor and patient placement

The Image receptor is placed in front of the patient and perpendicular to the midsaggital plane

The patients head is tilted upwards so that the canthomeatal line forms a 37-degree angle with the image receptor
• Position of the central X-ray beam

The central beam is perpendicular to the image receptor and centered in the area of the maxillary sinuses
• Resultant image

The midsagital plane should divide the skull images in two symmetric halves Postero-anterior Cephalometric projection
• Image receptor and patient placement

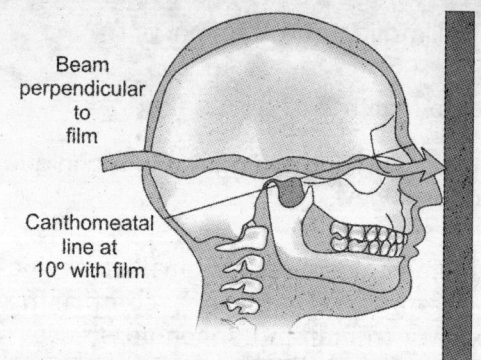

Fig. 10.3: Posteroanterior cephalometric projection

The image receptor is placed in front of the patient, perpendicular to the midsagital plane and parallel to coronal plane. The patient is placed so that canthomeatal line forms a 10-degree angle with the horizontal plane and Frankfurt plane perpendicular to image receptor.
• Position of the central X-ray beam

The central beam is perpendicular to image receptor, directed from posterior to anterior, parallel to patient's midsagital plane, and is centered at the level of bridge of nose
• Resultant image

The midsagital plane (represented by an imaginary line extending from the inter-proximal space of the maxillary central incisors through the nasal septum and the middle of bridge of nose) should divide the skull image in two symmetric halves.

SHORT ANSWERS

Q9 Eagle's Syndrome

Ans. Refer to Q7 of September 2001

Q10 Clinical features of erosive lichen planus.

Ans.

Refer to Q3.1 of September 1998.

Q11 Radiographic appearance of amelo-blastoma

Ans.

Refer to Q2 of March 2000

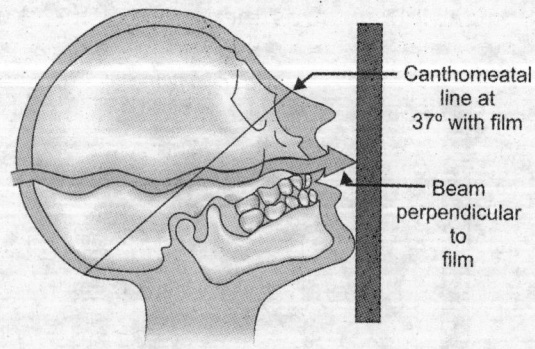

Fig. 10.2: Water's projection

Q12 Hutchinson's triad
Ans.

Hutchinson's triad includes

a. Hypoplasia of incisors and molar teeth.

b. Eighth nerve deafness

c. Interstitial keratitis.

The Hutchinson's triad is the pathagnomonic feature of the congenital syphilis. Congenital syphilis is transmitted to offspring only by an infected mother and is not inherited.

The patients inherit great variety of lesions in congenital syphilis which includes

i. Frontal bossing,

ii. Short maxilla,

iii. High palatal arch,

iv. Saddle nose,

v. Mulberry molars,

vi. Irregular thickening of sternoclavicular portion of clavicle,

vii. Protuberance of mandible.

Q13 Sturge-Weber syndrome
Ans.

(Encephalofacial or Encephalotrigeminal Angiomatosis)

It is characterized by angiomatosis of the face with a variable distribution sometimes matching the dermatomes of one or more trigeminal nerve divisions, leptomeningeal angiomas particularly of parietal and occipital lobes of brain with associated characteristic intracranial calcifications, contralateral hemiplegia, and one or more neurologic syndrome.

Oral Changes

- Include massive growth of gingiva
- Asymmetric jaw growth
- Tooth eruption sequence is altered.
- Intraoral lesions occur on same side of the body as other angiomas occur in the patient.

Q14 Indications for bitewing radiographs
Ans.

Bitewing radiographs: Show only the crowns of teeth and adjacent alveolar crests

Bitewing Radiography

This is also called as interproximal radiograph

- Horizontal bitewing films
- Vertical bitewing films

Residual alveolar crests in the maxilla and the mandible will be recorded on the radiograph

Uses/Indications

- In the diagnosis of interproximal caries
- To study the height of pulp chamber
- To study the occlusion of the teeth
- In the diagnosis of pulp stones
- To study height of alveolar bone or assessment of bone loss
- In diagnosis of secondary caries
- To detect interproximal calculus, foreign bodies and subgingival calculus.

Q15 Enumerate four differences between pemphigus vulgaris and benign mucous membrane pemphigoid
Ans.

Table. 10.1

Q16 Anodontia
Ans.

Refer to Q18 of March 2002

Q17 Name four drugs causing gingival enlargement.
Ans.

Refer Q.18. March 2000 for detailed explanation

1. Nifedipine–Calcium channel blocker
2. Phenytion–Antiepileptic drug.
3. Dilantin sodium–Anticonvulsant drug.
4. Cyclosporin–Immunosuppressant.

Table 10.1

Pemphigus vulgaris	Benign mucous membrane pemphigoid
Location: Anywhere on oral mucosa.	Oral mucosa and conjunctiva
Age/sex of occurrence: 40–70 years; either sex	Over 40 years; either sex
Clinical features: Oral lesions consists of multiple bullae that may precede, accompany, or follow skin lesions painful ulcers; Nikolsky's sign is positive.	Bullous lesions that become ulcers, patients in general good health, involvement of other mucous membrane is common.
Microscopical features: Intraepithelial accumulation of fluid,degeneration of epithelial cells; mild subvesicular oedema and inflammation; Tzank cell is seen in bullae.	Intraepithelial and subepithelial accumulation of fluid.
Treatment: Symptomatic only; cortisone of temporary value	Symptomatic
Prognosis-poor, disease fatal in >50% cases	Good, but eye lesions may cause blindness.

Q18 Shimmer's Test

Ans.

Objective

This test is done to evaluate salivary gland function in suspected Sjogren's syndrome patients.

Technique

The schirmer's test consists of placing a strip of filter paper in the lower conjunctival sac.

Inference

Normal patients will wet 15 mm of filter paper in 5 minutes but Patients with Sjogren's syndrome will wet less than 5 mm of filter paper in 5 minutes.

This indicates the abnormality in the lacrimal gland secretion Sjogren's syndrome consists of Xerostomia, Xerophthalmia (primary Sjogren's syndrome) and connective tissue disease such as Rheumatoid arthritis, progressive systemic sclerosis, systemic lupus erythematosis or polymyositis(secondary Sjogren's syndrome).

Uses

In similar manner, function of submandibular, sublingual and parotid gland can be analyzed with the help of this test.

QUESTION PAPER

Long Essays

1. Define autoimmune diseases and enumerate autoimmune diseases that have indirect and direct effect on oral cavity. Give the clinical features and investigations of pemphigus vulgaris.
2. What are the indications for occlusal radiographs? Describe the radiographic techniques in taking maxillary and mandibular cross-sectional occlusal radiographs.

Short Essays

3. Pathogenesis and management of Osteoradionecrosis
4. Etiology and signs and symptoms of Bell's palsy.
5. Classification and uses of penicillin.
6. Types and uses of Grids
7. Indications and contraindications of sialography.
8. Priciple and Indications for Clark's technique/ Shift cone technique.

Short Answers

9. Plummer vinson syndrome
10. Lipshutz bodies.
11. Radiographic appearance of Fibrous dysplasia.
12. Four differences between Pemphigus Vulgaris and Benign mucous membrane Pemphigoid.
13. Turner's tooth
14. Auspitz sign
15. Name two conditions that show elevated serum alkaline phosphatase level.
16. Sturge-Weber syndrome
17. Exfoliative cytology.
18. Postherpetic neuralgia

SOLUTIONS

LONG ESSAYS

Q1 Define autoimmune diseases and enumerate autoimmune diseases that have indirect and direct effect on oral cavity. Give the clinical features and investigations of pemphigus vulgaris.

Ans.

Definition

It is a condition in which structural or functional damage is produced by the action of immunologically competent cells or antibodies against the normal components of the body.

Enumeration of Autoimmune diseases that have indirect and direct effect on oral cavity

Classification

1. Haemocytolytic autoimmune disease
   - Autoimmune haemolytic anemia.
   - Autoimmune thrombocytopenia
   - Autoimmune leukoplakia

2. Localized (organ specific) autoimmune disease
   - Autoimmune disease of thyroid gland – Hashimoto's disease.
   - Thyrotoxicosis (Grave's disease)
   - Addison's disease
   - Autoimmune orchitis
   - Autoimmune disease of nervous system
   - Myasthenia gravis
   - Pernicious anemia

3. Systemic (or non-organ specific)
   - Systemic lupus erythematosis
   - Rheumatoid arthritis
   - Polyarthritis nodosa
   - *Sjogren's syndrome:* Triad of conjunctivitis sicca, dryness of mouth withsalivary gland enlargement and rheumatoid arthritis.

4. Transitory autoimmune process
   - Anemia
   - Thrombocytopenia
   - Nephritis following infection

The autoimmune diseases classification 2 according to Burkitt:

1. Primary immune disease
2. Secondary immune disease
3. Acquired immune deficiency syndrome
4. The connective tissue disease
5. Allergy

Clinical Features

- Pemphigus vulgaris is an autoimmune disease.

- The classical lesion of pemphigus is a thin-walled bullae arising on otherwise normal skin or mucosa.

- The bullae rapidly breaks but continues to extend peripherally, eventually leaving large areas devoided of skin.

- A charactristic sign of the disease may be obtained by application of pressure to an intact bulla In patients with pemphigus vulgaris the bullae will enlarge by extensions to an apparently normal surface.

- Another characteristic feature of the disease is that pressure to an apparently normal area will result in formation of a new lesion. This phenomenon is called as the "Nikolsky's sign", results from upper layers of skin pulling away from the basal layer. This is caused due to the prevesicular edema which disrupts the epidermal junction.

- The course of pemphigus is variable. The disease terminating in death or recovery within few days or weeks or being prolonged for months or years.

Oral Manifestations

Lesion starts on the buccal mucosa, often on areas of trauma along the occlusal plane. The palate and gingiva are common sites. Oral lesions are present up to four months before the skin lesions appear.

Investigations

- Biopsies are taken from an intact vesicle or bulla which is less than 24 hours old, especially from the advancing edge.
- Cytologic examination of the Tzanck smear is helpful in diagnosing pemphigus vulgaris
- Indirect immunofluorescent antibody test distinguishes pemphigus from pemphigoid and other chronic oral lesion. Technique: Serum from a patient is placed over prepared slide of an epidermal structure such as guinea pig's oesophagus. Then the slide is overlaid with fluorescein tagged anti human gamma globulin.
- Patients with pemphigus vulgaris will have antibodies against intercellular substance that will show up under a fluorescent microscope.
- Direct immunofluorescent test: Specimens of patients own skin or mucous is used directly. This is more sensitive and done in early stages of pemphigus. In this technique, fluorescein tagged antihuman gamma globulin is placed over the patients tissue specimen and viewed under fluorescent microscope.

Q2 What are the indications for Occlusal Radiographs? Describe the radiographic techniques in taking maxillary and mandibular cross sectional Occlusal Radiographs.

Ans.

Indications of Occlusal Radiographs Refer Q6.1 of September 1998

Cross Sectional Maxillary Occlusal Radiograph

- *Image field:* This projection shows the palate, zygomatic process of the maxilla, anteroinferior aspects of each antrum, nasolacrimal canals, teeth from second molar to second molar and nasal septum.
- *Film placement:* Seat the patient upright with the sagittal plane perpendicular to the floor and occlusal plane horizontal. Place the film, with its long dimension perpendicular to the sagittal plane, crosswise in the mouth. Gently push the film in backward until it contacts the anterior border of the mandibular rami. The patient stabilizes the film by gently closing the mouth.
- *Projection of the central ray:* Direct the central ray at a vertical angulation of +65° and a horizontal angulation of 0° to the bridge of nose just below the nasion, towards the middle of the film.

Cross Sectional Mandibular Occlusal Radiograph (Figs 11.1 and 11.2)

- *Image field:* This projection includes the soft tissue of the floor of mouth and reveals the lingual and buccal plates of mandible from second molar to second molar. When this view is made to examine the floor of the mouth (eg. for sialolith), the exposure time should be reduced to one half the time used to create an image of the mandible.

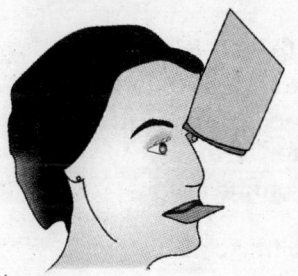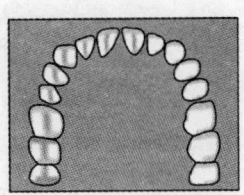

Fig. 11.1: Cross sectional maxillary occlusal projection

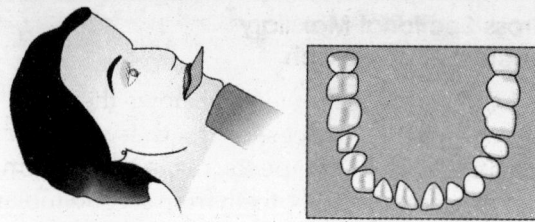

Fig. 11.2: Cross sectional mandibular occlusal projection

- *Film placement:* Seat the patient in a semi-reclining position with the head tilted back so that the ala tragus line is almost perpendicular to the floor.

  Place the film in the mouth with its long axis perpendicular to the sagittal plane and with the tube side towards the mandible.

  The anterior border of the film should be approximately 1cm beyond the mandibular central incisor. Ask the patient to bite gently on the film to hold it in position.

- *Projection of the central ray:* Direct the central ray at the midline through the floor of mouth approximately 3 cm below the chin at right angles to the center of film.

SHORT ESSAYS

Q3 Pathogenesis and management of Osteoradionecrosis.
Ans.
Refer to Q5 of September 2000.

Q4 Etiology and signs and symptoms of Bell's palsy.
Ans.

Etiology
Etiology of Bell's palsy is idiopathic. Facial palsy may result due to thrombosis, hematosis /hamartoma, Parkinson, hemiplegia or lesions involving 'Lower Motor Neuron'.

- With in the pons- Pontine lesions

Lesions involve Facial Muscles
1. Acute/chronic degenerative lesions of facial nerve
2. Other pontine lesions
3. Poliomyelitis
4. Multiple Sclerosis
5. Tumor

Lesions with in the Posterior Cranial Fossa
Facial nerve is in close proximity to nervus intermedius and eighth nerve.
1. Acoustic neuroma.
2. Pontine cerebro-angle tumour.

Lesions within Temporal Bone
1. Fracture/trauma
2. Infections of middle ear at the level of mastoid.
3. Surgical operations at the ear
4. Mastoidectomy.
5. Tumor of bone
6. Jame's Ramsay-Hunt Syndrome
   Herpes Zoster of geniculate ganglion causes facial paralysis through secondary involvement of motor fibers.
7. Hemorrhage into facial canal- Hypertension, Leukemia.

After Emergence
1. Parotitis
2. Malignant tumor
3. Melkerson's Rosenthal syndrome
4. Reidforth's syndrome
5. Traumatic use of forceps.

Clinical Features
Refer to Q 18.September 2002

Q5 Classification and uses of Penicillin.
Ans.

Classification
Semisynthetic Penicillins

1. Acid resistant alternative to penicillin G Phenoxymethyl Penicillin

2. Penicillinase resistant penicillins
   - Methicillin
   - Oxacillin
   - Cloxacillin
   - Naficillin
   - Flucloxacillin
   - Dicloxacillin
3. Extended spectrum penicillins
   - Amino penicillins
     - Ampicillin
     - Bacampicillin
     - Amoxicillin
   - Carboxypenicillins
     - Carbenicillin
     - Carbenicillin Indanyl
     - Carbenicillin Phenyl
     - Ticarcillin
   - Ureidopenicillins
     - Mezlocillin
     - Piperacillin
   - Mecillinam
4. Beta-Lactamase Inhibitors
   - Clavulonic Acid
   - Sulbactam

Natural Penicillins

Uses of penicillins.

Dental uses of Oral Penicillins

1. Periodontal abscess
2. Periapical abscess
3. Acute suppurative pulpitis
4. Ludwig's angina
5. Vincent's angina- suppurative infection of salivary gland
6. Postoperative and post traumatic infections, injury

Medical uses of Oral Penicillin

1. Sinusitis
2. Meningitis
3. Syphilis
4. Tonsillitis
5. Pharyngitis
6. Gonorrhea
7. Diphtheria
8. Tetanus
9. Anthrax
10. Actinomycosis
11. Skin, bone, soft tissue infections.

Side effects of Penicillin's

1. Anaphylactic shock
2. Skin rash, serum sickness like syndrome
3. Bone marrow depression
4. GI upset-Diarrhea is common with Ampicillin
5. Angioedema
6. J-H Reaction in Syphilis when pencillin is given.
   {Referred from Tripathi Pharmacology text}

Q6 Types and uses of Grids
Ans.

Refer to Q6 of September 2002.

Q7 Indications and contraindications of Sialography
Ans.

Sialogram is a radiograph which is taken by a technique in which radiopaque dye is injected in the salivary glands and radiographs are taken to study the normal anatomy, physiology or pathologic condition in relation to gland.

This is a useful diagnostic adjunct for detection of salivary gland disease.

Indications

Refer Q2 of September 20ns

Contraindications

1. If patient is allergic to or hypersensitive to iodine

2. In cases of fulminating ascending infection of gland from duct opening

3. Acute inflammation of salivary gland as it causes retrograde dissemination. Example: in acute suppurative sialadenitis.

4. If the patient has to get immediate thyroid function test the sialography is contra-indicated as absorption of iodine present in contrast medium, across glandular mucosa may interfere studies.

Q8 Principle and Indications for Clark's technique/Shift Cone Technique.
Ans.

Principle (Fig. 11.3)

The relative positions of radiographic images of two separate objects change when the projection angle at which the images made is changed.

- The position of an object may be determined with respect to reference structures using the tube shift technique. The fig shows two radiographs of an object exposed at different angles. Compare the position of the object in question on each radiograph with the reference structures.

- If the tube is shifted and directed at the reference object (Example: The apex of a tooth) from a more mesial angulation and the object in question also moves mesially with respect to the reference object, the object lies lingual to the reference object.

- Alternatively, if the tube is shifted mesially and the object in question appears to move distally, it lies on the buccal aspect of reference object.

These relations can be easily remembered by the acronym SLOB: Same lingual opposite buccal.

Thus the object in question appears to move in same direction with respect to the reference structures as does the X-ray tube, it is on the lingual aspect of the reference object; if it appears to move in the opposite direction as the X-ray tube, it is on the buccal aspect. If it does not move with respect to the reference object, it lies at the same depth (in the same vertical plane) as the reference object.

Indications for Clark's Technique

- Object localization
- Location of a foreign object or an impacted tooth within the jaw
- Location of normal anatomical landmarks and comparison of anatomy displayed on images helps distinguish changes in horizontal or vertical angulation
- The buccal or lingual location of impacted tooth can be identified.

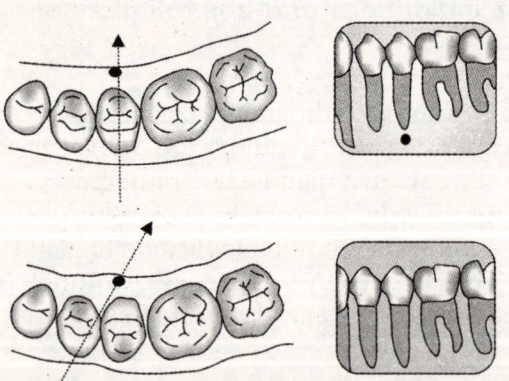

Fig. 11.3: An object on the lingual surface of the mandible may appear apical to the second premolar. When another radiograph is made of this region angulated from the mesial side, the object appears to have moved mesially with respect to the second premolar apex (same lingual is acronym SLOB)

SHORT ANSWERS

Q9 Plummer-Vinson syndrome
Ans.
Refer Q2 of September 1998.

Q10 Lipshutz Bodies
Ans.
Refer Q11.Sept 2002

Q11 Radiographic appearance of Fibrous Dysplasia.
Ans.
Location
- Posterior aspect of maxilla
- Lesions are unilateral expect for rare cases.

Periphery
Defined with gradual blending of normal trabecular bone into an abnormal trabecular pattern.

Internal Structure
- Abnormal trabeculae are shorter, thinner, irregularly shaped, and more numerous than normal trabeculae.
- Fibrous dysplasia have a granular appearance or ground glass appearance resembling small fragments of shattered windshield in early stage.
- A pattern resembling the surface of an orange i.e. peau-d-orange.
- A wispy arrangement-cotton wool appearance
- An amorphous dense pattern
- A distinctive characteristic is organization of abnormal trabaculae into a swirling

Effects on surrounding Structures
There is expansion with maintenance of a thinned outer cortex.

Q12 Four differences between Pemphigus Vulgaris and Benign Mucous membrane Pemphigoid
Ans.
Refer to Q15 of March 2003.

Q13 Turner's Tooth
Ans.
Turner's tooth is a type of hypoplasia involving a single tooth most commonly maxillary permanent incisor, maxillary or mandibular premolar.

Clinical Features
The hypoplasia may be of any degree ranging from mild brownish discoloration of the enamel to severe pitting and irregularity of the tooth crown.

Etiology
1. Bacterial infection involving periapical tissue of deciduous tooth may disturb the ameloblastic layer of permanent tooth and result in a hypoplastic crown.
2. Trauma to deciduous teeth when it has been driven into alveolus and has disturbed the permanent tooth bud.

Treatment
- Veneering, composite restoration
- Pulpally involved tooth is RCT treated and restored with crown.
- Bleaching can be done for mild cases of discoloration.
  (Referred from White and Phoroah-Radiology text)

Q14 Auspitz sign
Ans.
Auspitz sign is a characteristic feature of Psoriasis. Psoriasis is a chronic inflammatory dermatologic disease characterized by occurrences of small, sharply delineated, dry papules, each covered by delicate silvery scale.

If deep scales are removed, one or more tiny bleeding points are disclosed, a characteristic feature termed as Auspitz sign.

After removal of scale the surface of skin is red and dusky in appearance.

Histologic Features
Uniform parakeratosis, absence of stratum granulosum and elongation and clubbing of rete pegs.

The epithelium over connective tissue papillae is thinned and it is from these points that bleeding occurs when scales are peeled off.

Tortuous, dilated capillaries extending high in papillae are prominent.

Q15 Name two conditions that show elevated serum alkaline phosphatase levels.

Ans.

- Hyperparathyroidism
- Fibrous dysplasia
- Paget's disease
- Osteoporosis

Q16 Sturge-Weber Syndrome

Ans.

Refer Q13 March 2003

Q17 Exfoliative Cytology

Ans.

Refer Q12.Sept 2002.

Q18 Postherpetic Neuralgia

Ans.

This is a persistent neuralgia that continues after the acute herpes zoster lesion has healed. Acute herpes zoster is recurrent infection and the neurotropic virus travels along the involved nerve, causing a neuritis and eventually vesicular disease of skin or mucous membrane.

Clinical Features

- Pain is more common in individuals older than 60 years, although it can occur at any age.
- Episodes of severe lancinating or burning pain occur at the site of a former eruption, usually accompanied by hyperalgesia of healed scars
- There is no trigger zone.

Treatment

Short term, high dose systemic corticosteroid
- Tricyclic antidepressant therapy
- Local anaesthetic block– Topical capsaicin.

RGUHS March 2004

QUESTION PAPER

Long Essays

1. Define ulcers. Classify ulcers of oral cavity. Write the clinical features and managememt of Erythema multiforme.

2. What are the parts of X-ray tube? Describe the working of X-ray tube and add a note on Bremsstrahlung radiation.

Short Essays

3. Pathogenesis and management of oral leukoplakia.

4. Etiology and signs and symptoms of trigeminal neuralgia.

5. Indications and contraindications of corticosteroid therapy in dentistry.

6. Composition and function of developing solution.

7. Types and uses of filtration.

8. Composition and uses of intensifying screen.

Short Answers

9. Toluidine blue staining

10. Talon's cusp

11. Four causes of a dark radiograph

12. Radiographic appearance of ameloblastoma

13. Ascher's syndrome

14. Bell's sign

15. Radiographic appearance of periapical granuloma

16. Four oral manifestations of Aplastic Anemia.

17. Four causes for trismus.

18. Two differences between direct and indirect immunofluorescence.

SOLUTIONS

LONG ESSAYS

Q1 Define ulcers. Classify ulcers of oral cavity. Write the clinical features and management of Erythema Multiforme.

Ans.

Definition

An ulcer is defined as a break in the continuity of the covering epithelium, skin or mucous membrane. It may either follow molecular death of the surface epithelium or its traumatic removal.

Classification of ulcers of the oral cavity

Refer to Q1 of march 2000.

Clinical Features

General Findings

EM is seen most frequently in children and young adults and is rare after 50 years of age.

It has acute or an explosive onset. A patient may be asymptotic and in less than 24 hours have extensive lesions of skin and mucosa.

Erythema Multiforme Simplex

Least severe form of disease is characterized by macules and papules 0.5–2 cm in diameter, appearing in a symmetric distribution.

Area's Involved

- Hands, feet and extensor surfaces of elbows and knees. The face and neck are commonly involved, but only severe cases will affect the trunk.
- Typical skin lesion may be non-specific macules and papules and vesicles.
- More typical skin lesions contain petechiae in the center of lesion.
- 'Pathagnomonic lesion' is the target or is a lesion which consists of central bulla or pale clearing area surrounded by edema and bands of erythema.

Stevens-Johnson's Syndrome

- It is a Severe Vesiculobullous form of Disease
- A very severe form of EM with widespread involvement typically including skin, oral cavity, eyes and genitalia.
- It commences with the abrupt occurrence of fever, malaria, photophobia and eruptions of oral mucosa, genitalia and skin.
- The mucocutaneous lesions are hemorrhagic and often vesicular/bullous
- *Oral mucous membrane lesions:* Extremely severe and so painful that mastication is impossible. Mucosal vesicles/bullae occur which rupture and leave surfaces covered with a thick white or yellow exudates. The patient drools blood tinged saliva.
- Erosions on pharynx are common.
- Lips may exhibit ulcerations with bloody crusting lips are extensively eroded and painful.
- *Eye lesions:* Photophobia, a characteristic of disease is conjunctivitis corneal ulceration and panophthalmitis keratoconjunctivitis sicca may occur or blindness may result from bacterial infection
- *Genital lesions:* Non-specific urethritis, balanitis and or vaginal ulcers.
- *Others:* Tracheobronchial ulceration and pneumonia

TENS (Toxic Epidermal Necrolysis)

This is secondary to drug reaction, and results in sloughing of the skin and mucosa in large sheets.

Morbidity is high from secondary infection, fluid and electrolyte imbalance or involvement of lung, liver or kidney.

Management

1. EM simplex- mild cases of oral EM are treated with supportive measures only.
   - Topical anesthetic mouthwash
   - Soft and liquid diet
2. Moderate to severe cases
   - Systemic corticosteroids for short course
     - Dexamethasone
     - Prednisone

   Only clinicians familiar with side effects should use this. Initial dose of 30 mg/day to 50 mg/day prednisone or methyl pre-dnisolone for several days and then tapered is considered helpful in shortening the healing time.
3. Severe cases: Higher doses of steroids are necessary. Prophylactic acyclovir can be used to prevent HSV- related EM.
4. TENS is treated in burn centers where necrotic skin is removed and general anesthetic and healing takes place under sheets of porcine xenografts.

Q2 What are the parts of X-ray tube? Describe the working of X-ray Tube and add a note on Bremsstrahlung Radiation.

Ans.

Parts of X-ray tube (Fig. 12.1)

1. *Cathode:* An X-ray tube consists of a filament and a focusing cup. The filament is the source of electrons within the X-ray tube.

   The filament lies in focusing cup, a negatively charged concave reflector made of molybdenum.
2. *Anode:* This consists of a tungsten target embedded in a copper stem. Focal spot is the area on target to which focusing cup directs the electrons from filament.
3. *Evacuated glass envelop or tube:* The cathode and anode lie within an evacuated glass tube.

Working of X-ray Tube

Function of cathode

- Cathode consists of filament and focusing cup. The filament is a coil of tungsten wire about 2 mm in diameter and 1 cm or less in

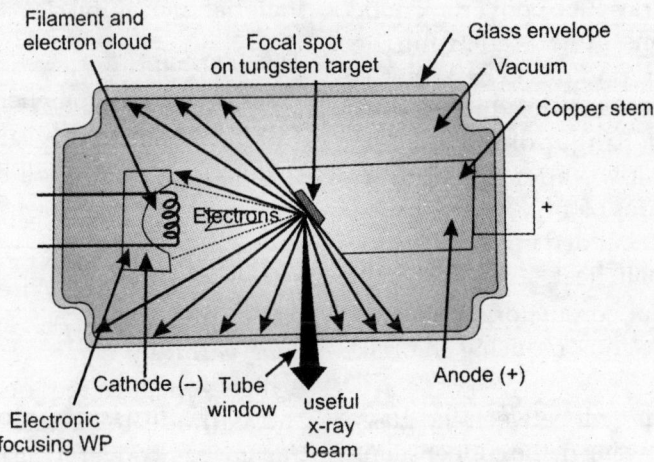

Fig. 12.1: X-ray tube with the major components

length which is mounted on two stiff wires that support it and carry the electric current.

- These two mounting wires lead through the glass envelope and connect to both the high and low voltage electrical sources.
- The filament is heated to incandescence by the flow of current through the low-voltage source and units electrons at a rate proportional to the temperature of filament.
- Filament is the source of electrons within the X-ray tube. The filament lies in a focusing cup, a negatively charged concave reflector made of molybdenum. The focusing cup electro statically focuses the electrons emitted by the incandescent filament into a narrow beam directed at a small rectangular area on anode called the focal spot.
- The electrons move in this direction because they are separated by the negatively charged cathode and attracted to positively charged anode.
- The X-ray tube is evacuated to prevent collision of moving electrons with gas molecules, which would significantly reduce their speed. This also prevents oxidation and 'burnout' of the filament.

Function of Anode

- The target is an X-ray tube converts kinetic energy of electrons generated from the filament into X-ray photons. The target is made up of tungsten as it has high atomic number, high melting point, thermal conductivity and low vapor pressure at working temperatures of an X-ray tube. The tungsten target is embedded in a 'large block of copper' to dissipate heat.
- Copper is a thermal conductor, dissipates heat from tungsten, thus reducing the risk of target melting.
- In addition, insulating oil between the glass envelope and the housing of the copper stem. This type of anode is stationary anode.

- Focal spot is the area on the target to which the focusing cup directs the electrons from the filament.
- Effective focal spot, i.e. the projection of focal spot perpendicular to the electron beam is smaller than the actual size of focal spot. So the target is inclined at 20° to the central ray of X-ray beam to increase in sharpness of the image with a larger focal spot for heat dissipation from a small apparent source of X-rays.
- Another method of dissipating the heat from small focal spot is to use rotating anode. The tungsten target will be in form of beveled disk that rotates when the tube is in operation and the heat is distributed over the expanded area.

Power Supply of X-ray Tube

- Provide a low voltage current to heat the X-ray tube filament by use of a step-down transformer.
- Generate a high potential difference between anode and cathode by use of a high voltage transformer.

These transformer and the X-ray tube lie within an electrically grounded metal housing called the head of X-ray machine. An insulating material such as, oil surrounds the transformer.

Tube current

The flow of electrons here is from filament to anode and then back to the filament through the wiring of power supply.

$$\text{Filament} \underset{\text{Wire}}{\overset{\text{Electrons}}{\rightleftarrows}} \text{Anode}$$

Tube voltage

A high voltage is required between the anode and cathode to generate X-rays. An auto-transformer converts the primary voltage from the input source into the secondary voltage.

The secondary voltage regulated by kilovolts peak (kVp) selector dial. So kVp controls the voltage between the anode and the cathode of the Xray tube. The high voltage transformer provides high voltage of 60–100 kv required by X-ray tube to accelerate electrons from cathode to anode and generate X-rays. Intensity of radiation produced at anode increases as anode voltage increases.

Timer

Timer controls the duration of X-ray exposure and length of time that high voltage is applied to the tube and therefore the time during which tube current flows and X-rays are produced.

Production of X-rays (Fig. 12.2)

Electrons traveling from the filament to the target convert some of their kinetic energy into X-ray photons by the formation of bremstrahlung and characteristic radiation.

Bremsstrahlung Radiation (Fig. 12.3)

1. The primary source of X-ray photons from an X-ray tube, are produced by the sudden stopping or slowing of high-speed electrons at the target (braking radiation)

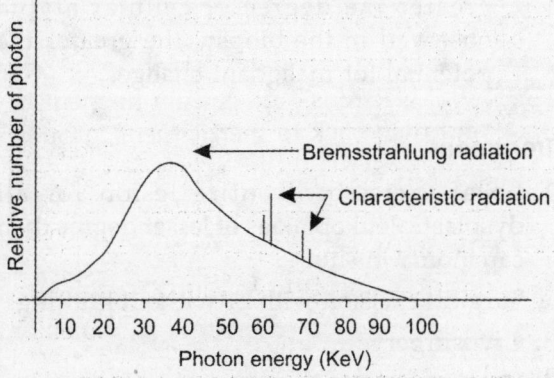

Fig. 12.2: Spectrum of photons emitted from an X-ray beam generated at 100 kVp. The vast preponderance of radiation in Bremsstrahlung, with a minor addition of characteristic radiation

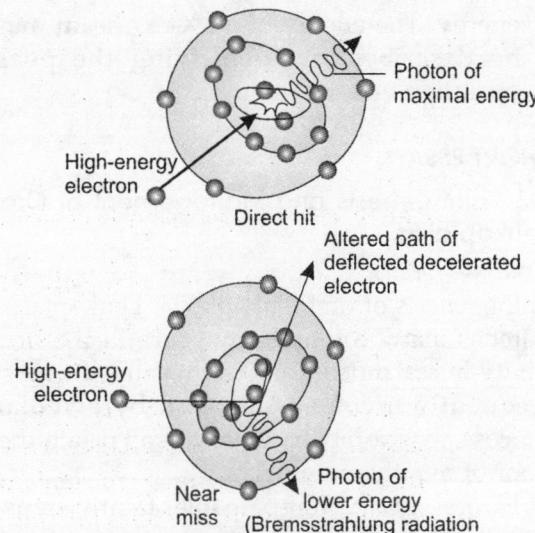

Fig. 12.3: Bremsstrahlung radiation is produced by the direct hit of electrons on the nucleus in the target (A) or by the passage of electrons near the nucleus, which results in electrons being deflected and decelerated (B).

2. When electrons from the filament strike the tungsten target, X-ray photons are created. The electrons hit a target nucleus directly or if their path takes them close to a nucleus.

3. If a high-speed electron directly hits the nucleus of a target atom, all its kinetic energy is transformed into a single X-ray photon.

4. The energy of the resultant photon is numerically equal to energy of the electron.

5. In these interactions, a negatively charged high-speed electron is attracted towards the positively charged nuclei and loses some of its velocity. This deceleration causes the electron to lose some kinetic energy, which is given off in the form of many new photons.

6. The closer the high-speed electron approaches the nuclei, the greater is the electrostatic attraction on the electron, the braking effect, and the energy of the resulting Bremsstrahlung photons.

7. The Bremsstrahlung interaction generates X-ray photons with a continuous spectrum of

energy. The energy of an X-ray beam may be described by identifying the peak operation voltage (KVp).

SHORT ESSAYS

Q3 Pathogenesis and Management of Oral Leukoplakia.

Ans.

Pathogenesis of oral leukoplakia. Leukoplakia patches may be found anywhere in the oral cavity-buccal mucosa and commisures are most frequently involved followed by alveolar mucosa, tongue, lip, hard palate, soft palate and floor of mouth and gingiva.

Earliest lesion: Non-palpable, faintly translucent, white discoloration.

Later: Localized or diffuse, slightly elevated plaques of irregular outlines develop. These are opaque, white and may have fine granular texture. The lesion progresses to thickened white lesion, showing indurations, fissuring and ulcer formation.

Histopathologically, the lesion represents features of epithelial dysplasia which may be mild to moderate.

Management of Oral Leukoplakia

1. Initial treatment of suspected Leukoplakia
   - Eliminate all possible local irritants.
   - Eliminate any identified systemic predisposing factors.
   - Topical anti-fungal is administered for 1–2 weeks and a specific appointment made for follow-up evaluation at the end of that period.
2. Second appointment
   - If the lesion is not subsided or responded to treatment biopsy is done.
   - Patient's habitually abused tobacco and alcohol should be made to eliminate by counseling and medical treatment.
   - Subsequent treatment of lesions depends on the outcome of biopsy.

3. Third appointment after results
   - If no evidence of dysplasia is found and the biopsy site is felt to be representative of entire lesion, conservative treatment is acceptable.
   - Small lesions are completely excised and annually checked for recurrence of lesion and patient is instructed to report any apparent recurrences.
   - Larger lesions with out dysplasia (verrucous or nodular type)
     - Removal of lesions surgically
     - Follow up evaluation
     - With or without local medication
     - Systemic vitamin A has been recommended as an adjunctive treatment for extensive leukoplakia that can't be removed entirely by surgery.
   - For extensive lesion, systemic administration 13-cis retinoic acid or alltrans retinoic acid.
     - Topical administration of vitamin A is also helpful.
   - In dysplastic forms of lekoplakia

The lesion has greater potential for undergoing malignant change. The greater the degree of cellular atypia observed in the biopsy, the greater the potential for malignant change.

Treatment

1. Local excision of entire lesion for all dysplastic leukoplakias of lesser degree than carcinoma in-situ.
2. Surgical excision with or without grafting.
3. Cryosurgery
4. Laser obliteration.
5. Topical application of anticancer chemotherapy bleomycin in dimethyl sulphoxide and human fibroblast interferon.

Q4 Etiology and signs and symptoms of trigeminal neuralgia.

Ans.

Definition

Trigeminal neuralgia is defined as sudden, usually unilateral severe, brief, stabbing, lancinating, recurring pain in the distribution of one or more branches of trigeminal nerve.

Etiology

1. Vascular factors

   Transient ischemia and autoimmune hypersensitivity responses leads to demyelination of nerve.

2. Idiopathic causes

   The defect in the sensory nucleus of 5th cranial nerve

   - Trigeminal gasserian ganglion
   - Any nerve may lose myelin sheath

3. Secondary causes

   - Trauma
   - CNS lesions

4. *Mechanical factors:* Pressure of aneurysm of intrapetrous portion of internal carotid artery.

5. Anomaly of superior cerebellar artery as it lies in contact with sensory root of trigeminal neuralgia and its elevation has reduced pain.

6. Dental cause

7. Infection

8. Jaw bone cavities

9. Multiple Sclerosis

10. Petrous ridge compression

11. Post-traumatic neuralgia.

12. Intracranial tumor

13. Intra cranial vascular abnormality

14. Viral etiology- post herpetic neuralgia.

Clinical Features

Signs

- Trigeminal neuralgia occurs in late middle age in persons with no abnormal neurological deficit as loss of corneal reflex, anesthesia, paraesthesia, and muscular atrophy/weakness.

- Intermittent paroxysmal, lancinating shock like pain, elicited by slight touching superficially.

- Trigger points are there depending on the division of nerve is involved

  V1–Supraorbital ridge of affected side

  V2–Skin of upper lip, ala of nose/cheek of upper gums

  V3–Trigger points are on lower lip, teeth/gums.

- Pain rarely cross the midline

- Refractory period is there between attacks but dull aching persists.

- The paroxysms occur in cycles, each cycle lasting for weeks or months and with time, cycle appears closer and closer. With each attack pain seems to become more intense and intolerable.

- In extreme cases frozen or mask like face is seen.

Symptoms

- Patient complains of sudden, unilateral intermittent paroxysmal, sharp, shooting pain, elicited suddenly by touching or cold breeze or while brushing.

- Patient always complains of dull aching pain.

- During an attack of 1–10 min, the patient grimaces with pain, clutches his hands over affected side of the face, avoids touching the area.

- Oral hygiene is poor

- Patient will lead a poor quality of life, as he will always be scared of getting pain.

Q5 Indications and contraindications of corticosteroid therapy in dentistry.
Ans.

Indications
In Dentistry

1. Apthous ulcer.
2. Dentine hypersensitivity.
3. Desquamitive gingivitis.
4. Oral lichen planus.
5. Oral pharyngitis
6. Pulp capping.
7. Pulpotomy.
8. Post extraction pain, trismus and edema.
9. TMJ arthritis.
10. Oral submucous fibrosis.

In Medicine

- Replacement therapy
- Primary/secondary adrenal insufficiency.
- Anti inflammatory in rheumatoid arthritis, osteoarthritis, bronchial asthma.
- Leukemia.
- Immune suppression in organ transplants, bell's palsy, cerebral edema.
- Anti inflammatory effect.
- Collagen diseases.
- Mixed connective disease syndrome.
- Polymyositis.
- Poly arthritis nodosa
- Granulomatous poly arthritis
- Systemic lupus erythematosus

Contraindications

- Hypertension or cardiovascular disease
- Peptic ulcer
- Osteoporosis
- Diabetes mellitus
- Tuberculosis or other infections
- Psychological difficulties
- Glaucoma
- Pregnancy
- Young patients

Q6 Composition and function of developing solution.
Ans.
Refer to Q6.2 of September 1998.

Q7 Types and uses of filtration
Ans.
An X-ray consists of a spectrum of X-ray photons of different energies. Only photons with sufficient energy to penetrate through anatomic structures reach the image receptor (usually film) are useful for diagnostic radiology.

Those that are of low energy (long wavelength) contribute to patient exposure (and risk) but do not have enough energy to reach the film. Consequently, to reduce patient dose, the less penetrating photons should be removed. This can be accomplished by filtration. Types and uses Refer to Q8 of March 2002.

Q8 Composition and function of Intensifying Screen.
Ans.
Refer to Q6.2 of October 1999.

SHORT ANSWERS
Q9 Toluidine blue staining
Ans.

Indications

- To diagnose early carcinomatous or premalignant lesions such as leukoplakia, erythroplakia.
- To differentiate between different inflammatory and dysplastic disorders.
- Lesions, which are not indicated for biopsy.

Composition of Toluidine Blue Solution

- Toluidine blue 1 gm
- Acetic acid 10 cc
- Absolute alcohol 4.2 cc
- Distilled water 86 cc
- The pH is adjusted to 4.5.

Procedure

- Isolate and dry the area which has lesions
- Apply 1% acetic acid with camel hair brush
- Wait for 20 sec and rinse with water
- Apply Toluidine blue solution 1% with fresh brush
- Wait for 10–20 sec
- Decolorize with 2% acetic acid
- Apply Lugol's iodine solution
- Area is photographed and biopsy is planned

Disadvantage

False negative and false positive results are common. So biopsy is necessary for confirmation.

Q10 Talon's Cusp

Ans.
Definition

An anomalous structure resembling an eagle's talon which projects lingually from clingulum areas of mandibular and maxillary central incisors.

Clinical Features

- The cusp looks as T-shaped when viewed from incisal region
- Talon's cusp is seen in either sex and both primary and permanent dentition.
- It is covered by normal enamel and dentin.
- It contains a horn of pulp

Associated Syndrome

Rubinstein Taybi Syndrome: Developmental retardation, broad thumb, great toes, characteristic facial features, delayed or incomplete descent of testes in males, stature head circumference and bone, age below 50th percentile.

Complications

- Talon's cusp is more prone for food lodgment calculus deposition and causes halitosis.
- Due to attrition of the cusp, pulp exposure can occur.

Treatment

Oral prophylaxis, reduction of the cusp to normal tooth contour and restoration with crown after endodontic treatment.

Q11 Four causes of a Dark Radiograph

Ans.

A. Processing error
- Over development
- Developer concentration too high
- Inadequate fixation
- Accidental exposure to light

B. Over exposure
- Excessive mA
- Excessive KVp
- Insufficient film source distance
- Excessive time

Q12 Radiographic appearance of Ameloblastoma

Ans.
Refer to Q2 of March 2000

Q13 Ascher's Syndrome

Ans.

Ascher's syndrome is associated with acquired double lip with blepherochalasis and non toxic thyroid enlargement.

Clinical Features
Double Lip

It is an anomaly characterized by a fold of excess tissue on the inner mucosal aspect of lip.

- More predilection for upper lip
- When the upper lip is tensed double lip resembles a cupid's bow.

Blepherochalasis: It is the drooping of the tissue between the eyebrow and edge of the upper eyelid so that it hangs loosely over the margin of the lid.

- It is caused by relaxation of the supratarsal fold as a result of atrophy and thinning of skin of eyelid.
- Thyroid enlargement is not constant and may appear until several years after eyelid involvement.

Treatment

- Cosmetic purpose or functions involving speech and mastication
- Surgical excision of excessive tissue

Q14 Bell's Sign
Ans.
In facial paralysis due to dysfunction of upper part, there is inability to wrinkle the forehead and raise the eyebrow. There may also be slight drop of eyebrow. When the patient closes the eye, the globe turns upwards and there is slight movement of upper eyelid. This is known as Bell's Sign.

Complication
There may be exposure keratitis because of inability to close the eyelid. The patient is unable to wink and maintain oral hygiene. There will be food lodgment and halitosis.

Treatment
Medical therapy: Steroids such as betamethasone 0.5 mg is given

Multivitamin Tablets
Physiotherapy: Facial massage is helpful in relieving the paralysis

Surgical treatment: If facial paralysis remains more than 6 weeks, then surgical treatment is advised.

Significance of Bell Sign
To diagnose upper or lower motor neuron paralysis in cases of trauma.

Q15 Radiographic appearance of Peri-apical Granuloma
Ans.
A Periapical Granuloma also known as Pyogenic Granuloma is defined as a growth of granulomatous tissue continuous with the periodontal ligament resulting from death of pulp and diffusion of bacteria and bacterial toxins from root canal into the surrounding periradicular tissues through the apical and lateral foramina.

Radiographic Features
1. *Location*
   Epicenter is at apex of involved tooth or at another region of tooth root.

2. *Periphery*
   The periphery of periapical granuloma is well defined, with a sharp transition zone. The area of rarefaction is well defined with lack of continuity of lamina dura.

3. *Internal structure*
   Radiolucency in the periapical region detectable of change in bone density, resulting in widening of periodontal ligament space.

4. *Surrounding structure*
   It is affected by resorption of bone and loss of lamina dura.

Q16 Four oral manifestations of Aplastic Anemia.
Ans.
Aplastic anemia is a disease characterized by general lack of bone marrow activity, it may

affect RBC, WBC and platelets resulting in pancytopenia.

Oral Manifestations

1. Petechiae, purpuric spot or frank hematoma of oral mucosa at any site.
2. Spontaneous gingival hemorrhage
3. Neutropenia leads to lack of resistance to infection and results in development of ulcerated lesions of oral mucosa and pharynx. Severe cases result in gangrene.
4. Due to thrombocytopenia, prolonged bleeding time occurs and clot retraction is poor, healing of extraction socket is delayed.

Q17 Four causes for Trismus.
Ans.
1. Due to infection
   - Pericoronitis
   - Ludwig's Angina
2. Due to trauma
   - Fracture of zygomatic arch
   - Fracture of mandible
3. Due to tetany
   - Carpopedal spasm is seen in hypocalcemia
4. Due to tetanus
   - Following acute infection of clostridium tetani the lock jaw symptoms are seen
5. Extra articular fibrosis
6. Myositis Ossificans
7. Due to TMJ inflammation
   - Myositis
   - Synovitis
   - Osteoarthritis.

Q18 Two differences between direct and indirect Immunofluorescence.
Ans. Table 12.1

Table 12.1

Direct immuno fluorescence (One step procedure)	Indirect immuno fluorescence (Two-step procedure)
Antiserum to microorganism is conjugated with flourocein. When the conjugate is incubated on a clinical smear containing the microorganism and washed off. The antigen(Ag)-antibody(Ab) reaction takes place. The organism is visualized by its fluorescent outline in fluorescent microscopy. Antibody in patient's serum for microorganism $\downarrow$ Conjugated $\downarrow$ Antigen-antibody reaction $\downarrow$ Organism visualized	Antiserum to microorganism is incubated on clinical A smear of lesion. It is washed off and then a conjugate of fluorescent dye and an antiserum to 1st antiserum are incubated and then again washed off. Antibody-1 is incubated Fluorescent + Antibody-2 is incubated with Antibody-1 Organism is visualized.
Directly the fluorescein tagged antihuman gammaglobulin is placed over the patient's tissue having lesion like pemphigus vulgaris and viewed under fluorescent microscope.	Serum from the patient is placed over the epidermal structure and then slide is overlaid with the fluorescent tagged antihuman gamma globulin.Antibodies against against the antihuman gamma globulin shows pemphigus vulgaris under fluorescent microscope.

QUESTION PAPER

Long Essays

1. Define pain. Enumerate the causes of facial pain. Write clinical features and management of myofacial pain dysfunction syndrome
2. Enumerate the effects of radiation on oral tissues. Discuss the measures of radiation protection in dental radiology

Short Essays

3. Classification and Management of Recurrent aphthous stomatitis
4. Differential diagnosis of non-scrapable white patch on tongue
5. Etiology and management of Oral submucous fibrosis
6. Oral manifestations and dental considerations in diabetes mellitus
7. Types and uses of intraoral radiographs
8. Principle and indications of Panoramic radiographs

Short Answers

9. Albright's syndrome
10. Radiographic appearance of mandibular fracture
11. Tzanck smear
12. Four differences between leukoplakia and lichen planus
13. Pink tooth of mummery
14. Nikolsky's sign
15. Name four conditions showing onion peel appearance
16. Brush biopsy
17. Carcinoma in-situ
18. Name two investigations to be carried out in suspected HIV infection.

LONG ESSAYS

Q1 Define pain. Enumerate the causes of facial pain. Write clinical features and management of myofacial pain dysfunction syndrome

Ans.

Definition of Pain

According to Monheims: Pain is defined as an unpleasant emotional experience initiated by noxious stimulus and transmitted over specialized or specific neural network to central nervous system where it is interpreted as such

According to Burkitt: Pain is defined as an unpleasant sensory and emotional experience associated with actual or potential tissue damage or described in terms of such damage

Causes of Facial Pain

- Regional Classification of Orofacial Pain
  - Cutaneous and Mucogingival Pain
  - Mucosal pain of pharynx, nose and Para nasal sinus
  - Pain of dental origin
  - Pain of musculoskeletal structure of face and mouth
  - Chronic facial pain syndrome
  - Pain caused due to neuralgias
- According to clinical characteristics
  - Somatic Pain
  - Neurogenic Pain
  - Psychogenic Pain
- According to origin
  - Dental Pain
  - Pulpal Pain
    a. Hyperactive pulpalgia
    Hypersensitivity
    Hyperemia

b. Acute Pulpalgia
Incipient
Moderate
Advanced
c. Chronic Pulpalgia
d. Necrotic pulp
e. Internal resorption of pulp
f. Traumatic Occlusion
g. Incomplete Fracture of tooth
- Periapical Pain
  a. Acute apical periodontitis
  b. Acute apical abscess
  c. Chronic apical periodontitis
    ♦ Cyst
    ♦ Granuloma
  d. Chronic apical abscess
- Periodontal Pain

Myofacial Pain Dysfunction Syndrome

Refer to March 2001 Q10

Q2 Enumerate the effects of radiation on oral tissues. Discuss the measures of radiation protection in dental radiology

Ans.

Effect of Radiation on Oral Tissues

Refer to march 2000 Q19

Measures of Radiation Protection

The guiding principle for use of diagnostic radiology in dentistry is to enhance the diagnostic benefits of dental radiographs minimize the associated radiation risks to patients and staff (Fig. 13.1).

Patient Selection

- Diagnostic radiography should be used only after clinical examination, consideration of patient's history and consideration of both

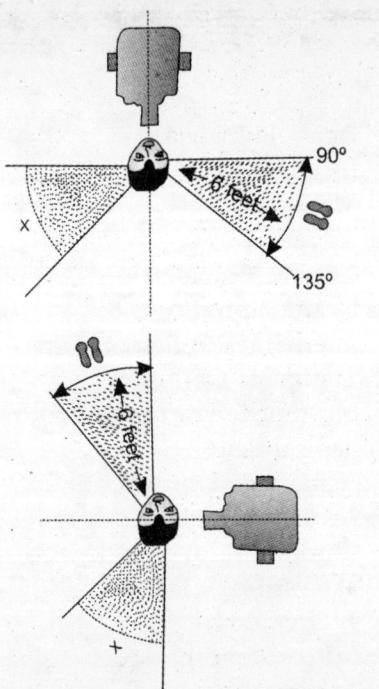

Fig. 13.1: *Position and distance rule:* If no barrier is available, the operator should stand at least 6 feet from the patient, at an angle of 900–1350 to central ray of the X-ray beam when the exposure is made

the dental and general health needs of the patient.

- High yield or referral criteria have to be considered i.e. the radiographic examination should provide information affecting their treatment or prognosis.

Conduct of Examination

Choice of Equipment

- *Selection of image receptor:* The basis for selecting film types, film intensifying screen combinations and other image receptors is to obtain the maximum sensitivity(speed) consistent with the image quality required for diagnostic task.
- *Intraoral image receptors:* Intraoral dental X-ray film is available in 3 speed groups-D, E and F. Group E is twice as fast as D and about

50 times as fast as regular dental X-ray film. Faster films are desirable from the standpoint of exposure reduction.

- *Intensifying screens:* Rare earth elements gadolinium and lanthanum decreases patient exposure by 50%.
- *Focal spot to film distance:* Combination of proper collimation and extended source patient distance (focal spot to film distance) will reduce the amount of radiation to patient. Longer FSFD results in increased resolution of radiograph.
- *Collimation:* The tissue area exposed to the primary X-ray beam should not exceed the minimum coverage consistent with meeting diagnostic requirements and clinical feasibility. Rectangular position indicating device (PID) may be attached to radiographic tube reduces 60% exposure.

Rectangular collimators may be used with round PID. Precision instrument, XCP instrument with rectangular collimator clipped to aiming ring.

- *Filtration:* The low energy photons, which have little penetrating power and are, absorbed by patient. So X- ray film is filtered with 3 mm of aluminium and rare earth elements like gadolinium, thulium-activated lanthanum oxybromide reduces patient exposure by 20–30%.
- Leaded aprons and collars leaded thyroid collars are strongly recommended to reduce patient eposure to radiation.

Choice of Intraoral Techniques

Operating the equipment kilovoltage: 70–100 kVp peaks as the kVp increases the radiographic contrast decreases.

Milliampere seconds: This should be decreased Photo timer is used to measure the quantity of radiation reaching the film and automatically terminates the exposure.

Protection of Personnel

The operatory should be so arranged so that the operator can stand at least 6 feet from the patient.

1. The operator can leave the room or take a position behind a suitable barrier or wall during exposure of film.
2. Operators should never hold the films in place.
3. Neither the operator nor patient should hold the radiographic tube housing during exposure.

   To ensure that personnel–monitoring devices are used which are referred to as "Film Badges", these devices provide a useful record of occupational exposure.

Quality Assurance

This may be defined as any planned activity to ensure that a dental office will consistently produce high quality images with a minimum exposure to patient and personnel.

Proper inspection should be done at suitable intervals, of the X-ray unit.

- Leakage radiation
- Verification of FSFD
- Stability of radiographic tube housing
- Dark Room
  - Light leaks
  - Safe Lighting
  - Cleanliness
- Ancillary Equipment

Continuing Education

Practitioners should stay informed about new information on radiation safety issues as well as developments in equipment, materials and techniques and adopt appropriate items to improve radiographic practices.

SHORT ESSAYS

Q3 Classification and management of Recurrent Aphthous Stomatitis (RAS)

Ans.

Refer to Q1 march 2000 solutions.

Q4 Differential Diagnosis of Non-scrapable White Patch on Tongue.

Ans.

Non-scrapable white lesions of oral mucosa which occur on tongue and also on other parts of mucosa like lips, cheek, floor of mouth are: Leukoplakia, Carcinoma In-Situ, Squamous Cell Carcinoma, White Sponge Nevus, Hereditary Benign Intra epithelial Dyskeratosis, Lichen Planus, White Hairy Tongue, Chemical Burn, Allergic Reaction, Dyskeratosis Congenita

Differential Diagnosis

A. An explanation for the patient's symptoms and identification of other significant disease process is done by differentiating the particular lesion from other similar lesions.

B. Non-scrapable white patch can be differentially diagnosed, according to various criteria like etiology, age/sex of occurrence, clinical features, microscopic features, etc. Differential diagnosis of non scrapable white patch on tongue (Table 13.1)

Q5 Etiology and Management of Oral Submucous Fibrosis

Ans.

Definition

Oral submucous fibrosis is a slowly progressive chronic fibrotic disease of oral cavity and oropharynx characterized by fibroelastic change and inflammation of mucosa, leading to a progressive inability to open the mouth, swallow or speak.

Etiology

OSMF may be caused due to direct stimulation from exogenous antigens like Areca alkaloids or changes in tissue antigenicity that may lead to an autoimmune response.

Pathogenesis: The inflammatory response releases cytokines and growth factors that

Table 13.1: Differential diagnosis of non scrapable white patch on tongue

Lesion	Age/sex	Clinical features	Microscopic features
Hereditary lesion			
White sponge Nevus	Childhood; either	Present in number of members of the same family; may appear in one area and then spread; asymptomatic; cannot be wiped off. Present as a bilaterally symmetrical white soft "spongy" or velvety thick plaques on buccal mucosa, ventral part of tongue, floor of mouth, labial mucosa, soft palate, alveolar mucosa.	Thickening of epithelial covering Superficial layers of epithelial cells are swollen and fail to stain.
Hereditary benign intra epithelialdyskeratosis	Childhood	White spongy mucosa, corners of mouth, lateral part of tongue, gingival palate and extra orally. White plaques on cornea and conjunctiva is seen.	Similar as above. Presence of benign dyskeratosis.
Dyskeratosis congenita	Childhood	It is a rare X-linked disorder characterized by atrophic leukoplakiaoral mucosa, with tongue and cheek severely affected. Dystrophicnails, hyper-pigmented skin.	—
Reactive and inflammatory lesions			
Frictional keratosis	—	White plaque with rough and frayed surface	Hyperkeratosis and acanthosis
Check chewing	Females after 35	Roughness or small tags of tissue. Lesions are poorly outlined whitich patches that are mixed with erythema and ulceration.	Hyperkeratosis and acanthosis
Chemical burn	—	Due to aspirin, silver nitrate, H_2O_2, dentifrices, etc. the injured area will be irregular in shape, white covered with pseudomembrane and very painful.	Non-keratinized tissue.
Infectious lesion			
Oral hairyleukoplakia (due to EBV, AIDSor severe immuno-deficiency)	Adulthood; Males	Lateral borders of the tongue is common. The lesion will be corrugated, shaggy or flared appearance or plaque like; often bilateral.	Hyperkeratosis with irregular surface, Acanthosis with superficial edema, koilocyticcels in spinous layer.
Lichen planus	5th decade; female	Clinically varied types are: reticular, erosive, bullous, whitish elevated lesions are seen which are lacy lesions associated with scaly papules on skin; oral lesion may precede skinlesion.	Saw tooth shaped epithelial-ridges, epithelium iskeratinized, connective tissueshows clear demarcated lymphocytic infiltration
White hairy tongue	Adulthood; Male	Long white hair like elongation of filiform papillae,asymptomatic or accompanied by pain, enlargement of tongue.	Marked elongation of filiform-papillae, inflammatory infiltrate of sub epithelial tissue.

promote fibrosis by inducing the proliferation of fibroblasts, up-regulating collagen synthesis and down-regulating collagenase production. So etiology includes

a. General nutritional and vitamin deficiencies.

b. Hypersensitivity to certain dietary constituents such as chilly, pepper, chewing tobacco etc.

c. Habitual betel chewing and nut of areca palm (areca catechu), the leaf of betel pepper (piper betel) and lime (calcium hydroxide). Betel chewing produces mild psychoactive and cholinergic effects. OSMF is a premalignant condition which may lead to leukoplakia and squamous cell carcinoma.

Management of OSMF

Refer March 2003 Q1

Q6 Oral manifestations and dental considerations in Diabetes Mellitus

Ans.

Oral Manifestations of Diabetes Mellitus

i. Dental decay is caused due to the increased concentrations of glucose in saliva and gingival crevicular fluid. Reduced buffering capacity of saliva leads to decalcification of tooth structure.

ii. *Periodontal disease:* Impaired chemotactic and phagocytic response to antigen. Altered neutrophil function are the causes of periodontal disease.

Greater proportions of gram negative organisms in gingival crevice causes altered host response.

iii. *Candidial infections:* Thrush is characterized by soft, white epithelial plaque invaded by fungal hyphae. It can be scraped off exposing the underlying erythematous mucosa.

　　– Uncontrolled diabetes is predisposing factor to oral candidiasis as it increases candidial colonization due to altered immune response iv) Lichen planus and oral lichenoid reaction is seen in patients with Sulphonylureas class of drugs (chlorpropamide etc.).

v. *Salivary gland and sialosis:* Diabetes mellitus is associated with painless enlargement of major salivary gland which is due to disorder of fat metabolism or an effect on gland parenchyma.

vi. *Xerostomia:* Patients who suffer from acute hypoglycemia have reduced flow rates of saliva due to dehydration and variations in drug therapy. Lesser degree of hyperglycemia may produce subjective symptoms of dry mouth called as 'burning mouth syndrome'.

vii. There will be alteration in taste sensation in NIDDM patients taking sulphonylureas.

viii. *Enamel hypoplasia:* Hypoglycemia affect the developing tooth bud.

ix. *Tongue and other pathologies:* Median Rhomboid Glossitis is one of the specific oral manifestations associated with diabetes but sometimes geographic tongue is also common. Median Rhomboid Glossitis is a well demarcated central non-ulcerated smooth pink or red area on middle third of the dorsum of tongue. Dry mucosal surfaces are irritated and are associated with burning tongue.

x. *Dry socket:* This is a painful condition in which there will be loss of clot after extraction leading to non healing socket with foul odour.

Dental considerations in Diabetes Mellitus

Patients with diabetes mellitus are managed in such a way as to minimize disturbances of metabolic balance. The physical and emotional stress, infection and surgical procedures may tend to alter the patients disease

• Appointment should be of short duration, especially in the morning.

- Patient should be encouraged to maintain their standard treatment regiments and patient's physician can be contacted in case of doubt
- Glucose drinks should be available in case of hypoglycemia
- Brittle diabetes needs recommendation from physician
- Regarding specific measures pertaining to dental treatment in diabetes, following should be considered.
  1. Local anesthetic without epinephrine is to be used in dental surgical procedures, as epinephrine can elevate the blood glucose concentration.
  2. Following extraction, suturing of the sockets has to be done to aid in hemostasis.
  3. Antibiotic prophylaxis before dental surgery is advised to prevent subsequent infection. Until stabilization of blood glucose level is achieved, complicated oral surgical procedures in dental emergencies should be avoided. Example: acute abscess should be treated by simple drainage and local anesthetic infiltration.

Q7 Types and uses of Intraoral Radiographs.
Ans.
Refer to March 1999 Q5

Q 8 Principle and indications of panoramic radiographs
Ans.
Principle of panoramic radiographs is based on the principle of tomography and scanography

Tomography is defined as the unobstructed crew of a structure in different directions without interference from structures above or below in that plane.

Scanography or narrow beam radiography refers to a narrow beam of radiation succe-ssively scanning different areas of tissue to cast image in the single film.

Principle of Panoramic Image Formation

1. Two adjacent disks rotate at the same speed in opposite directions and an X-ray beam passes through their centers of rotation.
2. Lead collimators in the shape of a slit, located at the X-ray source and at the image receptor, limit the central ray to a narrow vertical beam.
3. Radiograph objects A, B, C and D stand upright on the disk 1 and rotate past the slit.
4. Their images are recorded on the receptor, which also moves past the slit at the same time. The objects are displayed sharply on the receptor because they are moving past the slit at same rate and in the same direction as the receptor. This causes their moving shadows to appear stationary in relation to the moving receptor.
5. Any objects between the X-ray source and center of rotation of disk 1 move in opposite direction of the receptor, and their shadows are also blured on the receptor (Figs 13.2 and 13.3).
   - If disk 1 is held stationary and the X-ray source rotates so that the central ray constantly passes through the center of rotation of disk 1 and simultaneously, both disk 2 and lead collimator(Pb) rotate around the center of disk 1
   - When disk 2 moves, receptor on this disk also rotates past the slit.
   - To obtain optimal image definition, the speed of the receptor passing the

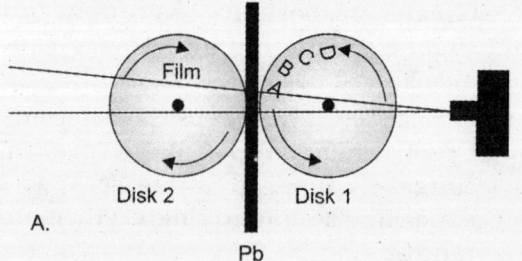

Fig. 13.2: Movement of the film and objects (A, B, C, D) about two fixed centres of rotation

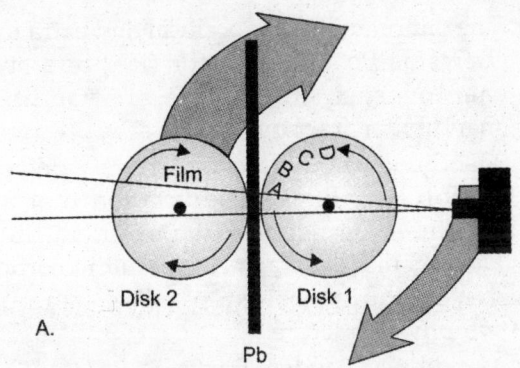

Fig. 13.3: Movement of film and X-ray source aobut one fixed center of roation.

collimator slit (Pb) be maintained equal to the speed at which the X-ray beam sweeps through objects of interest.

- When receptor is a charged-coupled device array, the image is electronically transmitted to the controlling computer as the X-ray beam hits it, and this transmission is continuous as the X-ray source and receptor travel around the patient.

- During the exposure cycle, the machine automatically shifts to one or more additional rotation centers.

- Structures near the X-ray source are so magnified (and their borders so blurred) that they are not seen as discrete images on the resultant image.

- These structures appear only as diffuse phantom or ghost images. Because of both these circumstances, only structures near the receptor are usefully captured on resultant image.

- Image layer is a three dimensional curved zone (focal trough) in which structures lying within the layer are reasonably well defined on final panoramic image.

- The image seen on radiograph is composed largely of anatomical structures located within focal trough.

- Objects in front of, or behind focal trough are blurred magnified/reduced in size and sometimes distorted to an extent of not being recognizable. Then focal trough is region in which structures will be revealed most sharply.

FOCAL TROUGH (Fig. 13.4)

Indications

1. OPG is indicated for visualization of all the teeth and surrounding structures.
2. OPG helps to visualize the relationship of TMJ to skull.
3. To visualize anterior view of sinuses at floor of nose.
4. To assess the depth of mandible and relationship of inferior dental canal with teeth or alveolar bone.
5. To demonstrate fracture of mandible from midline to neck of condyle.
6. To demonstrate periodontal disease in a general way.
7. To visualize ascending rami, coronoid and condylar process can be seen together.
8. To detect the impacted teeth and used for assessment of presence and the position of unerupted teeth in orthodontic treatment.
9. To demonstrate undiagnosed cysts, tumors or any other fibrous lesions.
10. OPG indicated when full month periapical radiography cannot be carried out especially in children, mentally handicapped patients, and in patients with trismus.

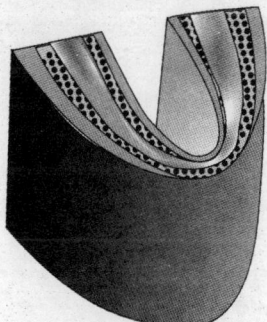

Fig. 13.4: The closer to the center of the trough (dark zone) and anatomic structures is positioned, the more clearly it is imaged on the resulting radiograph.

SHORT ANSWERS

Q9 Albright's Syndrome
Ans.

Definition

It is a severe form of fibrous dysplasia involving nearly all bones in the skeleton and accompanied by pigmented lesions of the skin, and also endocrine disturbances of varying types.

Clinical Features

It manifests early in life with an evident deformity, bowing or thickening of long bones, often unilateral in distribution.

- It's onset is insidious although aching recurrent bone pain is most common presenting skeletal symptoms
- The bones of face and skull are involved which may results in asymmetry
- Spontaneous fractures are common
- Café-au-lait spots i.e. skin lesions associated with disease consist of irregularly pigmented melanotic spots.
- More common in females.

Oral Manifestations

- Severe disturbance of bony tissue
- Lesions in the mandible
- Deformity of the jaws and eruption pattern of teeth is disturbed.

Radiographic Feature

- The medullary portions of bone are rarefied and irregular trabeculations are present, often a multilocular cystic appearance.
- The cortical bone is thinned and expanded.

Q10 Radiographic appearance of Mandibular Fracture
Ans.

The mandibular fracture sites are condyle, body and angle of the mandible

- The panoramic view, occlusal and extra oral views as Postero-anterior (PA) and sub-mentovertex skull views are useful in mandibular fracture.
- Mandibular body fracture: sharply defined radiolucent lines of separation that are confined to structure of mandible. Displacement of fragments result in cortical discontinuity or 'step'. For example symphysis fracture.
- Mandibular condyle fracture
  - Condylar neck
  - Condylar head

Outer cortical plate of posterior border of ramus condylar head, condylar notch on lateral and posteroanterior projections may reveal the presence of fractures.

- Deformities caused due to fracture are: Medial inclination of condyle, abnormal shape of condyle, shortening of neck, erosion and flattening.
- Fracture of alveolar process: number of cortical plates of alveolar process are apparent.
- The fracture direction indicates the type and severity of fracture. This helps in treatment and prognosis of fracture. For example horizontally favorable.

Q11 Tzanck Smear
Ans.

The Tzanck smear is prepared from intact (freshly opened) vesicles and smears stained by papanicolau or other stains giving good nuclear differentiation, will reveal characteristic Tzanck cells.

Tzanck cells are characterized particularly by degenerative changes which include swelling of nucleus and hyperchromatic staining.

Indications

- Pemphigus vulgaris
- Herpes simplex virus
- Genital herpes

- Cytologic examination of Tzanck smear is a supplemental; test for pemphigus.

Q12 Four differences between Leukoplakia and Lichen Planus.
Ans.
Table 13.2

Q13 Pink tooth of mummery
Ans.

Defination

It is an unusual form of tooth resorption that begins centrally within the tooth apparently initiated by a peculiar inflammatory hyperplasia of pulp.

Etiology

1. Caries exposure and accompanying pulp infection.
2. Invasion of pulp by granulation tissue arising in the periodontium.

Clinical Features

1. Pink hued area on crown of tooth which represents hyperplastic vascular pulp tissue filling the resorbed area and showing through the remaining overlying tooth substance.
2. Multiple tooth may be involved.

Radiographic Features

Round or ovoid radiolucent area in central portion of tooth associated with the pulp but not with external surface of tooth.

Treatment

- Root canal therapy
- Extraction of tooth.

Q14 Nikolsky's Sign
Ans.
Refer to march 2002 Q11.

Q15 Name four conditions showing Onion peel appearance.
Ans.
Laminar periosteal new bone formation has been reported to occur leading to onion peel appearance.
1. Garre's osteomyelitis
2. Ewing's sarcoma
3. Leukemia
4. Osteogenic sarcoma.

Table 13.2: Differences between Leukoplakia and Lichen Planus

Lichen planus	Leukoplakia
This is premalignant condition, i.e. generalized state of body which is associated with significally increased risk of cancer.	This is a premalignant lesion, i.e. morphologically altered tissues in which cancer is more likely to occur than it's apparent normal part.
The etiology is auto immune in nature, predisposing factors nervousness, emotional upset, over work, anxiety, malnutrition.	The etiology is mainly tobacco consumption. Smoking, alcohol, candidiasis, regional and systemic factors also play role in this lesion.
Saw tooth shaped rete pegs degeneration civiatte with liquefaction of bacteria bodies are seen in epithelium.	Histopathologically drop shaped rete pegs and Acanthosis is seen.
It affects younger age group. It affects skin and oral cavity. Types: Atrophic, Bullous, Ulcerative, Vesicular, Reticular, Plaque like.	Clinically, it affects older age group. It affects only oral cavity. Types: Homogeneous leukoplakia, Erosive, Speckled/nodular leukoplakia, Verrucous leukoplakia.

Q16 Brush Biopsy

Ans.

Brush biopsy is relatively a minor procedure carried out on tissues from living organisms to confirm the diagnosis histopatho-logically.

The epithelial cells of the lesion are brushed out on the slide and cytologic examination is carried out.

Indications

1. To diagnose true nature of lesion and to differentiate the lesion from malignant lesion.
2. For screening lesions whose gross appearance is such that biopsy, i.e. incision is not warranted.
3. Brush biopsy avoids the risk of seeding tumour cells in vascular lesions.

Advantages

- It takes little time.
- Minimal discomfort to the patient.

Q17 Carcinoma in-situ.

Ans.

Severe dysplastic changes in a red or white lesion indicate considerable risk for the development of cancer.

- The more severe grades of dysplasia merge with the condition referred to as carcinoma in situ, which implies that intra epithelial changes are the same as those seen in invasive cancers, even though there is no histologic evidence in the specimen submitted, that malignant cells have left the confines of epithelium.
- WHO has used the term carcinoma in situ only when the dysplastic change affects the whole or almost the whole thickness of epithelium involved.

Clinical Features

Shiny atrophic patches to leukoplakia to erythroplakia.

Treatment

Local excision with a wide border of normal tissue. *Example:* Bowen's disease is an intra epidermal squamous cell carcinoma that may progress to invasive carcinoma over time.

Q18 Name two investigations to be carried out in suspected HIV Infection.

Ans.

1. *ELISA tests for antibodies induced by specific HIV antigens*. Enzyme linked immunosorbent assay (ELISA)

   Procedure: An antigen is attached to a solid phase support and then bound to an enzyme. Serum or other solution containing the antibody being assayed is applied and excess antigen-enzyme complex is removed.

   Interpretation:The rate of substrate degradation determines the amount of antibody present. A substrate that yields a colored degradation product allows an easy spectrophotometric method of detection.

2. *Western blot test* is used to confirm all these samples which are positive to ELISA. This test detects antibodies to various components of HIV and hence is more specific.

3. *Polymerase chain reaction (PCR):* This is a gene amplification procedure.

14

RGUHS March 2005

QUESTION PAPER

Long Essays

1. Describe in detail sialography and its significance in various diseases of the salivary glands.
2. Classify oral ulceration with a suitable example of each condition. Describe the clinical feature and management of recurrent aphthous ulcers.

Short Essays

3. Collimation and filtration
4. Indications and radiographic technique for paranasal sinus view.
5. The general and oral manifestations of bismuthism.
6. Investigations and management of primary herpetic gingivostomatitis.
7. Composition and uses of intensifying screens.
8. Uses and side effects of oral penicillins.

Short Answers

9. Koplik's Spot
10. Eagle's syndrome
11. Ramsay Hunt syndrome
12. Carcinoma-in-situ
13. Radiographic appearance of hyperparathyroidism
14. Nikolsky's sign
15. Radiographic appearance of periapical cementoma
16. Anodontia
17. Paul-bunnel test
18. Erosive lichen planus.

SOLUTIONS

LONG ESSAYS

Q1 Describe in detail Sialography and its significance in various diseases of the salivary glands.

Ans.

Refer Q2 of September 2002.

Q2 Classify oral ulceration with a suitable example of each condition. Describe the clinical features and management of recurrent aphthous ulcers

Ans.

Refer to Q1 of March 2000.

SHORT ESSAYS

Q3 Collimation and Filtration

Ans.

Refer to March 2002 Q8

Q4 Indications and Radiographic Technique for Paranasal Sinus view

Ans.

Refer to March 2003 Q8

Q5 The general and oral manifestations of bismuthism.

Ans.

Refer to Q5 of march 2003

Q6 Investigations and management of primary herpetic gingivostomatitis.

Ans.

Refer to Q6 of march 2003

Q7 Composition and uses of intensifying screens

Ans.

Refer to Q6.2 of October 1999

Q8 Uses and side effects of oral penicillins

Ans.

Refer Q5 september 2003

SHORT ANSWERS

Q9 Koplik's Spot

Ans.

Refer Q16 March 2002

Q10 Eagle's Syndrome

Ans.

Refer Q7 september 2001

Q11 Ramsay Hunt Syndrome

Ans.

Refer Q19 March 2002

Q12 Carcinoma-in-situ

Ans.

Refer to Q17 of September 2004

Q13 Radiographic appearance of hyper-parathyroidism

Ans.

Refer to Q20 of March 2002

Q14 Nikolsky's Sign

Ans.

Refer to Q11 of march 2002

Q15 Radiographic appearance of Peri-apical Cementoma

Ans.

Refer Q4 March 2000 (also known as Periapical cemental dysplasia/cementoma)

Q16 Anodontia

Ans.

Refer to Q18 of March 2002

Q17 Paul Bunnel test

Ans.

Refer to Q13 of March 2002

Q18 Erosive Lichen Planus

Ans.

Refer Q1 October 1999

15

RGUHS August 2005

QUESTION PAPER

Long Essays

1. Describe the principle, indications and limitations of panoramic radiography.
2. Classify white lesions of oral cavity. Describe the etiology, clinical features and management of leukoplakia.

Short Essays

3. Laboratory investigations for anaemia.
4. Types of osteomyelitis and their features.
5. Oral manifestations of HIV.
6. Properties of X-rays.
7. Indications for paranasal sinus view.
8. Management of myofacial pain dysfunction syndrome.

Short Answers

9. Gray
10. Tzank test.
11. Fordyce's granules
12. Radiographic appearance of osteosarcoma
13. Collimation of X-ray beam
14. Types of radiation caries.
15. Ramsay Hunt syndrome
16. Brachytherapy
17. Auspitz sign
18. Causes of angular chelitis

LONG ESSAY

Q1 Describe the principle, indications and limitations of panoramic radiography.

Ans.

Refer Q8 of September 2004 for principles and indications.

Limitations of Panoramic Radiography

- The images do not display the fine anatomic details available on intraoral periapical radiographs. Thus panoramic radiographs are not useful for detecting small carious lesions, fine structure of marginal peri-dontium or periapical disease.

- The proximal surfaces of premolars usually overlap so dental caries in proximal regions remain undetected.

- There will be unequal magnification and geometric distortion across the image. Occasionally presence of overlapping structures such as cervical spine can hide odontogenic lesions, particularly in incisor region.

- Clinically important objects may be situated outside the plane of focus (image layer) and may appear distorted or not present at all.

Q2 Classify white lesions of oral cavity. Describe the etiology, clinical features and management of leukoplakia.

Ans.

Classification of White Lesions of Oral Cavity

Refer to Q. 1 of October 1999 for classification

Leukoplakia

Etiology

- *Tobacco:* Chemical constituents of tobacco when (chewed or snuffed) and the end products of its combustion (when smoked), such as tars and resins are irritating substances which are capable of producing leukoplakic alterations of the oral mucosa.

- *Alcohol:* Irritates the mucosa

- *Chronic irritation:* Chronic repeated trauma or local chronic irritation like repeated dheek bites due to malocclusion, ill fitting dentures or sharp broken down teeth is considered to be extremely important in the etiology of leukoplakia as they constantly irritate the local mucosa

- *Syphilis:* Although rare but plays a role in causing leukoplakia

- *Vitamin deficiency:* Vitamin A deficiency is known to induce metaplasia and keratinization of certain epithelial structures especially of the glands and the respiratory mucosa. Vit. B deficiency causes chronic ulcers which can predispose to leukoplakia.

- *Hormones:* Keratogenic effects of both male and female sex hormones.

- Galvanism

- *Candidiasis:* The presence of candida albicans may bear responsibility for initial development of leukoplakia.

Clinical Features

- *Site:* Anywhere on the mucosa but in descending order they are found on alveolar mucosa, tongue, lip, hard and soft palates, floor of the mouth and gingiva

- The extent of involvement may vary from small well localized regular to irregular to diffuse lesions covering a considerable portion of oral mucosa

- Female predilection to males is seen

- On examination the patches may vary from a non palpable faintly transluscent white area to thick fissured, papillomatous and indurated lesions.

- The surface of the lesion is often finely wrinkled or shriveled in appearance and may feel rough on palpation
- The lesions are white gray or yellowish white but with heavy use of tobacco, it may assume a brownish colour.
- Histopathologically, the lesion represents features of epithelial dysplasia which may be mild to moderate

Management

Refer Q3 March 2004

SHORT ESSAYS

Q3 Laboratory investigations for anemia.
Ans.
Refer Q7 september 2002

Q4 Types of osteomyelitis and their features.
Ans.

Acute Suppurative Osteomyelitis
Clinical Features

- May involve either maxilla or mandible. In maxilla the disease usually remains fairly well localized to the area of initial infection. In mandible, bone involvement tends to be more diffuse and widespread.
- In infants this type is of hematogenous in origin, but other times it seems to be a result of local oral infection following some minor injury or abrasion.
- In adults, acute suppurative osteomyelitis manifests as severe pain with elevation in temperature and regional lymphadenopathy.
- Teeth involved are loose and sore so eating is difficult
- Periostitis develops leading to reddening or swelling of skin or mucosa.
- Paraesthesia or anaesthesia of lip is common

Radiographic Features

Individual trabeculae become fuzzy and indistinct and radiolucent areas begin to appear.

Chronic Suppurative Osteomyelitis

- May develop after acute phase of the disease has subsided
- The pain is less severe, mild temperature elevation is seen and also slight elevation in the leukocyte count
- Acute exacerbation of chronic disease may occur periodically.

Chronic Focal Sclerosing Osteomyelitis (Condensing osteitis)

- Occurs in young persons before age of 20 years.
- Mandibular 1st molar is most commonly involved which presents large carious lesion
- Mild pain may be present.

Radiologic Features

Pathognomonic well circumscribed radiographic mass of sclerotic bone surrounding and extending below the apex of one or both roots.

Entire root outline is nearly always visible. It is reaction of bone to a mild bacterial infection entering the bone through carious tooth in persons who have high degree of tissue reactivity.

Chronic Diffuse Sclerosing Osteomyelitis

This represents proliferative reaction of the bone to a low grade infection.

- Occur at any age but common in older persons, especially edentulous mandibular jaws.
- There will be acute exacerbation of the dormant chronic infection, resulting in mild suppuration, many times with the spontaneous formation of a fistula opening

onto the mucosal surface to establish drainage.

- Vague pain and bad taste in mouth.

Radiologic Features

Radiopaque lesion may be extensive and is bilateral.

The border between the normal and the sclerosed bone is often indistinct.

Chronic Nonsuppurative Osteitis (Chronic osteomyelitis with proliferative periostitis or Garre's osteomyelitis)

- Occur in young persons before the age of 25 years
- Anterior surface of tibia is the most common site
- High opportunity for the infection to enter maxilla or the mandible than any other bone
- Patient presents with toothache or jaw pain and bony hard swelling on the outer surface of the jaw.
- The mass is usually of several weeks duration.

Q5 Oral manifestations of HIV.
Ans.
Refer to Q1 of September 2000.

Q6 Properties of X-rays.
Ans.
Refer to Q5 of September 2001.

Q7 Indications for paranasal sinus view.
Ans.
Refer to March 2003 Q8.

Q8 Management of myofacial pain dysfunction syndrome.
Ans.
Refer to March 2001 Q10.

SHORT ANSWERS

Q9 Gray
Ans.
Gray is the SI unit of absorbed dose. 1 Gray = 1 joule/kg.

Absorbed dose is a measure of the energy absorbed by any type of ionizing radiation per unit mass of any type of matter.

Traditional unit of absorbed dose is rad. 1 gray = 100 rads. 1 rad = 0.01Gy. The severity of deterministic damage seen in irradiated tissues or organs depends on the amount of radiation received. All individuals receiving doses above the threshold level show damage in proportion to the dose.

Acute Radiation Syndrome

Radiation in gray	Symptoms
1–2	Prodromal
2–4	Mild hematopoetic
4–7	Severe hematopoetic
7–15	Gastrointestinal hematopoetic
50	Cardiovascular and CNS

Q10 Tzanck Test
Ans.
This is a diagnostic test done by preparing Tzanck smear. The Tzanck smear is prepared from intact (freshly opened) vesicles and smears stained by papanicolau or other stains giving good nuclear differentiation, will reveal characteristic Tzanck cells.

Tzanck cells are characterized particularly by degenerative changes which include swelling of nucleus (ballooning degeneration), hyperchromatic staining and typical lipschutz bodies. Characteristic multinucleated giant cels are seen in recurrent herpes simplex infection.

Indications

- Pemphigus vulgaris

- Herpes simplex virus
- Genital herpes

Cytologic examination of Tzank smear is a supplemental test for pemphigus. Skin lesions and oral lesions in particular may be easily identified as viral diseases by cytologic smears and its typical findings.

Q11 Fordyce's granules
Ans.

Fordyce's granule is a developmental anomaly characterized by heterotropic collections of sebaceous glands at various sites in the oral cavity.

Etiology

Occurrence of sebaceous glands in the mouth may result from inclusion in the oral cavity of ectoderm having some of the potentialities of skin in the course of development of maxillary and mandibular processes.

Clinical Features

- Appear as small yellow spots, either discretely separated or forming relatively large plaques, often projecting slightly above the surface of the tissue.
- They are found most frequently in bilaterally symmetrical pattern on the mucosa of the cheeks opposite the molar teeth but can also occur on the inner surfaces of lips in the retromolar region lateral to the anterior faucial pillar.
- Occasionally it may also form on tongue, gingiva, frenulum and palate

Treatment

Requires no treatment and it has no functional significance. Benign sebaceous gland adenoma may form from these intraoral structures. Keratin filled pseudocysts can develop from the ducts of these sebaceous glands. These may sometimes equire excision.

Q12 Radiographic appearance of osteo-sarcoma
Ans.
Refer to Q4 of September 2002 solution.

Q13 Collimation of X-ray beam
Ans.
Refer to March 2002 Q8

Q14 Types of radiation caries.
Ans.
Refer to Q2. Of September 2004

Q15 Ramsay Hunt syndrome
Ans.
Refer to Q19 of March 2002

Q16 Brachytherapy
Ans.
Radiation therapy has an advantage of treating the disease in situ and avoiding the need for the removal of tissue and it may be the treatment of choice for many T1 and T2 tumours. Radiation may be administered to a localized lesion by using implant techniques or to a region of head and neck by using external beam radiation.

Interstitial and intra cavitary implants are used to treat primary cancers in head and neck. Isotopes used include gold, cesium and iridium.

Indications

- Primary treatment modality for localized tumors in anterior 2/3rd of the oral cavity
- Boosted doses of radiation to specific sites
- For treatment following recurrences.

Procedure

- Directly implanted sources may be used to deliver radiation or an after loading technique may be used in which the radiation source is placed by using previously inserted guide tubes.

- The frequency of the tissue necrosis is related to the treated volume and to the proximity of the implant to the bone.
- Tissue deflectors are used to deflect tongue. These devices can be fabricated using a double layer of flexible mouth guard material or by using heat cured acrylic. (Refer Fig. 8.31, page 212, Burket's 10th edition). Lead foil can be applied to the surface of the deflector.
- Devices can be made to keep radiation from superficial treatment of lip from affecting alveolar base.

- Lead cutouts can be made and placed on skin to isolate the lesion. These may be used in combination with an intraoral device that can shield the intraoral tissues.

Q17 Auspitz sign
Ans.
Refer to Q14 of September 2003.

Q18 Causes of angular chelitis
Ans.
Refer to Q3.1 of October 1999.

RGUHS March 2006 (OS)

QUESTION PAPER

Long Essays

1. What are the biologic effects of radiation in the oral cavity?
2. Classify Osteomyelitis. Write in detail about the etiology, clinical features, radiographic features and management of chronic suppurative osteomyelitis?

Short Essays

3. Occlusal radiography
4. Lichen planus
5. Enamel hypoplasia
6. Osteogenic sarcoma
7. Intensifying screens
8. Dental significance of hypertension

Short Answers

9. Jarisch-Herxheimer reaction
10. Pink tooth
11. Onion-skin appearance
12. Anaphylaxis
13. Temporomandibular joint ankylosis
14. Atypical facial pain
15. Fibroma
16. TNM staging
17. Benign migratory glossitis
18. Collimation

SOLUTIONS

LONG ESSAY

Q1 What are the biologic effects of radiation in the oral cavity?

Ans.

Refer to March 2000 Q19.

Q2 Classify Osteomyelitis. Write in detail about the etiology, clinical features, radiographic features and management of chronic suppurative osteomyelitis?

Ans.

Osteomyelitis is a medical term that describes an infection inside a bone. It's usually caused by a bacterial infection but the condition can also be the result of a fungal infection.

Types of Osteomyelitis

There are three main types of osteomyelitis:

- **Acute osteomyelitis,** where the bone infection develops within two weeks of an initial infection, injury or the onset of an underlying disease.

- **Sub-acute osteomyelitis,** where the bone infection develops within one ot two months of an initial infection, injury or onset of an underlying disease.

- **Chronic osteomyelitis,** where the bone infection develops two months or more after an initial infection, injury or onset of an underlying disease.

Acute osteomyelitis is more common in children than adults and usually develops as a complication of a pre-existing blood infection (haematogenous osteomyelitis).

Sub-acute and chronic osteomyelitis are more common in adults and usually develop as a result of an injury or trauma (contiguous osteomyelitis), such as a fractured bone.

Sub-acute and chronic osteomyelitis can also develop as a complication of a condition that affects the blood supply to the bones, such as diabetes, making the bones more vulnerable to infection.

Suppurative Osteomyelitis

Osteomyelitis is an inflammatory reaction of bone to infection which originates from either a tooth, fracture site, soft tissue wound or surgery site.

The dental infection may be from a root canal, a periodontal ligament or an extraction site.

Suppurative osteomyelitis can involve all three components of bone: periosteum, cortex, and marrow.

Usually there is an underlying predisposing factor like malnutrition, alcoholism, diabetes, leukemia or anemia.

Etiology

Predisposing factors are those that are characterized by the formation of avascular bone for example, therapeutically irradiated bone, osteopetrosis, Paget's disease, and florid osseous dysplasia.

Clinical Features

Osteomyelitis is more commonly observed in the mandible because of its poor blood supply as compared to the maxilla, and also because the dense mandibular cortical bone is more prone to damage and, therefore, to infection at the time of tooth extraction.

Clinical features include pain, pyrexia, painful lymphadenopathy, leukocytosis, and other signs and symptoms of acute infection. Later, after approximately two weeks, as the lesion progresses into the chronic stage, enough bone resorption takes place to show radiographic mottling and blurring of bone.

Management

Hyperbaric oxygen (HBO) has proven efficacious in the adjunct management

Radiographic Features

A sclerosed border called an involucrum forms around the affected area. The involucrum prevents blood supply from reaching the affected part. This results in the formation of pieces of sequestra or necrotic bone surrounded by pus. A fistulous tract may develop by the suppuration perforating the cortical bone and periosteum. The fistulous tract discharges pus onto the overlying skin or mucosa.

The radiopacity of the sequestra and the radiolucency of the pus give rise to the characteristic "worm-eaten" radiographic appearance. Radiographs also aid in locating the original site of infection such as an infected tooth, a fracture, or infected sinus.

Acute osteomyelitis is similar to an acute primary abscess in that the onset and course may be so rapid that bone resorption does not occur and, thus, a radiolucency may not be present on a radiograph.

SHORT ESSAY

Q3 Occlusal radiography
Ans.
Refer to September 1998 Q6.1.

Q4 Lichen planus
Ans.
Refer to march 2005 Q18.

Q5 Enamel hypoplasia
Ans.
Definition
Enamel hypoplasia may be defined as an incomplete or defective formation of the organic enamel matrix of teeth.

Types

1. Hereditary type (amelogenesis imperfecta)
2. Environmental

Classification
Hypoplastic

- Pitted, autosomal dominant(AD)
  - Local, AD
  - Smooth, AD
  - Rough, AD
  - Rough, autosomal recessive (AR)
- Smooth, X–linked dominant

Hypocalcified

Autosomal dominant and autosomal recessive.

Hypomaturation

- With taurodontism, AD
- X–linked recessive
- Pigmented, AR
- Snow–capped teeth

Clinical Features

- *Hypoplastic*–enamel has not formed to full normal thickness on newly erupted developing teeth
- *Hypocalcified*–enamel is so soft that it can be removed by a prophylaxis instrument
- *Hypomaturation*–enamel can be pierced by an explorer point under firm pressure and can be lost by chipping away from the underlying normal appearing dentin.
- All teeth of both dentitions are affected to some degree
- Crowns may or may not show discolouration (yellow to dark brown)
- Contact points between teeth are often open and occlusal surfaces and insical edges are frequently abraded
- Histology shows disturbance in the differentiation or viability of ameloblasts resulting in defective matrix formation.

Radiographic Features

- Complete absene of enamel or when present, is very thin chiefly over the tips of the cusps and on interproximal surfaces

Classification

Causes are:

- Nutritional deficiency (Vit. A, C, and D)
- Exanthematous diseases (measles, chicken pox and scarlet fever)
- Congenital syphilis (Hutchinson's teeth)
- Hypocalcemia
- Birth injury, prematurity
- Local infection or trauma (Turner's teeth or Turner's hypoplasia)
- Chemical ingestion (fluoride)
- Idiopathic

Pathogenesis

Disturbance of ameloblasts during the formative stages of tooth development. Fluoride interferes with normal calcification process.

Clinical Features

- Unlike the hereditary variety, teeth of both dentitions are not affected
- Specific features depend upon the cause
- Syphilis–Hutchinson's teeth, mulberry molar or Moon's molars or Fournier's molars
- In mild environmental there may be only few grooves or pits or fissures on the enamel surface.
- In moderate cases there are rows of deep pits arranged horizontally across the surface of the tooth
- In severe cases a considerable portion of enamel may be completely absent

Treatment is aimed only at improving the cosmetic appearance.

Q6 Osteogenic sarcoma

Ans.

Refer to September 2002 Q4.

Q7 Intensifying screens

Ans.

Refer to Q4 of September 2001.

Q8 Dental significance of hypertension

Ans.

Dental management in hypertensive patients can be complicated, since any procedure causing stress can further increase the blood pressure and can precipitate acute complications such as a cardiac arrest or a cerebrovascular accident. Chronic complications of hypertension, especially impaired renal function, can affect dental management.

Management

Dentists have a unique opportunity to detect cases of hypertension since patient visits at routine intervals are encouraged. It is a professional responsibility of a dental clinician to inform the patient of their hypertensive state and to offer medical advice, including appropriate referrals.

There are no recognized oral manifestations of hypertension but antihypertensive drugs can often cause side-effects, such as:

- Xerostomia,
- Gingival overgrowth,
- Salivary gland swelling or pain,
- Lichenoid drug reactions,
- Erythema multiforme,
- Taste sense alteration, and
- Paresthesia.

Dental clinician must focus on the actions, interactions and adverse effects of the antihypertensive medications, as well as the overall management of blood pressure of the patient in the dental chair.

The appropriate modifications for differing stages of hypertension is outlined in the algorithm presented below. There are, however, several areas of general dental management to be considered in the hyper-tensive patients.

Anesthesia

Local Anesthesia

Dental patients with hypertension are best treated under local anesthesia being sure that the anesthesia is complete so that no anxiety induced elevation of blood pressure occurs. The use of vasoconstrictors such as epinephrine in local anesthetic agents is known to have negligible influences on blood pressure in hypertensive patients, according to numerous clinical studies. Data in regard to epinephrine-containing local anesthetics has consistently shown that blood pressure and heart rate are minimally affected by the typically low dose and short duration of the drug use in dentistry, both in healthy and those with existing cardiovascular conditions. Nonetheless, the use of epinephrine-containing anesthetics in patients with uncontrolled hypertension, and elective dental procedures are contraindicated.

Anxiety Control

The anxiety and stress associated with dental treatment typically causes a rise in blood pressure and may precipitate cardiac arrest or a cerebrovascular accident. Preoperative reassurance and oral sedation may help in alleviating anxiety related rise in pressure. Use of sedatives the night before a procedure may also be used.

Relative analgesia technique using nitrous oxide (N_2O) can also reduce both systolic and diastolic pressure by up to 10–15 mm Hg, after approximately 10 minutes of use, preoperatively.

Timing of Dental Appointments

The increase of blood pressure in hypertensive patient is associated with the hours surrounding awakening that peaks by midmorning. This fluctuation of blood pressure tends to be less likely in the afternoon. Afternoon appointments are recommended over mornings for this reason.

Orthostatic Hypotension

Orthostatic hypotension may be a problem in patients using antihypertensive agents that reduce sympathetic outflow or peripheral vasodilatory actions, such as centrally acting a-2-adrenergic agonists, post-ganglionic adrenergic inhibitors, α-1-adrenergic antagonists, and diuretics. Management of orthostatic hypotension includes avoiding sudden postural changes, such as return to sitting position from the supine operating position. The patient should also be instructed to stay seated for a short period until such time that adequate cerebral perfusion has occured.

Other Dental Concerns

Aspirin is now commonly taken by patients with hypertension to decrease associated coronary or cerebral vascular thrombotic disease, and aspirin may cause bleeding problems. Many patients with hypertension develop systolic heart murmurs, in which case *prophylaxis for endocarditis* should be given.

SHORT ANSWERS

Q9 Jarisch-Herxheimer reaction

Ans.

The Herxheimer reaction (also known as Jarisch-Herxheimer or Herx) occurs when large quantities of toxins are released into the body as bacteria (typically spirochetes) die during antibiotic treatment.

Typically the death of these bacteria and the associated release of endotoxins occurs faster than the body can remove the toxins. It is manifested by fever, chills, headache, myalgia (muscle pain), and exacerbation of skin lesions. Duration in syphilis is normally only a few hours. The intensity of the reaction reflects the intensity of inflammation present.

The Herxheimer reaction has shown an increase in inflammatory cytokines during the period of exacerbation, including tumor necrosis factor alpha, interleukin 6 and interleukin-8. The reaction is also seen in other diseases, such as borreliosis (Lyme disease and tick-borne relapsing, fever, bartonellosis, brucellosis, typhoid fever, Myalgic encephalomyelitis, and trichinellosis, Q fever, and cat scratch disease.

Q10 Pink tooth
Ans.
Refer to Q13 of September 2004.

Q11 Onion-skin appearance
Ans.
Refer to Q15 of September 2004.

Q12 Anaphylaxis
Ans.
Anaphylaxis is an acute multi-system severe type I hypersensitivity reaction. Anaphylaxis can present with many different symptoms due to the systemic effects of histamine release. These usually develop over minutes to hours. The most common areas affected include: skin (80% to 90%), respiratory (70%), gastrointestinal (30% to 45%), heart and vasculature (10% to 45%), and central nervous system (10% to 15%)

Skin
Skin involvement may include generalized hives, itchiness, flushing, and swelling of the lips, tongue or throat.

Respiratory
Respiratory symptoms may include shortness of breath, wheezes or stridor, and low oxygen.

Gastrointestinal
Gastrointestinal symptoms may include crampy abdominal pain, diarrhea, and vomiting.

Cardiovascular
Due to the presence of histamine releasing cells in the heart coronary artery spasm may occur with subsequent myocardial infarction or dysrhythmia.

Nervous System
A drop in blood pressure may result in a feeling of lightheadedness and loss of consciousness. There may be a loss of bladder control and muscle tone. and a feeling of anxiety and "impending doom".

Causes
Anaphylaxis can occur in response to any allergen. Common triggers include insect bites or stings, foods, medication and latex rubber.

Food
Many foods can trigger anaphylaxis. The most common are peanut, tree nuts, shellfish, fish, milk, and egg. Severe cases are usually the result of ingesting the allergen.

Medication
Any medication may potentially trigger anaphylaxis. The most common to do so include antibiotics (β-lactam antibiotics in particular), aspirin, ibuprofen, and other analgesics. Some drugs (polymyxin, morphine, X-ray contrast and others) may cause an "anaphylactoid" reaction (anaphylactic-like reaction) on the *first exposure*. This is usually due to a toxic reaction, rather than the immune system mechanism that occurs with "true" anaphylaxis. The symptoms, risk for complica-

tions without treatment, and treatment are the same, however, for both types of reactions. Some vaccinations are also known to cause "anaphylactoid" reactions.

Venom

Venom from stinging or biting insects such as Hymenoptera or Hemiptera may induce anaphylaxis in susceptible people.

Q13 Temporomandibular joint ankylosis
Ans.

This is a condition in which condylar movement is limited by a mechanical problem in the joint ("true ankylosis") or by a mechanical cause not related to joint components ("false" ankylosis).

- True ankylosis–bony or fibrous
  - *Bony:* In this the condyle or ramus is attached to the temporal bone by an osseous bridge.
  - *Fibrous:* A soft tissue (fibrous) union of joint component appear normal.
- False ankylosis–may result from conditions that inhibit condylar movement such as muscle spasm, myositis ossificans, or coronoid process hyperplasia.

Clinical Features

- Mostly caused by mandibular trauma or infection.
- Common cause of TMJ ankylosis is rheumatoid arthritis and in rare cases bilateral fractures may be the cause.
- Most cases in infancy occur secondary to birth injury.
- Patients have a history of progressively restricted jaw opening or limited opening.
- Some degree of mandibular opening is possible through flexing of the mandible.

Radiographic Features

In fibrous ankylosis:
- Articulating surfaces are irregular because of erosions.

- The joint space is very narrow and two irregular surfaces may appear to fit one other like a jigsaw puzzle.
- Radiograpic signs of remodeling occa-sionally are visible as the joint components adapt to repeated openings at mandibular opening.

In Bony Ankylosis

- The joint space may be partly or completely obliterated by the osseous bridge, which vary form a slender segment of bone, which may be difficult to locate, to a large bony mass.
- Often morphologic changes occur – compensatory progressive elongation of the coronoid process and deepening of the antegonial notch in the mandibular ramus on the affected side as a result of muscle function during attempted mandibular opening.
- Coronal CT images are the best diagnostic imaging method to evaluate ankylosis.

Treatment

- Joint mobility is improved by surgical removal of the osseous bridge or creation of a pseudarthrosis.

Q14 Atypical facial pain
Ans.

- This constitutes a group of conditions in which there is a vague, deep, poorly localized pain in the regions supplied by the fifth and ninth cranial nerves and the second and third cervical nerves.
- The pain is not associated with trigeminal neuralgia, glossopharyngeal neuralgia, post-herpetic neuralgia, or with diseases of the teeth, throat, nose, sinuses, eyes or the ears, and the distribution of this pain is unanatomic. Since it involves portions of a sensory supply of two or more nerves and may cross the mid line.
- This pain, lacks a trigger zone, is constant and persists for weeks, months or years.

Q15 Fibroma

Ans.

This is a benign tumor of connective tissue origin and is the most common soft tissue neoplasm occurring in the oral cavity.

Clinical Features

- Appears as an elevated lesion of normal colour with smooth surface and a sessile or sometimes a pedunculated base.
- Well defined slowly growing lesion occurring at any age but most common in 3rd to 5th decades
- Originates from gingiva, buccal mucosa, tongue, lips and palate
- Histology shows bundles of interlacing collagenous fibers interspersed with varying numbers of fibroblasts or fibrocytes and small blood vessels.

Treatment

Surgical excision. Recurrence after complete excision is very very rare.

Q16 TNM staging

Ans.

Definition of TNM Categories of Malignant tumors about the Oral Cavity

T – Primary Tumor

- T1S - Carcinoma in situ.
- T1 - Tumor 2 cm. or less in greater diameter.
- T2 - Tumor greater then 2 cm but not greater than 4 cm in greater diameter.
- T3 - Tumor greater than 4 cm in greater diameter.

N- Regional Lymph Nodes

- N0-No clinically palpable cervical lymph node(s); or palpable node(s) but metastasis not suspected.
- N1-Clinically palpable homolateral cervical lymph node(s) that are not fixed, metastasis not suspected.
- N2-Clinically palpable contralateral or bilateral cervical lymph node(s) that are not fixed, metastasis suspected.
- N3-Clinically palpable lymph node(s) that are fixed, metastasis suspected.

M- Distant Metastasis

- M0-No distant metastasis.
- M1-Clinical and/or radiographic evidence of metastasis other than to cervical lymph nodes.

Clinical Stage- Grouping of Carcinoma of the Oral Cavity

Stage I: T1 N0 M0
Stage II: T2 N0 M0
Stage III: T3 N0 M0
          T1 N1 M0
          T2 N1 M0
          T3 N1 M0
Stage IV: T1 N2 M0   T1 N3 M0
          T2 N2 M0   T2 N3 M0
          T3 N3 M0   T3 N3 M0

Or any T or N category with M1.

Q17 Benign migratory glossitis

Ans.

It is also called as geographic tongue.

Geographic tongue is a condition of the tongue affecting approximately 3% of the population. It is characterized by painful, discolored regions of taste buds. The condition is usually chronic, but only manifests after eating specific exacerbating foods. It is also known by other names like "Glossitis areata exfoliativa," "Glossitis areata migrans," "Lingua geographica," "Stomatitis areata migrans," and "Transitory benign plaques of the tongue."

Symptoms (Fig. 16.1)

- The top side of the tongue is covered in small protrusions called papillae. In a tongue

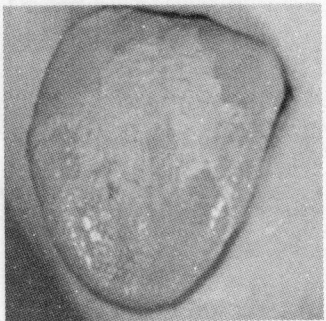

Fig. 16.1: Geographic tongue

affected by geographic tongue, there are red patches on the surface of the tongue bordered by grayish white.

- The papillae are missing from the reddish areas and overcrowded in the grayish white borders. The small patches may disappear and reappear in a short period of time (hours or days), and change in shape or size.
- While it is not common for the condition to cause pain, it may cause a burning or stinging sensation, especially after contact with certain foods.
- Foods that sometimes cause irritation, burning or slight swelling of the tongue include tomato, eggplant, walnuts, sharp cheeses, spicy foods, sour foods, candy and citrus. Geographic tongue may also cause numbness.
- Coexistence of fissures of the tongue is often noticed. Chemicals, such as mouth washes and teeth whiteners, can also aggravate the condition.

Causes

Its cause is uncertain, though tends to run in families and is associated with several different genes, though studies show family association may also be caused by similar diets.

Geographic tongue is more commonly found in people who are affected by environmental sensitivity, such as allergies, eczema, and asthma.

Its prevalence also varies by nationality (0.6% of Americans, 4% of young Iraqis, 2% of young Finns) and gender (females affected three times more than males).

Vitamin B deficiencies, allergies, and hormonal changes. Geographic tongue is said to occur more often in women, especially during high hormonal times such as during ovulation or pregnancy, and while taking birth control (generally around the 17th day).

Histopathology

Irregular areas of dekeratinized and desquamated filiform papillae (red in color) are surrounded by elevated whitish or yellow margins due to acantholysis and hyperkeratosis. Neutrophils migrate into the epithelial layer, creating what are termed Munro's abscesses.

Treatment

While there is no known cure or commonly prescribed treatment for geographic tongue, there are several ways to suppress the condition, including avoiding foods that exacerbate the problem. Some individuals report relief from chewing mint leaves or sucking on a mint candy or gum during a flare up.

Zinc supplements has resulted in a dramatic reduction in the incidence of the condition. Some people affected by geographic tongue also report that taking Vitamin B supplements causes the condition to go away temporarily.

Anti-inflammatory steroids applied topically clears the patches. Burning may also be reduced by taking antihistamines. The condition is usually asymptomatic and insignificant; persistent pain is rare.

Q18 Collimation
Ans.
Refer to March 2002 Q8.

QUESTION PAPER

Long Essays

1. What are the effects of radiation in the oral cavity? Write in detail about osteoradionecrosis.
2. Classify Oro facial pain. Write in detail about the etiology, clinical features and management of trigeminal neuralgia.

Short Essays

3. Postero anterior water's view
4. Exfoliative cytology
5. Enamel hypoplasia
6. Localization technique
7. Myositis ossificans
8. Herpangina
9. Burning mouth syndrome
10. Properties of X-rays
11. Syncope
12. Radiographic features of fractures of the teeth

Short Answers

13. Concrescence
14. White sponge nevus
15. Principle of panoramic radiography.
16. Id reaction
17. Sturge-Weber syndrome
18. Fixing solution
19. Residual cyst
20. Nikolsky's sign
21. Desquamative gingivitis
22. Lichenoid reaction

LONG ESSAY

Q1 What are the effects of radiation in the oral cavity? Write in detail about osteo-radionecrosis.

Ans.

Refer to March 2000 Q19

Q2 Classify Orofacial pain. Write in detail about the etiology, clinical features and management of trigeminal neuralgia.

Ans.

Refer to September 2004 Q1 and March 2004 Q4.

Trigeminal Neuralgia

Refer to Q1 of September 1998 and Q2 of October 1999

SHORT ESSAYS

Q3 Postero anterior water's view

Ans.

Refer to March 2003 Q8.

Q4 Exfoliative cytology

Ans.

Refer to September 2003 Q17.

Q5 Enamel hypoplasia

Ans.

Refer to Q5 March 2006 (OS).

Q6 Localization technique

Ans.

A method of identifying the buccolingual dimension of a tooth by taking a second radiographic image at an angle of 90 degrees to the first. The technique is also useful for identifying the position of subgingival anomalies. Also called **right-angle technique**; *SLOB rule*, which stands for **S**ame **L**ingual, **O**pposite **B**uccal.

Q7 Myositis ossificans

Ans.

A very rare progressive disorder involving calcification of muscles, tendons and ligaments.

Symptoms of Myositis Ossificans

The list of signs and symptoms mentioned in various sources for Myositis ossificans includes the 14 symptoms listed below:

- Muscle weakness
- Rigid muscles
- Tendon weakness
- Rigid tendons
- Calcium deposits in muscles
- Movement pain
- Tenderness
- Skin swelling over calcified site
- Shortened digits
- Skeletal malformations
- Malformed fingers
- Malformed toes
- Limited joint movement
- Skin swelling-over calcified site.

Q8 Herpangina

Ans.

Herpangina is also called aphthous pharyngitis or vesicular pharyngitis is a specific viral infection. Coxsackie group A viruses are the cause with types 1, 6, 8, 10, 16 and 22 as well as other enteroviruses being isolated at various times.

Clinical Features

- Sporadic outbreaks commonly seen in older children.
- Summer disease
- Generally mild sore throat with low grade fever along with headache and sometimes vomiting

- Prostration and abdominal pain
- Later small ulcer with gray base and an inflamed periphery on the anterior faucial pillars and sometimes on the hard and soft palates, posterior pharyngeal wall, buccal mucosa and tongue. These ulcers are preceeded by numerous small vesicles which are often overlooked.
- Transmitted through contact with an incubation period of 2–10 days.

Laboratory Findings

Herpangina is a clinical diagnosis. Laboratory studies are generally not indicated because herpangina is a mild and self-limited illness.

- Investigate the salient features of the history and physical examination, including the following:
  - Season (depending on the latitude)
  - Age
  - Exposure history
  - Clinical symptoms
  - The WBC count is usually within the reference range.
- Isolation of enterovirus in cell culture remains the criterion standard for diagnosis.[6] To isolate the virus, obtain cultures from swabs of the nasopharynx. Other specimens that may produce an isolate include stool and rectal swabs, urine, serum, and CSF.
- Serum antibodies to coxsackievirus may be measured after the onset of clinical symptoms. The antibody titer should show a 4-fold rise in serial samples performed 2–3 weeks apart.
- Polymerase chain reaction can be performed for enteroviral RNA of the throat, blood, CSF, urine, feces, and tissue specimens.

The offending virus can usually be isolated in suckling mice or hamsters by inoculation of scrapings from the throat lesions or stool specimen of nearly all the patients who manifest the clinical signs and symptoms.

Histologic Findings

No histopathologic findings are specific to herpangina.

Treatment

No treatment is necessary as the disease appears to be self limiting and presents with few complications. Those reported consists of acute parotitis, meningitis, hemolytic anaemia and hemorrhagic diathesis.

Q9 Burning mouth syndrome

Ans.

Burning mouth syndrome (BMS) is a painful, frustrating condition often described as a scalding sensation in the tongue, lips, palate, or throughout the mouth. Although BMS can affect anyone, it occurs most commonly in middle-aged or older women.

BMS often occurs with a range of medical and dental conditions, from nutritional deficiencies and menopause to dry mouth and allergies. But their connection is unclear, and the exact cause of burning mouth syndrome cannot always be identified with certainty.

Signs and Symptoms

Moderate to severe burning in the mouth is the main symptom of BMS and can persist for months or years. For many people, the burning sensation begins in late morning, builds to a peak by evening, and often subsides at night. Some feel constant pain; for others, pain comes and goes. Anxiety and depression are common in people with burning mouth syndrome and may result from their chronic pain. Other symptoms of BMS include:

- Tingling or numbness on the tip of the tongue or in the mouth
- Bitter or metallic changes in taste
- Dry or sore mouth.

Causes

There are a number of possible causes of burning mouth syndrome, including:

- Damage to nerves that control pain and taste
- Hormonal changes
- Dry mouth, which can be caused by many medicines and disorders such as Sjögren's syndrome or diabetes
- Nutritional deficiencies
- Oral candidiasis, a fungal infection in the mouth
- Acid reflux
- Poorly-fitting dentures or allergies to denture materials
- Anxiety and depression.

In some people, burning mouth syndrome may have more than one cause. But for many, the exact cause of their symptoms cannot be found.

Diagnosis

A review of your medical history, a thorough oral examination, and a general medical examination may help identify the source of your burning mouth. Tests may include:

- Blood work to look for infection, nutritional deficiencies, and disorders associated with BMS such as diabetes or thyroid problems
- Oral swab to check for oral candidiasis
- Allergy testing for denture materials, certain foods, or other substances that may be causing your symptoms.

Treatment

Treatment should be tailored to individual needs.

- Adjusting or replacing irritating dentures
- Treating existing disorders such as diabetes, Sjögren's syndrome, or a thyroid problem to improve burning mouth symptoms
- Recommending supplements for nutritional deficiencies

- Switching medicine, where possible, if a drug you are taking is causing your burning mouth
- Prescribing medications to
  - Relieve dry mouth
  - Treat oral candidiasis
  - Help control pain from nerve damage
  - Relieve anxiety and depression.

When no underlying cause can be found, treatment is aimed at the symptoms to try to reduce the pain associated with burning mouth syndrome.

Self-care tips to help ease the pain of burning mouth syndrome.

- Sip water frequently.
- Suck on ice chips.
- Avoid irritating substances like hot, spicy foods; mouthwashes that contain alcohol; and products high in acid, like citrus fruits and juices.
- Chew sugarless gum.
- Brush your teeth/dentures with baking soda and water.
- Avoid alcohol and tobacco products.

Q10 Properties of X-rays

Ans.

Refer to September 2001 Q5.

Q11 Syncope

Ans.

Partial or complete loss of consciousness with interruption of awareness of oneself and ones surroundings. When the loss of consciousness is temporary and there is spontaneous recovery, it is referred to as syncope or, in nonmedical quarters, fainting. Syncope accounts for one in every 30 visits to an emergency room. It is pronounced sin-ko-pea.

Syncope is due to a temporary reduction in blood flow and therefore a shortage of oxygen to the brain. This leads to lightheadedness or a "black out" episode, a loss of consciousness.

Temporary impairment of the blood supply to the brain can be caused by heart conditions and by conditions that do not directly involve the heart.

Non-cardiac Causes

Syncope is most commonly caused by conditions that do not directly involve the heart. These conditions include:

- *Postural (orthostatic) hypotension:* Drop in blood pressure due to changing body position to a more vertical position after lying or sitting;
- Dehydration causing a decrease in blood volume.
- Blood pressure medications leading to low blood pressure.
- Diseases of the nerves to the legs in older people (especially with diabetes or Parkinson's disease) when poor tone of the nerves of the legs draws blood into the legs from the brain.
- High altitude.
- Brain stroke or "near-stroke" (transient ischemic attack).
- A migraine attack.
- Fainting after certain situations (situational syncope) such as:
  - Blood drawing,
  - Urinating (micturition syncope),
  - Defecating (defecation syncope),
  - Swallowing (swallowing syncope), or
  - Coughing (cough syncope) that trigger a reflex of the involuntary nervous system (the vasovagal reaction) that slows the heart and dilates blood vessels in the legs and cause one to feel nausea, sweating, or weakness just before losing fainting.

Decreased blood flow to the brain can occur because:

1. The heart fails to pump the blood;
2. The blood vessels don't have enough tone to maintain blood pressure to deliver the blood to the brain;
3. There is not enough blood or fluid within the blood vessels; or
4. A combination of reasons one, two, or three above.

Q12 Radiographic features of fractures of the teeth

Ans.

Radiographic Signs

1. The presence of a.radiolucent line (usually sharply defined with in the anatomic boundaries of the structure.
2. A change in the normal anatomic outline or shape of the structure.
3. A defect in the outer cortical boundary, which may appear as a deviation in the smooth outline,a gap in the outer cortical bone, or a step like defect.
4. An increase in the density of the bone, which may be caused by the overlapping of two fragments of the bone.

Fractures of the Teeth

Dental Crown Fractures

- Fractures that involve only the enamel without the loss of enamel substance (infraction of the crown or crack)
- Fractures that involve enamel or enamel and dentin with loss of tooth substance but without pulpal involvement (uncomplicated fracture)
- Fractures that pass through enamel, dentin, and pulp with loss of tooth substance (complicated fracture)
- Radigraph provides information regarding the location and extent of the fracture and the relationship of the pulp chamber as well as the stage of root development of the involved tooth.

Dental Root Fracture

R/F: Dental root fracture may occur at any level and involve one or all the roots of multirooted teeth. Most fractures occur in middle third of root fracture appears as sharply defined radiolucent line or increase in periodontal ligament space adjacent to fracture site.

Vertical Root Fractures

They run lengthwise from the crown toward the apex of the tooth.usually both sides of the root is involved. Crack is usually oriented in the facio-lingual plane in both anterior and posterior teeth. Vertical apical root fractures occur with the tip of the root, and can cause severe to intense pain

Radiographic features a radiolucent line is seen and in later stages development of inflammatory lesion, bone loss positioned more coronally towards the alveolar crest,widening of periodontal membrane space

Crown Root Fractures

Fractue involving both crown and the root involving pulp. Direct trauma is the cause of anterior teeth fracture and large restorations or caries is the cause in posterior teeth fracture.These fractures are not usually seen on the radiograph.

SHORT ANSWERS

Q13 Concrescence

Ans. Concrescence is a condition of teeth where the cementum overlying the roots of at least two teeth join together or roots of two or more teeth are united by cementum. It may involve either primary or secondary teeth.

Causes

The cause can sometimes be attributed to trauma or crowding of teeth, excessive occlusal force, local infection.

If condition occurs during development, it is called true concrescence. If later, it is acquired concrescence.

Clinical Features

Maxillary molars are involved more frequently esp a third molar and supernumerary tooth. Involved teeth may fail to erupt or may erupt incompletely.

Radiographic Features

Concrescence and the superimposed teeth has to be distinguished.

Treatment

Surgical separation of the teeth may be necessary if one is to be extracted.

Q14 White sponge nevus
Ans.

White sponge nevus, also known as Cannon's disease, Hereditary leukokeratosis of mucosa, and White sponge nevus of Cannon appears to follow a hereditary pattern as an autosomal dominant trait. Although it is congenital in most cases, it can occur in childhood or adolescence.

Pathophysiology

It is caused by a mutation of the keratin 4 and keratin 13 genes. White sponge nevus has an autosomal dominant pattern of inheritance

Presentation (Fig. 17.1)

It presents in the mouth, most frequently as a thick bilateral white plaque with a spongy texture, usually on the buccal mucosa, but sometimes on the labial mucosa, alveolar ridge or floor of the mouth. The gingival margin and dorsum of the tongue are almost never affected.

Although this condition is perfectly benign, it is often mistaken for leukoplakia. Occasional lesions are less thickened and reveal a "watery" or semitransparent appearance. Lesions are usually well demarcated from the surrounding normal mucosa, as opposed to the poor demarcation of leukoedema and smokeless tobacco keratosis. The plaques do not change

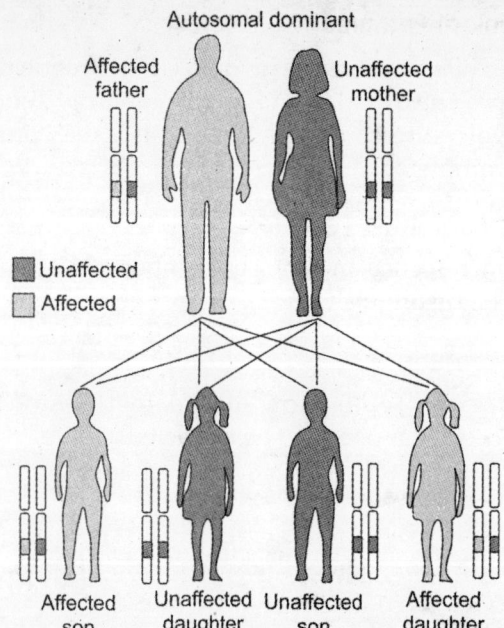

Fig. 17.1: Pattern of inheritance

significantly when the cheeks are stretched and, rarely, the plaques are small, multiple and scattered about the affected mucosa rather than being a single more diffuse keratosis.

Treatment and Prognosis

White sponge nevus remains essentially unchanged after the first few months of onset. The occasional mildly symptomatic case may respond to topical applications of tetracycline. There is no malignant potential and it does not interfere with normal masticatory functions, and so no treatment is required except for the rare example of a plaque which extends onto the lip vermilion and is surgically removed for aesthetic reasons.

Q15 Principle of Panoramic Radiography
Ans.

General Principles of Panoramic Imaging

- Employs scanography (slit beam) and tomography

- Tomography allows radiographing in one plane of an object while blurring or eliminating images from structures in other planes.
- "Tomo" is Greek for section
- View sections or radiographic slices

Tomography

- Used extensively in medicine
- Basis for CT (computed tomography) and MRI (magnetic resonance imaging)

Tomogram

- Client remains stationary while xray source and film move in opposite directions in a fixed relationship through one or a series of rotation points (Figs 17.2 to 17.5). Rotation points can be inside or outside of the focal trough

Focal trough in tomogram or "plane of acceptable detail," or "image layer," is the plane that is not blurred on the radiograph
- Focal trough in pantomogram
  - Width and thickness governed by many factors
  - Objects lying within the focal spot are shown clearly; objects outside are blurred

A panoramic radiograph or pantomogram is produced using *curved-surface* tomography.

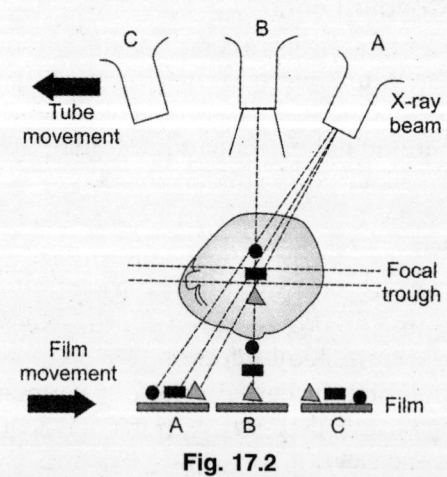

Fig. 17.2

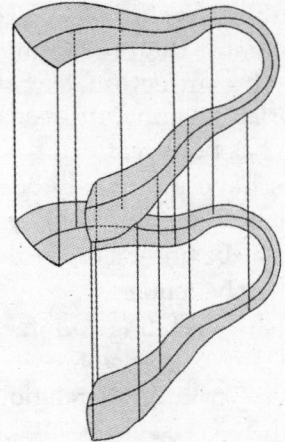

Fig. 17.3

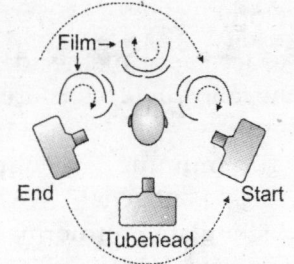

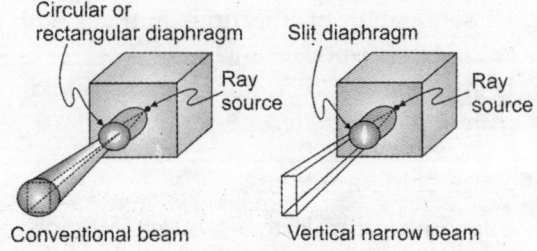

Fig. 17.5

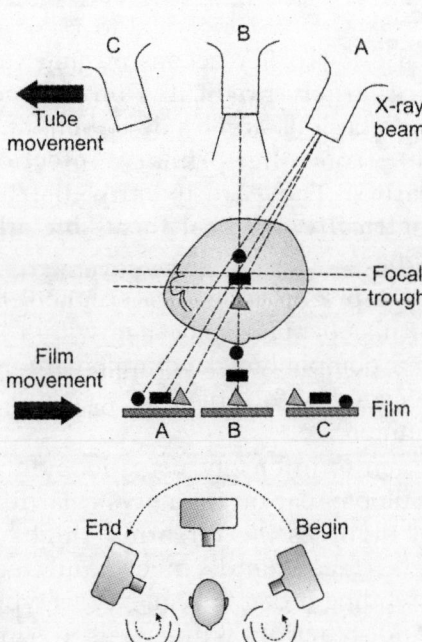

Fig. 17.4

- Rotational panoramic radiography is accomplished by rotating a narrow beam of radiation in the *horizontal plane* around an invisible pivot point/axis positioned intraorally.

- Film and tube travel in opposite directions around the client
- Client remains stationary as xray tube and film cassette-holder (which are connected) both rotate around the client
- The pivot point/axis is called the *rotation center*
- The center of rotation changes as the film and tubehead rotate which allows the image layer to conform to the elliptical shape of the dental arches

Q16 Id reaction
Ans.

Id reaction, or autoeczematization, is a generalized acute cutaneous reaction to a variety of stimuli, including infectious and inflammatory skin conditions. The pruritic rash that characterizes the id reaction, which is considered immunologic in origin, has been referred to as dermatophytid, pediculid, or bacterid when associated with a corresponding infectious process. Clinical and histopathological manifestations are variable and depend on the etiology of the eruption.

Pathophysiology

While the exact cause of the id reaction is unknown, the following factors are thought to be responsible:

1. Abnormal immune recognition of autologous skin antigens
2. Increased stimulation of normal T cells by altered skin constituents
3. Lowering of the irritation threshold
4. Dissemination of infectious antigen with a secondary response, and
5. Hematogenous dissemination of cytokines from a primary site.

Etiology of Id Reactions

- Infections with dermatophytes, pulmonary histoplasmosis, mycobacteria, viruses, bacteria, or parasites (pediculosis)
- Contact dermatitis, stasis dermatitis, or other eczematous dermatoses
- Papulonecrotic tuberculid, and some other tuberculids, are now thought to be true cutaneous forms of tuberculosis and not id reactions because of the identification (by polymerase chain reaction) of *Mycobacterium tuberculosis* in lesions.

Clinical Features

Id reactions result from a variety of stimuli, including infectious entities and inflammatory skin conditions. Dermatological manifestations vary and depend on the etiology of the eruption. General history may include the following:

- Varying degrees of pruritus are typically noted.
- An acute onset of an extremely pruritic, erythematous, maculopapular, or papulo-vesicular eruption occurs 1–2 weeks after primary infection or dermatitis. Id reactions associated with stasis dermatitis are usually symmetrical and, in descending order of frequency, involve the forearms, thighs, legs, trunk, face, hands, neck, and feet.
- Id reactions are usually preceded by exacerbation of the preexisting dermatitis induced by infection, scratching, or inappropriate therapy. (Id reaction to tinea incognito has been reported)
- Reactions have previously been reported after radiation treatment of tinea capitis.
- Vesicles may be present on the hands or feet.
- Fingers may be tender.
- Travel history relating to infectious agent exposure may be relevant.
- A history of cultural or religious practices may indicate possible contact allergens leading to an id reaction.

Physical

Clinical lesions of id reactions are quite variable and are largely predicated on the inciting etiology. Lesions are, by definition, at a site distant from the primary infection or dermatitis. They are usually distributed symmetrically. Clinical forms include the following:

- A widespread, symmetrical eruption of small follicular papules associated with a kerion and a pompholyx like eruption are usually associated with inflammatory tinea pedis (common).
- An acute, intensely pruritic, symmetric maculopapular or papulovesicular reaction that involves the forearms, thighs, legs, trunk, face, hands, neck, and feet (in descending order of frequency) is typical of the id reaction with stasis dermatitis (common).
- Erysipelaslike eruption on the anterior leg secondary to a dermatophytosis may occur (less common).
- Extracutaneous manifestations include fever, anorexia, generalized adenopathy, splenomegaly, and leukocytosis (uncommon).
- The clinical picture may rarely mimic erythema multiforme.

Q17 Sturge-Weber syndrome
Ans.
Refer to September 2003 Q16.

Q18 Fixing solution
Ans.
Refer to September 1998 Q6.2.

Q19 Residual cyst
Ans.
Residual cyst is an odontogenic cyst that remains in the jaw after the removal of a tooth. A residual cyst arises as a consequence of an improper surgical elimination of a radicular cyst. Its clinical and histological characteristics are identical to those of a radicular cyst. Radiologically it will be seen as a radiolucency of variable size at the site of a previous tooth extraction. Large residual cysts may be treated by marsupialization (Fig. 17.6).

The radiograph to the left shows a well delineated radiolucency with a markedly radiopaque periphery. This lesion is not related to the neighboring premolar. Note the roof of the cyst elevating the floor of the maxillary sinus. After surgical removal and biopsy the lesion proved to be a cyst. This cyst was a consequence to caries in the first maxillary molar. That molar was extracted and portions

of the cystic wall were left within bone. Those rests gave rise to a so-called residual cyst. Therefore, any cyst must be carefully removed in order to avoid recurrences.

Fig. 17.7 is another example of a residual cyst. It is important to remember that on X-ray this lesion is a radiolucency and that the radiographic differential diagnosis should include a variety of lesions which can present as a radiolucid image such as: non-odontogenic benign neoplasms (i.e.: hemangiomas, neurolemmo-mas, etc.), odontogenic benign neoplasms (i.e. unicystic ameloblastoma, adenomatoid odontogenic tumor, etc.) or other lesions primary to bone like Langerhans cell histiocytosis. Therefore a biopsy is imperative to establish the proper diagnosis.

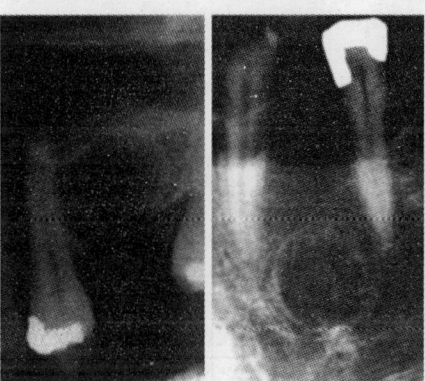

Fig. 17.7

Q20 Nikolsky's sign
Ans.
Refer to Q 11 march 2002.

Q21 Desquamative gingivitis
Ans.
Desquamative gingivitis is a cutaneous condition characterized by diffuse gingival erythema with varying degrees of mucosal sloughing and erosion.

Desquamative gingivitis is a serious condition in which the outer layers of the gums

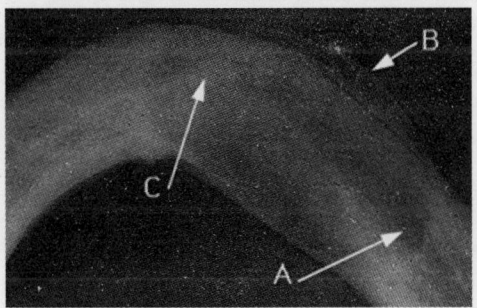

Fig. 17.6: This large residual cyst has been present for many years in the mandible of a 67 year-old man. Arrow A points to the mandibular canal. Arrow B points to the expansion of the labial cortical plate produced by the cyst. Arrow C points to a radicular rest.

separate from the underlying tissue, exposing nerve endings. The gums become so loose that the outer layers can actually be rubbed away with as little as a cotton swab.

Desquamative gingivitis occurs mainly in postmenopausal women. Women over the age of 45 should watch their mouths carefully for signs of gingivitis, especially changes in gum color or appearance and tenderness. Symptoms of desquamative gingivitis include red gums that are painful to the touch with white patches or coating and loose tissue. Knowing the signs of desquamative gingivitis will help you catch the disease early, and diligent oral hygiene can greatly reduce the effects and spread of the disease.

Treatment is based on eliminating bacteria from the oral cavity; therefore, oral practices is the principal stage. It's vital to brush and floss each day, and to consult the dental professional for standard cleanings regularly, also.

Q22 Lichenoid reaction
Ans.

Lichenoid tissue reaction (LTR) is characterised by epidermal basal cell damage which takes the form of liquefaction degeneration or cell death either apoptosis or necrosis with an associated cascade of histologic events in epidermis and dermis.

Drug-induced lichenoid reactions are skin eruptions that occur after ingestion, contact, or inhalation of certain chemicals, with the most common inducers being gold salts, beta blockers, antimalarials, thiazide diuretics, furosemide, spironolactone, and penicillamine.

For further knowledge this implication in dentistry is given:

Lichenoid amalgam reaction, also known as amalgam associated oral lichenoid reaction, is an uncommon allergic reaction following long exposure to dental amalgam filling(s).

The clinical clues that it may suggest this diagnosis are close proximity to a dental amalgam filling, localised lesion, asymmetrical. The buccal mucosa (inside of the cheek) is the most common site affected, with the border of the tongue the next commonest. Oral lichenoid lesions have been classified into three groups based on the relationship to the amalgam filling:

• Group I – lesion is limited to the area in direct contact with the amalgam filling
• Group II – the lesion exceeds the area of contact ·
• Group III – the lesion shows no contact with an amalgam filling.

As with idiopathic oral lichen planus, there are four clinical patterns – reticular, erosive, atrophic and plaque-like, with the reticular pattern seen most commonly.

The lesion may be asymptomatic or show symptoms such as pain or sensitivity to eating hot or spicy foods.

Diagnosis of lichenoid reaction is done by clinical examination and following :

• A biopsy of the lesion
• Immunofluorescence may be done to exclude autoimmune diseases of the mouth, and again is the same as for idiopathic oral lichen planus.
• Patch testing

18

RGUHS March 2007 (OS)

QUESTION PAPER

Long Essays

1. Define Leukoplakia. Discuss the etiopathogenesis, clinical features and treatment of oral leukoplakia
2. Enumerate the types of intraoral radiographs. Describe briefly the technique of obtaining intraoral periapical radiograph of maxillary central incisors

Short Essays

3. Indications and interpretation of Clark's technique
4. Classification and clinical significance of endogenous pigmentation
5. Clinical features and investigations of submandibular Sialolithiasis
6. Clinical features and treatment of acute suppurative osteomyelitis
7. Clinical features and management of degenerative arthritis of TMJ
8. Types and indications of biopsy in oral medicine

Short Answers

9. Requirements of darkroom
10. Two indications and contraindications of sialography
11. Four differences between recurrent aphthous and recurrent intraoral herpes ulcers
12. Four causes of Macroglossia
13. Taurodontism
14. Papillon Lefèvre syndrome
15. Name four conditions showing soap bubble appearance on skull radiograph
16. Composition of X-ray film
17. Western blot test
18. Name four indications for bitewing radiograph

SOLUTIONS

LONG ESSAYS

Q1 Define Leukoplakia. Discuss the etiopathogenesis, clinical features and treatment of oral leukoplakia.

Ans.

Leukoplakia is defined as a whitish patch or plaque which cannot be characterized clinically or pathologically as any other disease entity and whose occurrence is not associated with any physical or chemical causative agents except for the use of tobacco.

Refer to March 2004 Q3 solution for the second part of the question.

Q2 Enumerate the types of intraoral radiographs. Describe briefly the technique of obtaining intraoral periapical radiograph of maxillary central incisors

Ans.

Types of intraoral radiographs Refer to march 1999 Q4

Technique of obtaining intraoral periapical radiograph of maxillary central incisors. Refer September 1998 Ques. 5.

SHORT ESSAYS

Q3 Indications and interpretation of Clark's technique

Ans.

Refer to Q8 of September 2003.

Q4 Classification and clinical significance of endogenous pigmentation

Ans.

Refer to Q1 of September 2001.

Q5 Clinical features and investigations of submandibular Sialolithiasis

Ans.

Refer to Q7 of March 2001.

Q6 Clinical features and treatment of acute suppurative osteomyelitis

Ans.

It is an infection of bone marrow which principally is via the hematogenous route.

Clinical Features

- Affects all ages and has a strong male predilection
- Common in mandible because of poorer vascular supply
- Rapid onset, pain, swelling of adjacent soft tissues
- Fever, lymphadenopathy and leukocytosis
- Associated teeth may be mobile and sensitive to percussion
- Purulent drainage may be present
- Paraesthesia of lower lip is not uncommon

Radiologic examination in addition to complete examination with plain radiographs, the following additional modalities may be employed

- 2 phase nuclear medicine study composed of a Tc99 bone scan followed by a gallium citrate scan may help to confirm the diagnosis.
- Computed tomography reveals more bone surface for detecting sequestra or periosteal new bone.
- MRI with T2W images displays abnormal marrow oedema

Radiographic Features

- Very early – no changes identified
- Location – posterior body of mandible
- Ill defined periphery
- Internal structure – slight decrease in the density of involved bone with loss of sharpness of existing trabeculae, in time the

bone destruction becomes more profound leading to area of radiolucency. Later appearance of sclerotic lesion and sequestra.

- Surrounding structures – it can stimulate bone resorption or formation. A radiolucent band separates the periosteal new bone from the bone surface.

Treatment

Removal of the source of inflammation is the primary goal of the therapy. Antibiotic treatment is the mainstay along with establishing drainage which may entail removal of tooth, RCT or surgical incision and drainage.

Medicinal therapy – massive antibiotic therapy should be started as early as possible. Culture and sensitivity tests should be carried out. Intravenous fluids should be given. Blood transfusion recommended if Hb falls.

High protein and multivitamin diet is advised.

Surgical therapy – is always carried out under the cover of antibiotics. Incision and drainage of the pus is the treatment of choice. Glove drain can be left in place. Wound should be irrigated with normal saline or antibiotic solution thrice daily.

Q7 Clinical features and management of degenerative arthritis of TMJ

Ans.

Degenerative joint disease (DJD) is a noninflamatory disorder of joints characterized by joint deterioration and proliferation. Joint deterioration is characterized by loss of articular cartilage and bone erosion and the proliferative component is characterized by new bone formation at the articular surface and in the subchondral region.

In acute cases deterioration predominates whilst in chronic cases proliferative changes predominate. DJD is thought to occur when the ability of the joint to adapt to excessive forces is exceeded.

Etiology

Primary DJD has unknown causative factors while in secondary DJD many factors have a role to play including congenital diseases, storage disorders, acute trauma, hypermobility and loading of the joint such as those occurring in parafunction and internal derangements.

Clinical Features

- Occurs at any age
- Female preponderance
- Pain and tenderness on palpation- unilateral pain directly overlying the condyle
- Crepitus felt on intraauricular and pretragus palpation with deviation of mandible to the painful side
- Limitation of motion and muscle spasm-restricted mandibular opening
- Feeling of stiffness after a period of inactivity
- Anterior open bite may be a feature

Radiographic Features

- In maximal intercuspation joint space may be narrow or absent which often correlates with an internal derangement and frequently with the perforation of the disc or posterior attachments resulting in bone to bone contact of joint components.
- Signs of previous remodeling such as flattening and subchondral sclerosis may be evident
- Loss of cortex or erosions of the articular surfaces of TMjoint are the cahrecteristics
- In some cases Ely cysts are visible (they are not true cysts but areas of degeneration that contain fibrous tissue, granulation tissue and osteoid).
- Bony proliferation at the periphery of articular surfaces (called osteophytes), typically seen over the anterosuperior aspect of the condyle, lateral aspect of the temporal bone or both. In severe cases osteophytes extend from articular eminence to condylar head.

- Joint mice are loose intraarticular free osteophytes
- Glenoid fossa may be enlarged in severe DJD, also seen are erosion of condylar head

Differential Diagnosis
- Rheumatoid arthritis
- Osteoid osteoma

Treatment

Conservative treatment for 6 months to 1 year with NSAID's, heat, soft diet, rest and occlusal splints that allow free movement of the mandible

Intraarticular steroids in acute conditions.

Arthroplasty to remove the erosive surfaces is also an option.

Artificial TMJ's to treat patients with advanced degenerative changes.

Q8 Types and indications of biopsy in oral medicine
Ans.

Biopsy is a relatively minor surgical procedure carried out on tissues removed from living organisms to confirm the diagnosis histopathologically.

Types
- Incisional done in lesions that are too large to excise initially without an established diagnosis
- Excisional lesions that are small can be excised en masse and sent for histopathological examination
- Aspirational a large bore needle (18G) is used to aspirate at the most fluctuant point of the lesion and contents sent for examination
- Punch–has very little role in oral surgery and may be used in mass sereening of cancer patients
- Exfoliative is an adjunct to the surgical biopsy. It is a quick, simple, painless and bloodless procedure. It helps in checking the false negative biopsies. Used for follow up detection of recurrent carcinoma in previously treated cases. Valuable for screening lesions whose gross appearance is such that biopsy is not warranted.
- FNAC takes little time and has minimal discomfort to the patient. Advantages are that it is rapid, relatively safe and cost effective while the disadvantages are that there is a risk of tumor cell seeding along the track and utility of only positive findings giving any information.

Indications of Biopsy
- Useful to diagnose the true nature of the lesion
- Doubtful malignant lesions
- Cystic lesions
- Oral cancer screening
- Prognostic indicator in the cysts of jaws

SHORT ANSWERS

Q9 Requirements of darkroom
Ans.

The dark room should be convenient to the x ray machines and dental operatories and should be atleast 4 × 5 feet.
- Lightproof-a light-tight door or doorless maze is used. Door should have a lock to prevent accidental opening.
- The room should be well ventilated
- An exhaust fan is to be used
- Room temperature should be controlled as temperatures of 90 deg farenhite or higher can cause fogging of films
- Safe lighting is low intensity illumination of relatively long wavelength. Red GBX2 filter is recommended in the dark rooms for safelighting.
- Manual processing tanks should be kept albeit as back up for an automatic processor or digital imaging system.
- Thermometer–to constantly monitor the temperature of developing, fixing and washing

solutions. This thermometer should not contain mercury as it could break and contaminate the processor or the solution, instead it should contain alcohol or other metal.

Q10 Two indications and contraindications of sialography
Ans.
Refer Q2 of September 2002.

Q11 Four differences between recurrent aphthous and recurrent intraoral herpes ulcers
Ans.

Criteria	Aphthous ulcer	Herpetic ulcer
Cause	Idiopathic/multi aetiologic	Herpes simplex virus infection
Nature	Aphthous ulcer single or multiple will be covered by gray membrane with well circum-scribed margin and surrounded by a halo	Involves almost whole mucous membrane and produce characteristic vesicles
Lipshutz bodies	Absent	Present
After healing	No symptoms	May have post herpetic neuralgia

Q12 Four causes of Macroglossia
Ans.
Macroglossia is the for unusual enlargement of the tongue. Severe enlargement of the tongue can cause cosmetic and functional difficulties including in speaking, eating, swallowing and sleeping.

Amyloid Disorders
Amyloidosis is an accumulation of insoluble proteins in tissues that impedes normal function.
1. Primary amyloidosis
2. Myeloma associated amyloidosis
3. Lubarsch pick syndrome
4. Immunoglobulinemic amyloidosis

Hypothyroid Macroglossia
Macroglossia is also a clinical feature in Hypothyroid disorders which include
1. Congenital hypothyroidism
2. Young Simpson syndrome
3. Zadik Barak Levin syndrome
4. Athyreotic cretinism
5. Kocher-Debre-Semelaigne syndrome

Overgrowth Disorders
1. Beckwith-Wiedemann syndrome
2. Simpson-Golabi-Behmel syndrome
3. Acromegaly

Chromosomal Disorders
1. Triploid syndrome
2. Chromosome 4, trisomy 4p

Other Miscellaneous
1. Mucopolysaccharidosis
2. Mannosidosis, Alpha B, lysosomal
3. Glycogen storage disease type 2, or Pompe's disease
4. Fucosidosis
Apparent macroglossia can also occur in Down syndrome.

Q13 Taurodontism
Ans.
Taurodontism is a condition found in molar teeth where the body of the tooth and pulp chamber is enlarged vertically at the expense of the roots. As a result, the floor of the pulp and the furcation of the tooth is moved apically down the root. The underlying mechanism of taurodontism is the failure or

late invagination of Hertwig's root sheath, which is responsible for root formation and shaping causing an apical shift of the root furcation. The constriction at the amelo-cemental junction is usually reduced or absent. Taurodontism is most commonly found in permanent dentition although the term is traditionally applied to molar teeth. In some cases taurodontism seems to follow an autosomal dominant type of inheritance. Taurodontism is found in association with amelogenesis imperfecta, ectodermal dysplasia and tricho-dento-osseous syndrome. The term means "bull like" teeth derived from similarity of these teeth to those of ungulate or cud-chewing animals.

According to Shaw these can be classified as:

- Hypotaurodont
- Hypertaurodont
- Mesotaurodont.

According to mangion taurodontism may be:
- A retrograde character
- A primitive pattern
- Mendelian recessive character
- Atavistic feature
- A mutation.

The condition is of anthropological importance as it was seen in Neanderthals. It has also been reported in Klinefelter's syndrome. The teeth involved are invariably molars, sometimes single and at the other times multiple teeth may be involved. The teeth themselves may look normal and do not have any particular anatomical character on clinical examination.

On a dental radiograph, the involved tooth looks rectangular in shape without apical taper. The pulp chamber is extremely large and the furcations may be only a few millimeters long at times.

Q14 Papillon Lefèvre syndrome
Ans.

Papillon–Lefèvre syndrome (also known as "Palmoplantar keratoderma with periodontitis") is an autosomal recessive genetic disorder caused by a deficiency in cathepsin C.

PLS is characterized by periodontitis and palmoplantar keratoderma. The severe destruction of periodontium results in loss of most primary teeth by the age of 4 and most permanent teeth by age 14. Hyperkeratosis of palms and soles of feet appear in first few years of life. Gorlin, et al. have suggested that calcification of the dura mater is a third component of the syndrome.

Eruption of the primary dentition into the oral cavity is accompanied by severe gingival inflammation and a generalized aggressive periodontitis, resulting in tooth mobility. By the age 4 or 5 years, the primary teeth frequently become loose and exfoliate. After exfoliation of the primary dentition, the gingival inflammation resolves. As the permanent teeth erupt, the same sequence of events recur and, without intervention, most of the permanent teeth are lost by 15–17 years of age.

Severe resorption of alveolar bone gives the teeth a 'floating-in-air' appearance on dental radiographs.

Retinoids and antibiotics have been used for treating the condition. Dentures have to be given to most patients who loose their teeth. Osseointegrated implants are an option for the future and can have a great impact psycho-socially by restoring esthetics as well as function.

Q15 Name four conditions showing soap bubble appearance on skull radiograph
Ans.

The conditions that can present with soap bubble appearance are:
- Ameloblastama,
- Adenocystic carcinoma
- Aneurysmal bone cyst

Q16 Composition of X-ray film
Ans.

The answer given here is very descriptive. For short answer type questions, write only what is asked. This answer can be used as a short note (Fig. 18.1).

The **film base** provides the structural strength for the film. However, the base must be flexible for ease of processing, essentially be transparent to light and be dimensionally stable over time. Early base materials were glass and cellulose nitrate, but more recently cellulose triacetate and polyester have been adopted. A thin layer of adhesive is then applied to the base and this binds the emulsion layer. Covering the emulsion is a thin supercoat that serves to protect the emulsion from mechanical damage.

The two most important ingredients of a **photographic emulsion are gelatin and silver halide.** With most X-ray film the emulsion is coated on both sides of the film but its thickness varies with the nature and type of the film, but is usually no thicker than 10 mm. Photographic gelatin is made from bone and is ideal as a suspension medium in that it prevents clumping of grains. In addition, processing chemicals can penetrate gelatin rapidly without destroying its strength or permanence.

Silver halide is the light sensitive material in the emulsion. In X-ray film, sensitivity is increased by having a mixture of between 1% and 10% silver iodide and 90 to 99% silver bromide. In photographic emulsion the silver halide is suspended in the gelatin as small crystals (called grains). Grain size might average one to 2.3 mm in diameter with up to a billion silver ions per grain and billions of grains per ml of emulsion. In its pure form the silver halide crystal has low photographic sensitivity. The emulsion is sensitised by heating it under controlled conditions with a reducing agent containing sulphur. This results in the production of silver sulphide at a site on the surface of the crystal referred to as a sensitivity speck. It is the sensitivity speck that traps electrons to begin formation of the latent image centres.

Silver bromide is cream coloured and absorbs ultraviolet and blue light, but reflects green and red light. Historically, this was fine since the principle emission from calcium tungstate screens is blue light. Films for photography of image intensifier images and films for use with rare earth screens need to have their spectral sensitivity broadened to encompass the longer wavelengths associated with the emissions from these screens. This is accomplished by the addition of suitable dyes. Thus, we have green sensitive orthochromatic film and red sensitive panchromatic film.

Q17 Western blot test
Ans.

The western blot (alternatively, protein immunoblot) is an analytical technique used to detect specific proteins in a given sample of tissue homogenate or extract. It uses gel electrophoresis to separate native or denatured proteins by the length of the polypeptide (denaturing conditions) or by the 3-D structure of the protein (native/non-denaturing conditions). The proteins are then transferred to a membrane (typically nitrocellulose or PVDF), where they are probed (detected) using antibodies specific to the target protein. Steps in a western blot

- Tissue preparation
- Gel electrophoresis

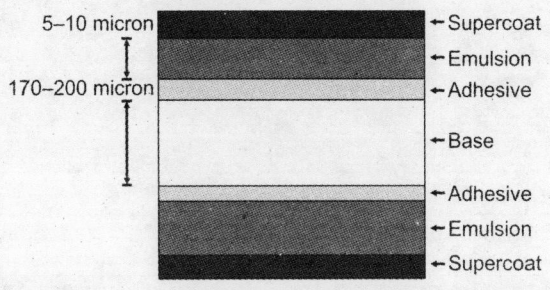

Fig. 18.1: X-ray film

5–10 micron ← Supercoat
← Emulsion
170–200 micron ← Adhesive
← Base
← Adhesive
← Emulsion
← Supercoat

- Transfer
- Blocking
- Detection
  Two step
  One step
- Analysis
  - Colorimetric detection
  - Chemiluminescent detection
  - Radioactive detection
  - Fluorescent detection
- Secondary probing

Q18 Name four indications for bitewing radiograph
Ans.
Refer to March 1999 Q5.

19

RGUHS February 2007 (OS)

QUESTION PAPER
Long Essays

1. Describe the normal anatomical landmarks in intraoral radiographs.
2. Classify vesiculobullous lesions. Write in detail about the etiology, clinical features and management of pemphigus vulgaris.

Short Essays

3. Biological effects of radiation in oral cavity
4. Periapical radio-opacities
5. Peutz-Jegher syndrome
6. Types of X-ray film processing
7. Dental significance of diabetes mellitus
8. Hypervitaminosis A

Short Answers

9. Fordyce granules
10. Polycythemia rubra vera
11. Fibromatosis gingivae
12. Adenomatoid odontogenic tumour
13. Replenisher
14. Ectodermal dysplasia
15. Psoriatic arthritis
16. Discoid lupus erythematosus
17. Uremic stomatitis
18. Drug-induced gingival hyperplasia

LONG ESSAYS

Q1 Describe the normal anatomical landmarks in intraoral radiographs.
Ans.

Appearance of the "Normal" Tooth on Periapical Radiographs

X-ray images rely on the physical attenuation of the X-ray beam to form an image on film. The denser the tissue, the more radiation it will absorb. The more radiation absorbed by the tissues, the less reaches the film. The more radiation that passes through the tissue and reaches the film, the darker the area will be on the image.

The most dense area of a normal tooth is the enamel cap, which typically appears more radiopaque (white) than the other tissues. The dentin is less dense and appears as a uniform grey area. The junction between the enamel and dentin is very distinct. The layer of cementum on the root surface is nearly the same density as the dentin, thus it is usually not apparent radiographically. The soft tissues of the pulp are much less dense than the other tooth structures and typically appear radiolucent. In normal, fully-formed teeth the root canal may be apparent extending to the apex of the root with a recognizable apical foramen.

Supporting structures of the tooth that are visible radiographically include the lamina dura, the alveolar crest, the periodontal ligament space, and the cancellous bone. When the X-ray beam is projected directly through the long axis of the lamina dura, it is seen clearly as a thin, white line. If the beam passes through at an angle, the lamina dura may appear more diffuse or not be visible at all. The radiographic appearance of the alveolar crest varies from a dense layer of cortical bone to a smooth surface without cortical bone. The level of the bony crest is considered normal when it is not more than 1.5 mm from the cementoenamel junction of the adjacent teeth. The periodontal ligament space appears as a radiolucent space between the root and lamina dura, beginning at the alveolar crest, extending around the portion of the root within the alveolus, and returning to the alveolar crest on the opposite side. The width of the PDL varies from tooth to tooth, although it is typically thinner in the middle of the root and wider near the alveolar crest and root apex. Cancellous bone lies between the cortical plates of both jaws and shows many small radiolucent pockets of marrow which create the trabecular pattern we see on the film. The trabecular pattern varies considerably from patient to patient and even within the same patient. The trabeculae in the maxillar are typically small and form a dense granular pattern while the trabecular pattern of the mandible is larger and coarser.

Normal Maxillary Radiographic Anatomy

The normal maxillary anatomical landmarks:
- Intermaxillary suture
- Anterior nasal spine
- Nasal fossa and nasal septum
- Incisive foramen
- Superior foramina of nasopalatine canal
- Lateral fossa
- Nose
- Nasolacrimal canal
- Maxillary sinus
- Zygoma and zygomatic process of maxilla
- Nasolabial fold
- Pterygoid plates

The borders of the maxillary sinus are formed of thin cortical bone which appear as thin radiopaque lines on periapical radiographs. The size of the maxillary sinus varies considerably although the right and left sinuses are typically symmetrical. The floor of the sinus is seen on periapical radiographs near the apices of the molars and premolars, and may extend down as far as the crest of the alveolar ridge, particularly in edentulous areas. Radiopaque lines traversing the sinus either horizontally or vertically are septae, bony projections from the floor and wall of the antrum. Septae give the sinus the appearance of being divided into compartments, although this is not the case. The radiolucent compartments formed by the septae sometimes mimic periapical pathoses.

Occasionally small bone nodules on the floor of the maxillary sinus may imitate root tips. One way to differentiate the two is to look for trabecular pattern; a nodule will show trabecular pattern while a root tip will not.

The zygoma appears as a U-shaped radiopaque line with the round portion superimposing the area of the first and second molars. Depending on the angle in which the X-ray beam passes through the zygoma, it will vary in size, width, and definition.

The nasolabial fold may appear as an oblique line traversing the premolar region. The line of contrast is well-defined and the area of increased radiopacity is caused by the superimposition of the cheek tissue. This feature increases with age and can be used to identify the side of the maxilla if the area is edentulous.

The medial and lateral pterygoid plates lying immediately posterior to the maxillary tuberosities have a variable appearance (another view of the pterygoid plates), often not being visible at all. Typical appearance is a single radiopaque shadow with no trabecular pattern. The hamulus may be seen extending inferiorly from the medial pterygoid plate and does show trabecular pattern.

Normal Mandibular Radiographic Anatomy

On periapical radiographs of the central incisors the mental fossa appears as a radiolucent depression extending laterally from the midline and between the alveolar ridge and the mental ridge. Due to the thinness of the bone in the area, the mental fossa appears slightly radiolucent compared to adjacent bone and may be mistaken for periapical disease.

The mental foramen is seen on some periapical radiographs and has a varying appearance; sometimes round or oblong, sometimes slitlike. Typically it is positioned halfway between the lower border of the mandible and the alveolar crest, in the region of the apex of the second premolar. It may appear over the apex of a tooth, mimicking periapical pathoses. A second radiograph from another angle will likely cause the appearance of the foramen to shift in relation to the apex and confirm its identity.

The mandibular canal appears inconsistently and is seen as a dark linear shadow with thin radiopaque borders. The canal extends radiographically from the mandibular foramen to the mental foramen.

Nutrient canals appear in a small number of patients as radiolucent lines extending vertically from the inferior dental canal to the interdental space between the mandibular incisors. Occasionally the canals may appear as small round radiolucencies perpendicular to the cortex and can be mistaken for pathology.

The mylohyoid ridge appears as a radiopaque line running from the area of the third molars to the premolar region, occasionally superimposing the molar roots. The margin of the ridge is varies and is often not well defined.

The submandibular gland fossa is located below the mylohyoid ridge in the molar area and appears as a radiolucent area with a sparse trabecular pattern.

The external oblique ridge is the continuation of the anterior border of the mandibular ramus which disappears in the area of the first molar. On periapical radiographs it appears superior to the mylohyoid ridge, running nearly parallel to it. Radiographically it appears as a radiopaque line with varying width, density, and length.

The coronoid process is often seen in the molar region and appears as a triangular opacity superimposed on the area of the third molar. Trabecular pattern may or may not be visible.

Q2 Classify vesiculobullous lesions. Write in detail about the etiology, clinical features and management of pemphigus vulgaris.
Ans.
Classification
Refer to Q1 of March 2000. Etiology, clinical features and management of pemphigus vulgaris. Refer to Q1 of September 2003 and Q9 of September 2000.

SHORT ESSAYS
Q3 Biological effects of radiation in oral cavity
Ans.
Refer to march 2000 Q19 solution.

Q4 Periapical radio-opacities
Ans.
Refer to march 2001 Q2 solution.

Q5 Peutz-Jeghers syndrome
Ans.
Peutz-Jeghers Syndrome
(Hereditary Intestinal Polyposis Syndrome)
It consists of familial generalized intestinal polyposis and pigmented spots on the face, oral cavity and sometimes the hand and feet.

The polyposis and the pigmentation appear to be due to single pleiotropic gene and not to linked genes.

Only about 50 percent of the reported patients have a familial history of the syndrome; the remainders are isolated cases resulting from sporadic mutations.

Clinical Features
1. The melanin pigmentation of the lips and oral mucosa is usually present from birth and appears as small brown macules measuring 1 to 5 mm in diameter.
2. Interaorally, the buccal mucosa is most frequently involved with the gingiva and hard palate next.
3. On the face the spots tend to be grouped around the eyes, nostrils and lips. the mucosal surface of the lips, particularly the lower lips , is almost invariably involved.
4. Facial pigmentation tends to fade later in life.
5. Intestinal polyps manifest themselves clinically in the small intestine. Thus patients may have episodes of abdominal pain and signs of minor obstruction.
The role of dentist in detecting this syndrome is important, since the intestinal condition may be recognized early through a tentative diagnosis based on the oral and paraoral manifestations.

Q6 Types of X-ray film Processing
Ans.
Types of X-ray film Processing
Manual Processing
- *Replenish solution:* Adding fresh developer and fixer
- Stir solution
- Mount films on the hanger
- Set timer
- Develop
- Rinse
- Fix
- Wash and dry

Rapid-Processing Chemicals

These solution develop well in 15 sec and fix them in15 sec at room temperature .They have same general formulation but contain higher concentration of hydroquinone and more alkaline PH then conventional solutions.

Used in endodontics and in emergency situations.

Automatic Film Processing

Equipment is available. Depending on the equipment and the temperature of the operation an automatic processor requires only 4 to 6 mins to develop, fix, wash, and dry a film.

When extraoral films are processed, the light shielded compartment is removed to provide room for feeding the larger film into the processor.

Weather automatic processor equipment is appropriate for a specific practice depends on the dentist and the nature and volume of practice.

Mechanism: This consists of a transport mechanism that picks up the unwrapped films and passes it through the developing , fixing, washing, and drying section.

The transport system most often used is a series of rollers driven by a constant speed motor that operates through gears belts or chains. Rolleres consists of independent assemblies of multiple rollers in a rack with 1 rack for each step in the operation. Rollers move the film through the developing the processing solutions. Top rollers at the cross over point between the developer and fixer tanks remove the developing solutions, this helps in maintaining the uniformity of the processing chemicals.

Q7 Dental significance of diabetes mellitus
Ans.
Refer to September 2004 Q6 solution.

Q8 Hypervitaminosis A
Ans.
Definition
Hypervitaminosis A is having too much vitamin A in the body.
Alternative names: Vitamin A toxicity

Causes

There are two types of vitamin A hypervitaminosis:
- Acute–caused by taking too much vitamin A over a short period of time
- Chronic–occurs when too much of the vitamin is present over a longer period.

Chronic vitamin A toxicity develops after taking too much vitamin A for long periods.

Symptoms

- Abnormal softening of the skull bone (craniotabes — infants and children)
- Blurred vision
- Bone pain or swelling
- Bulging fontanelle (infants)
- Changes in consciousness
- Decreased appetite
- Dizziness
- Double vision (young children)
- Drowsiness
- Fatigue
- Headache
- Impotence and ejaculation failure
- Increased intracranial pressure
- Irritability
- Nausea
- Osteoporosis
- Poor weight gain (infants and children)
- Skin and hair changes
- Cracking at corners of the mouth
- Hair loss
- Higher sensitivity to sunlight
- Oily skin and hair (seborrhea)

- Skin peeling, itching
- Yellow discoloration of the skin
- Swelling of breast tissue in men (gynecomastia)
- Vision changes
- Vomiting

Examinations and Tests

- Bone hardening (calcification)
- High blood calcium levels
- High cholesterol
- High serum creatinine (suggesting kidney damage)
- Serum vitamin A levels

Treatment

Treatment involves simply stopping the use of too much vitamin A.

Outlook (Prognosis)

Most people fully recover. Possible complications

- Excessively high calcium levels
- Failure to thrive
- Kidney damage due to high calcium
- Liver damage
- Osteoporosis
- Prostate cancer

Recent studies show that taking too much vitamin A during pregnancy can cause abnormal development in the fetus.

Prevention

To avoid hypervitaminosis A, avoid taking more than the recommended daily allowance of this vitamin. Recent emphasis on vitamin A and beta carotene as anticancer vitamins may contribute to chronic hypervitaminosis A, if people take more than is recommended.

SHORT ANSWERS

Q9 Fordyces granules
Ans.

Refer to August 2005 Q11 solution.

Q10 Polycythemia rubra vera
Ans.

It is a chronic disease with an insidious onset characterized by an absolute increase in the number of red blood cells and in the total blood volume. This abnormality is of unknown origin but occasionally family history is positive.

Clinical Features

More common in males than females and in middle ages.

Headache or dizziness, weakness and lassitude, tinnitus, visual disturbances, mental confusion, slurring of speech and inability to concentrate.

Skin is flushed or diffusely reddened as a result of capillary engorgement, most obvious on head, neck and extremities

Splenomegaly is a constant feature and is often painful. Other gastric complaints such as gas pains, belching and peptic ulcers and bleeding from varices may occur.

Oral manifestations–deep purplish red mucosa, the gingiva and tongue being more severely affected. There is cyanosis due to high levels of reduced hemoglobin. Submucosal petechiae are also common.

Laboratory Findings

RBC count is elevated and may exceed 10,000,000 cells per cubic millimeter. Hemoglobin content is increased by 20 gm/dl color index is 1.0. Specific gravity and viscosity of the blood are increased. Leukocytosis is usual. There is hyperplasia of bone marrow. Bleeding and clotting time are normal.

Treatment

No specific treatment. The patient may be periodically bled or substances may be administered either to destroy blood (phenyl hydrazine) or to interfere with its formation.

Q11 Fibromatosis gingivae

Ans.

Fibromatosis gingivae is a diffuse fibrous overgrowth of gingival tissues. The condition is transmitted through a dominant autosomal gene. Many cases are sporadic without familial background.

Clinical Features

This condition manifested as a dense ,diffuse, smooth or nodular overgrowth of gingival tissues of one or both arch usually appearing about the time of eruption of permanent incisors. The tissue is usually not inflamed it is normal or even pale color. It is firm and dense that it may prevent the normal eruption of teeth. It is not painful and shows no tendency for hemorrhage.

The epithelium may be somewhat thickened with clongated rete pegs.The bulk of the tissue is composed of dense fibrous connective tissues. The bundle of collagen fibers are coarse and slow few interspersed fibroblast or blood vessels.

When tooth eruption is impeded, surgical removal of the excessive tissue and exposure of the teeth are indicated.

Q12 Adenomatoid odontogenic tumor

Ans.

Tumor is characterized by the formation of duct like structure by epithelial component of the lesion.

It is also categorized as a hamartomatous malformation or as an odontogenic cyst.

Clinical Features

The site of occurrence is greater in the maxilla (65%) than in the mandible (35%). The vast majority of the lesion measured between 1.5 and 3.0 cm, although large lesions exceeds 7.0 cm.

The large proportion of the tumor produced an obvious clinical swelling. There have been extaosseous occurrences.

Roentgenographic Feature

The dental roentgenogram reveals a destructive lesion of the jaw which may or may not be well circumscribed. The lesions are almost invariably unilocular radiolucencies but may contain faint to dense radiopaque foci.

Histological Features

The tumor is made up of epithelial cells, usually with only scanty storma of connective tissue.These epithelial cells, often polyhedral or even spindle shaped vary in their pattern from nests swords or cords to cells of a definite columnar or cuboidal variety arranged in duet like or adenomatoid fashion.

Q13 Replenisher

Ans.

Replenisher is a concentrated developing solution designed to maintain the active strength of developer through periodic addition to maintain original volume.

In the normal course of film processing, phenidone and hydroquinone are consumed, and bromide ions and other byproducts are released into solution. Developer also becomes inactivated by exposure to oxygen. These actions produce a "seasoned" solution, and the film speed and contrast stabilize. The developing solution of both manual and automatic developers should be replenished with fresh solution every morning to prolong the life of seasoned developer.

The recommended amount to be added daily is 8 ounces of fresh developer(replenisher) per gallon of developing solution. Some of the used solution may need to be removed to make the room for the replenisher.

Q14 Ectodermal dysplasia
Ans.

Ectodermal dysplasia is not a single disorder, but a group of syndromes all deriving from abnormalities of the ectodermal structures. Ectodermal dysplasias are described as "heritable conditions in which there are abnormalities of two or more ectodermal-structures such as the hair, teeth, nails, sweat glands, cranial-facial structure, digits and other parts of the body."

Presentation (Fig. 19.1)

- *Hair:* Individuals affected by an ED syndrome frequently have abnormalities of the hair follicles. Scalp and body hair may be thin, sparse, and very light in color
- *Nails:* Fingernails and toenails may be thick, abnormally shaped, discolored, ridged, slow-growing, or brittle. The cuticles may be prone to infections.
- *Skin:* The skin may be lightly pigmented. Skin sustaining injury may grow back permanently hypo-pigmented. In some cases, red or brown pigmentation may be present. Skin can be prone to rashes or infections and can be thick over the palms and soles. Care must be taken to prevent cracking, bleeding, and infection.
- *Other features:* People with ED often have certain cranial-facial features which can be distinctive, frontal bossing is common, longer or more pronounced chins are frequent, broader noses are also very commonSweat glands:Individuals affected by certain ED syndromes cannot perspire. Their sweat glands may function abnormally or may not have developed at all. Without normal sweat production, the body cannot regulate temperature properly. Therefore, overheating is a common problem, especially during hot weather. Access to cool environments is important.
- *Teeth:* In the development of tooth buds frequently result in congenitally absent teeth or in the growth of teeth that are peg-shaped or pointed. The enamel may also be defective.

Cosmetic dental treatment is almost always necessary and children may need dentures as early as two years of age. Multiple denture replacements are often needed as the child grows, and dental implants may be an option in adolescence. In other cases, teeth can be crowned. Orthodontic treatment also may be necessary. Because dental treatment is complex, a multi-disciplinary approach is best.

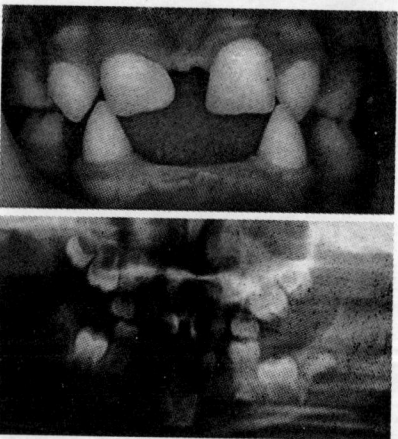

Fig. 19.1: Dental abnormalities in a 5-year-old girl who suffered from various symptoms of autosomal dominant hypohidrotic ectodermal dysplasia (HED) a) Intraoral view. Note that the upper incisors have been restored with composite material to disguise their original conical shape. b) Orthopantomogram showing absence of ten primary and eleven permanent teeth in the jaws of the same individual.

Q15 Psoriatic arthritis

Ans. Psoriatic arthritis is a type of inflammatory arthritis occur in people with chronic skin condition psoriasis. Psoriatic arthritis is said to be a seronegative spondyloarthropathy and therefore occurs more commonly in patients with tissue type HLA-B27.

Causes

The exact causes are not yet known, but several genetic associations have been identified.

Presentation

- As well as causing joint inflammation, psoriatic arthritis can cause tendinitis and a sausage-like swelling of the digits known as dactylitis.
- Radiology will give the appearance of "fluffy, new" bone.
- More than 80% of patients with psoriatic arthritis will have psoriatic nail lesions characterised by pitting of the nails, or more extremely, loss of the nail itself (onycholysis).
- Psoriatic arthritis can develop at any age, however on average it tends to appear about 10 years after the first signs of psoriasis.

Types of psoriatic arthritis:
- Symmetric
- Asymmetric
- Arthritis mutilans
- Spondylitis
- Distal interphalangeal predominant.

Treatment

- Treatment of psoriatic arthritis is similar to that of rheumatoid arthritis.The underlying process in psoriatic arthritis is inflammation, therefore treatments are directed at reducing and controlling inflammation. NSAIDs such as diclofenac and naproxen are usually the first line medication.
- Other treatment options for this disease include joint injections with corticosteroids - this is only practical if a few joints are affected.
- Second line treatments with immuno-suppressants

- A new class of therapeutics developed using recombinant DNA technology called tumor necrosis factor-alpha inhibitors.

Q16 Discoid lumpus erythematosus
Ans.

Discoid lupus erythematosus (DLE) is a chronic skin condition of sores with inflammation and scarring favoring the face, ears, and scalp and at times on other body areas. These lesions develop as a red, inflamed patch with a scaling and crusty appearance. The center areas may appear lighter in color with a rim darker than the normal skin.

Types

- *Localized:* It typically presents with skin lesions localized above the neck, with favored sites being the scalp, bridge of nose, cheeks, lower lip, and ears.
- Generalized discoid lupus erythematosus It involves the thorax and upper extremities in addition to the head and neck.
- Childhood discoid lupus erythematosus. It lacks a female predominance, has a low frequency of photosensitivity, and a higher progression to systemic lupus erythematosus.

Q17 Uremic Stomatitis
Ans.
Defination

Oral manifestation of uremia, consisting of varying degrees of erythema, exudation, ulceration, pseudomembrane formation, foul breath, and burning sensations.

Etiology

Its unknown but suggested that it may be due to raised level of ammonia compound. Ammonia is formed through the action of the bacterial ureases modifying salivary urea, which can be elevated in affected patients to 300 mg/ml. It may be due to hemorrhagic diathesis.

Clinical Features

Patients may have dysgeusia, i.e. altered perception to sweet and sour taste. Uremic stomatitis is characterized by the presence of painful plaques and crusts that are usually distributed on the buccal mucosa, dorsal or ventral surface of the tongue, gingiva, lips, and floor of the mouth.

Differential Diagnosis

Oral lichen planus and chronic hyperplastic candidiasis.

Treatment

Treatment consists of improvement of urea blood concentration and the underlying renal failure, supported by increased oral hygiene with antiseptic mouthwashes and anti-microbial/antifungal agents if nece-ssary.

Renal failure treatment and the oral mucosal lesions will resolve by hydrogen peroxide therapy.

Q18 Drug-induced gingival hyperplasia
Ans.

Refer to March 2003 Q17.

QUESTION PAPER
Long Essays

1. Describe Radiation protection measures
2. Classify candidiasis. Write in detail about the etiology, clinical features and management of oral thrush.

Short Essays

3. Albright's syndrome
4. Clark's rule
5. Drug-induced gingival hyperplasia
6. Dental considerations of pregnancy
7. Composition and action of developing and fixing solutions
8. Fibrous dysplasia
9. Electromagnetic spectrum
10. Renal rickets
11. Discoid lupus erythematosus
12. Hamartoma

Short Answers

13. Giant cells
14. Cotton wool appearance
15. Von Recklinghausen's disease
16. Tyre Track Appearance
17. Discolouration of teeth
18. Glossodynia
19. Oral manifestations of acquired immunodeficiency syndome
20. Indications of bite-wing radiographs
21. Agranulocytosis
22. Oral manifestations of syphilis

SOLUTIONS

LONG ESSAYS

Q1 Describe Radiation protection measures

Ans.

Refer to Q2 of September 2004.

Q2 Classify candidiasis. Write in detail about the etiology, clinical features and management of oral thrush.

Ans.

Refer to Q1 of September 2000, Q3 of September 2002.

SHORT ESSAYS

Q3 Albright's syndrome

Ans.

Refer to Q9 of September 2004.

Q4 Clark's rule

Ans.

Refer to Q8 of September 2003.

Q5 Drug-induced gingival hyperplasia

Ans.

Gingival overgrowth, also known as gingival hyperplasia secondary to drugs reported in epileptic children who were receiving therapy with phenytoin (Dilantin) for the treatment of seizures. Cyclosporine, a potent immuno-suppressant widely used since the early 1980s in organ transplant recipients and for psoriasis, and numerous calcium channel blocker agents, including nifedipine and amlodipine, have also been associated with gingival overgrowth. Nifedipine appears to have an additive effect when used together with cyclosporine in transplant recipients with hypertension. In addition, phenobarbital-induced gingival overgrowth has been reported but is rare and needs further evaluation.

Because not all patients on phenytoin, cyclosporine, and/or calcium antagonists develop gingival overgrowth, identifying patients at risk is important in order to take all the necessary measures to minimize the onset and severity of this condition.

Causes

Potential risk factors for drug-induced gingival overgrowth include the following:

- Poor oral hygiene
- Periodontal disease
- Periodontal pocket depth
- Gingival inflammation
- Degree of dental plaque
- Duration and dose of cyclosporine

Other intrinsic risk factors include the susceptibility of some subpopulations of fibroblasts and keratinocytes

Clinical Features

- The onset of drug-induced gingival overgrowth in susceptible individuals is insidious. Gingival overgrowth is asymptomatic, except in the presence of poor oral hygiene and dental plaque because patients may develop bleeding with tender and swollen gums. Patients with mal-positioned teeth, periodontal disease, and poor oral hygiene are at risk of developing gingival overgrowth. Severity varies depending on the oral health prior to the beginning of therapy; however, not all patients with poor oral hygiene develop drug-induced gingival overgrowth.
- Phenytoin-induced gingival overgrowth
- This is more likely to occur in patients with gingivitis and dental plaque.
- Increased dental plaque has been suggested to induce local inflammation and to serve as a reservoir for phenytoin.

- Cyclosporine-induced gingival overgrowth
- In susceptible patients (ie, presence of dental plaque, swollen gums, high dose of cyclosporine), gingival overgrowth may develop by the third month of therapy.
- Patients with poor oral hygiene and displaced teeth tend to develop bleeding gums upon probing.
- Aggressive plaque control and routine oral hygiene help in maintaining gums but may not prevent the onset of gingival overgrowth in susceptible individuals.
- Cyclosporine-induced gingival overgrowth is reversible once therapy is discontinued or when the dose is reduced.
- Cyclosporine and nifedipine-induced gingival overgrowth: Nifedipine potentiates the adverse effect (i.e. gingival overgrowth) of cyclosporine.
- Calcium antagonist–induced gingival overgrowth
- Oral hygiene plays a decisive role in the development of gingival enlargement.
- Substantial evidence in the dental literature indicates that gingival enlargement can be controlled successfully, even under the continuous administration of calcium antagonists, by meticulous professional and individual oral hygiene.

Physical

- Gingival enlargement occurs primarily on the labial gingival mucosa and in between the teeth (interdental papillae area).
- Gingival overgrowth is more pronounced on the labial aspect of the maxillary gingiva and in the interdental papillae.

Treatment

Medical Care

For dental care, refer patients to a general dentist and/or oral medicine specialist for evaluation.

Surgical Care

Gingivectomy with carbon dioxide or YAG laser is recommended for patients who have moderate-to-severe gingival enlargement that does not resolve when the dose is reduced, proper oral hygiene is maintained, or after a short course of antibiotics. In the majority of patients for whom drug discontinuation or substitution is not possible and for whom prophylactic measures have failed, surgical excision of gingival tissue remains the only treatment option.

Antibiotics

Azithromycin (Zithromax)

Used to treat mild-to-moderate oral microbial infections. Clinical studies comparing oral hygiene programs vs azithromycin indicate that azithromycin plus oral hygiene significantly reduces cyclosporine-induced gingival hyperplasia, while oral hygiene alone reduces oral symptoms but does not affect cyclosporine- induced gingival hyperplasia.

Mouthwash Antiseptics

Chlorhexidine Gluconate (Peridex)

Effective, safe, and reliable mouthwash antiseptic. Polybiguanide with bactericidal activity; usually is supplied as a gluconate salt. At physiologic pH, the salt dissociates to a cation that binds to bacterial cell walls.

Lysozyme, lactoferrin, glucose oxidase, lactoperoxidase (Biotene). Alcohol-free mouthwash antiseptic.

Q6 Dental considerations of pregnancy
Ans.

- Maternal concerns
- Fetal concerns
- Radiography
- Medication
- Summary

Maternal Concerns

Anatomic Change

- Uterus weight from 70 gm–1 kg
- Uterus volume from 10 ml–5000 ml
- Supine hypotensive syndrome
- Acute hypotensive episode
- Third trimeter 10–15%
- Compression of inferior vena cava and aorta
- Decrease venous return to heart
- Decrease uteroplacental perfusion and fetal distress
- Left lateral decubitus position
- Elevation the right hip 10–12 cm
- Sit up position
- Physiology changes
- Cardiovascular system
- Respiratory system
- Gastrointestinal system
- Renal system
- Hematological system

Psychological Changes

- Hypersensitivity regarding her size and appearance
- Fear of pain, disability, death and for baby
- Fear of dental procedures
- Sedation empathy and reassurance
- Minimize disturbance interruption and noises and to adjust room temperature and to minimize possible irritability

Fetal Concerns

- Avoidance of fetal hypoxia
- Avoidance of premature abortion
- Avoidance of teratogens

Radiography (Fig. 20.1)

- An adverse fetal effects is unlikely to result from exposure to less than 5 rads with lead apron in place over the female gonad. Dose from a single periapical radiograph is about 0.1 mrad.

- Make only the film absolutely essential for diagnosing the conditions
- Use lead-shielding
- Use long cone
- Use proper collimation and shielding
- Limited to affected tooth
- Extra care should be used while taking essential films to eliminate the need for repeated exposure

Medication

Local anesthesia: Local anesthesia are not teratogenic, and may administered to pregnancy patient is usual clinical doses. Large dose of prilocaine are known to cause methemoglobinemia which could cause maternal and fetal hypoxia

Local Vasoconstriction

- Delay uptake from the site of injection, Increase the effectiveness and duration,
- There is no specific contraindication to these vasoconstrictors in a pregnant patient although it is prudent to use minimal effective dose.

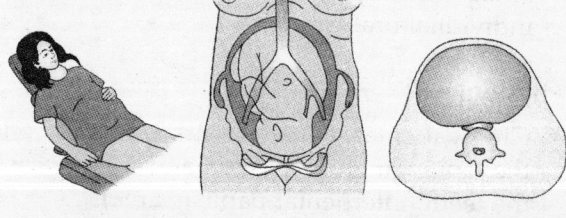

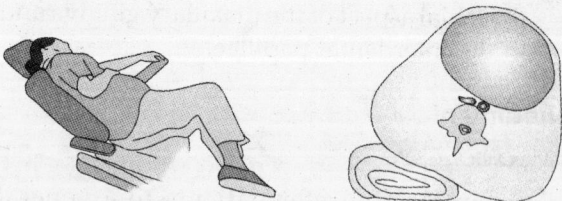

Fig. 20.1: Procedure in making radiographs for pregnancy patients

- Convulsion in a sensitized mother could also exert a teratogenic effect second to hypoxia
- The need for careful Hx taking and for aspiration and slow injected technique is obvious.
- Antibiotics penicillin is safe in all trimesters. aminoglycoside, chloramphenicol, tetracycline are contraindicated.
- Analgesics acetaminophen is safe aspirin, NSAIDs anti-inflammatory drugs are contraindicated.

Corticosteroids Contraindicated

Sedatives

The most care and consideration should be given to use of nonpharmalogical technique such as good patient management verbal sedation.

Obstetrical Emergences in Dental Office

- Syncope
- All trimester
- Hypotensive, dehydration, anemia, hypoglycemia and neurogenic disorder
- Not revived with ammonia
- Oxygen, vital sign, drinking fluid.
- Cardiac dysrhythmia
- Morning sickness
- Enhanced gag reflex and decreased gastric emptying time
- Aspiration of vomiting matter
- Oropharygeal suction
- Recumbent position
- Chest compression

Seizure

- *Bleeding and cramping:* Precedes miscarriage
- *Active bleeding or painful contraction:* On left site and oxygen, transfer
- Minor contraction not painful :on left site not an emergency

- If question arise regarding a particular patient status, consult the obstetrician before beginning treatment.

Summary

- Supine hypotensive syndrome
- Radiography minimal
- Medication penicillin, ACT
- Emergency A, B, C
- History taking, medical consultation, transfer.

Q7 Composition and action of developing and fixing solutions
Ans.
Refer to Q6.2 of September 1998.

Q8 Fibrous Dysplasia
Ans.
It is a benign bone tumor in which the normal osseous structures are replaced by fibrous tissues. Refer Q3 of this paper for additional details.

For radiographic features refer to Q11 of September 2003

Q9 Electromagnetic Spectrum
Ans.
The electromagnetic spectrum is the range of all possible frequencies of electromagnetic radiation. The "electromagnetic spectrum" of an object is the characteristic distribution of electromagnetic radiation emitted or absorbed by that particular object. Electromagnetic radiation interacts with matter in different ways in different parts of the spectrum. The types of interaction can be so different that it seems to be justified to refer to different types of radiation. At the same time, there is a continuum containing all these "different kinds" of electromagnetic radiation. Thus we refer to a spectrum, but divide it up based on the different interactions with matter.

Region of the spectrum	Main interactions with matter
Radio	Collective oscillation of charge carriers in bulk material (plasma oscillation). An example would be the oscillation of the electrons in an antenna.
Microwave through far infrared	Plasma oscillation, molecular rotation
Near infrared	Molecular vibration, plasma oscillation (in metals only)
Visible	Molecular electron excitation (including pigment molecules found in the human retina), plasma oscillations (in metals only)
Ultraviolet	Excitation of molecular and atomic valence electrons, including ejection of the electrons (photoelectric effect)
X-rays	Excitation and ejection of core atomic electrons, Compton scattering (for low atomic numbers)
Gamma rays	Energetic ejection of core electrons in heavy elements, Compton scattering (for all atomic numbers), excitation of atomic nuclei, including dissociation of nuclei
High energy gamma rays	Creation of particle-antiparticle pairs. At very high energies a single photon can create a shower of high energy particles and antiparticles upon interaction with matter.

Q10 Renal Rickets
Ans.

Renal Rickets

A bone disease where kidney dysfunction causes bone resorption and results in weak, soft bones. A disturbance marked by excessive excretion of phosphorus and calcium resulting from a lowered renal threshold of excretion of these mineral elements.

Symptoms of Renal Rickets

The list of signs and symptoms mentioned in various sources for renal rickets includes the 20 symptoms listed below:
- Weak bones
- Soft bones
- Fractures
- Kidney dysfunction
- Acidosis
- Bone resorption
- Hyperparathyroidism
- Skeletal deformity
- Bone pain
- Bowed legs
- Pigeon chest
- Bumps on rib cage
- Scoliosis
- Kyphosis
- Delayed tooth eruption
- Dental caries
- Weak teeth
- Short stature
- Impaired growth
- Muscle cramps

Causes:
- Kidney conditions
- Urinary system conditions
- Metabolic conditions
- Bone or skeletal conditions
- Musculoskeletal conditions

Q11 Discoid lupus erythematosus
Ans.
Refer Feb 2007 Q16

Q12 Hamartoma
Ans.
A hamartoma is a benign, focal malforma-tion that resembles a neoplasm in the tissue of its

origin. This is not a malignant tumor, and it grows at the same rate as the surrounding tissues. It is composed of tissue elements normally found at that site, but which are growing in a disorganized mass. They occur in many different parts of the body and are most often asymptomatic and undetected unless seen on an image taken for another reason.

Causes

Hamartomas result from an abnormal formation of normal tissue, although the underlying reasons for the abnormality are not fully understood. They grow along with, and at the same rate as, the organ from whose tissue they are made, and, unlike cancerous tumors, only rarely invade or compress surrounding structures significantly.

Types

Lung The most common hamartomas occur in the lungs.

Heart Cardiac rhabdomyomas are hamartomas composed of altered cardiac myocytes that contain large vacuoles and glycogen.

Hypothalamus One of the most troublesome hamartomas occurs on the hypothalamus. Unlike most such growths, a hypothalamic hamartoma is symptomatic; it most often causes gelastic seizures, and can cause visual problems, other seizures, rage disorders associated with hypothalamic diseases, and early onset of puberty.

Cowden syndrome is a serious genetic disorder characterized by multiple hamartomas. Usually skin hamartomas exist, and commonly (about 66% of cases) hamartoma of the thyroid gland exists. Additional growths can form in many parts of the body, especially in mucosa, the GI tract, bones, CNS, the eyes, and the genitourinary tract. The hamartomas themselves may cause symptoms or even death, but morbidity is more often associated with increased occurrence of malignancies, usually in the breast or thyroid.

Prognosis

Hamartomas, while generally benign, can cause problems due to their location. When located on the skin, especially the face or neck, they can be extremely disfiguring, as in the case of a man with a hamartoma the size of a small orange on his eyelid. They may obstruct practically any organ in the body, such as the eye, the colon, etc. They are particularly likely to cause major health issues when located in the hypothalamus, spleen or kidneys or lips.

SHORT ANSWERS

Q13 Giant Cells
Ans.

A giant cell is a mass formed by the union of several distinct cells (usually macrophages). It can arise in response to an infection or foreign body. Giant cells are transformed macrophages

Types

- Foreign-body giant cell
- Langhans giant cell
- Langhans giant cells are large cells found in granulomatous conditions.
- They are formed by the fusion of epithelioid cells (macrophages), and contain nuclei arranged in a horseshoe-shaped pattern in the cell periphery.
- Touton giant cells

Q14 Cotton wool appearance
Ans.

In the skull, the lytic phase (osteoporosis circumscripta) typically involves the frontal or occipital bones and progresses to a mixed pattern with multifocal sclerotic patches in the intermediate stage of the disease, referred to as a cotton wool appearance (Fig. 20.2).

Plain film of the skull reveals a large mottled area of radiolucency with small areas of increased density within it In the cranium, bone sclerosis may produce circular radiodense lesions in one area, whereas osteoporosis circumscripta is noted elsewhere. In the skull, the common region of involvement is the cranial vault. The osteolytic phase is called osteoporosis circumscripta and appears as multiple geographic, well-demarcated regions of bone resorption that may be mistaken for metastases. Focal radiodensities occur as pagetoid bone is formed. In the quiescent phase, there is a radiodense cotton-wool appearance with a thickened vault. Three phases of pagets disease:

- Active or osteolytic phase
- Aggressive bone resorption with lytic lesions
- Replacement of hematopoietic bone marrow by fibrous connective tissue with numerous large vascular channels
- Inactive or quiescent phase
- Decreased bone turnover with skeletal sclerosis and thickening of the cortex
- Mixed pattern
- Lytic and sclerotic phases frequently coexist

Q15 Von Recklinghausen' s disease
Ans.

Neurofibromatosis type I (NF-1), formerly known as von Recklinghausen diseaseafter the researcher who first documented the disorder, is a human genetic disorder. It is possibly the most common inherited disorder caused by a single gene. NF-1 is not to be confused with proteus syndrome (the syndrome which may have affectedThe Elephant Man), but

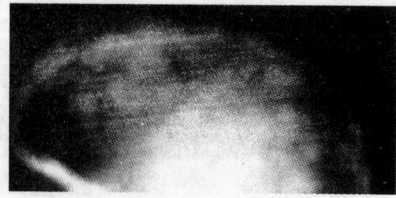

Fig. 20.2: Cotton wool appearance

rather is a separate disorder.

Clinical Findings

Peripheral Nervous System Lesions

A neurofibroma is a mass lesion of the peripheral nervous system. Its cellular lineage is uncertain, and may derive from Schwann cells, other perineural cell lines, or fibroblasts. Neurofibromas may arise sporadically, or in association with NF-1. A neurofibroma may arise at any point along a peripheral nerve. A cutaneous neurofibroma manifests as single or multiple firm, rubbery bumps of varying sizes on a person's skin. A solitary neurofibroma may also occur in a deeper nerve trunk, and only be seen on cross-sectional imaging (e.g. computed tomography or magnetic resonance) as a fusiform enlargement of a nerve.

Dermatologic manifestations flat pigmented lesions of the skin called café au lait spots.

Skeletal Lesions

Bones, especially the ribs, can develop chronic erosions (pits) from the constant pressure of adjacent neurofibromas and schwannomas. Similarly, the neural foramen of the spine can be widened due to the presence of a nerve root neurofibroma or schwannoma.

Treatment

There is no cure for the disorder itself. Instead, people with neurofibromatosis are followed by a team of specialists to manage symptoms or complications. Surgery may be needed when the tumors compress organs or other structures. Less than 8–12% people with neurofibromatosis develop cancerous growths; in these cases, chemotherapy can be tried.

Q16 Tyre Track Appearance
Ans.

In radiology tyre track appearance occurs due to reverse film position. If a film is placed in oral cavity in reverse way, i.e. non exposure side which contains lead foil, gets exposed resulting in lighter film because few X-ray photons get absorbed by the lead foil. The image of embossed pattern present on lead foil may be observed over the film, commonly called as Tyre track appearance.

Preventive Measures

Ensure convexity of embossed dot should face the X-ray tube.

Q17 Discolouration of Teeth
Ans.

Tooth discolouration is when the enamel (the hard, outer surface of the tooth) or the dentine (the layer below the enamel) become discoloured. Something as simple as food and drink may cause stains to appear on the teeth. Sometimes however, discolouration can indicate something more serious, such as exposure to substances that have harmed the teeth.

- *Foods/drinks:* Coffee, tea, colas, wines, and certain fruits and vegetables (for example, apples and potatoes) can stain your teeth.
- *Tobacco use:* Smoking or chewing tobacco can stain teeth.
- *Poor dental hygiene:* Inadequate brushing and flossing to remove plaque and stain-producing substances like coffee and tobacco can cause tooth discolouration.
- *Disease:* Several diseases that affect enamel (the hard surface of the teeth) and dentin (the underlying material under enamel) can lead to tooth discoloration. Treatments for certain conditions can also affect tooth color. For example, head and neck radiation and chemotherapy can cause teeth discoloration. In addition, certain infections in pregnant mothers can cause tooth discoloration in the infant by affecting enamel development.
- *Medications:* The antibiotics tetracycline and doxycycline are known to discolor teeth when given to children whose teeth are still developing (before the age of 8). Mouth rinses and washes containing chlorhexidine and cetylpyridinium chloride can also stain teeth. Antihistamines (like Benadryl), antipsychotic drugs, and drugs for high blood pressure also cause teeth discoloration.
- *Dental materials:* Some of the materials used in dentistry, such as amalgamrestorations, especially silver sulfide-containing materials, can cast a gray-black color to teeth.
- *Advancing age:* As you age, the outer layer of enamel on your teeth gets worn away revealing the natural yellow color of dentin.
- *Genetics:* Some people have naturally brighter or thicker enamel than others.
- *Environment:* Excessive fluoride either from environmental sources (naturally high fluoride levels in water) or from excessive use (fluoride applications, rinses,toothpaste, and fluoride supplements taken by mouth) can cause teeth discoloration.
- *Trauma:* For example, damage from a fall can disturb enamel formation in young children whose teeth are still developing. Trauma can also cause discoloration to adult teeth.

Treatment

The three most common remedies for tooth discoloration are:
- Whitening
- Veneers
- Caps (Crowns)

Q18 Glossodynia
Ans.

Glossodynia or burning mouth syndrome (BMS) (also known as "Burning tongue"and "Orodynia" is a condition characterized by a burning or tingling sensation on the lips, tongue, or entire mouth.

Causes

Possible causes include nutritional deficiencies, chronic anxiety or depression, type 2 diabetes, menopause, oral disorders such as thrush or dry mouth, or damaged nerves (specifically, cranial nerves associated with taste).

One cause of burning mouth pain, which may be often misdiagnosed as burning mouth syndrome, is a contact sensitivity Type IV hypersensitivity in the oral tissues to common substances such as sodium lauryl sulfate, a surfactant commonly used in household products, cinnamon aldehyde or dental materials. There are now several toothpastes on the market specifically withoutsodium lauryl sulfate or other preservatives which have been found to be associated with sensitivities.

Presentation

This condition appears more often in women, specifically women after menopause, than men. Pain typically is low or nonexistent in the morning and builds up over the course of the day.

Treatment

Low dosages of benzodiazepines, tricyclic antidepressants or anticonvulsants may prove to be an effective treatment.

Q19 Oral manifestations of acquired immunodeficiency syndrome
Ans.
Refer to Q1 of September 2000.

Q20 Indications of bite-wing radiographs
Ans.
Refer to Q11 of March 2000.

Q21 Agranulocytosis
Ans.
Refer to Q5 of March 2002.

Q22 Oral manifestations of syphilis
Ans.
Primary Syphilis

The mouth, perhaps surprisingly, is rarely the site of primary syphilis, and because of its transient nature, the oral ulceration of primary syphilis often goes unnoticed by the patient or by any unsuspicious clinician. Primary syphilis of the mouth manifests as a solitary ulcer usually of the lip or, more rarely, the tongue.

Ulceronodular Disease (Lues Maligna)

Ulceronodular disease is an explosive generalized form of secondary syphilis characterized by fever, headache, and myalgia, followed by a papulopustular eruption that rapidly transforms into necrotic, sharply demarcated ulcers with hemorrhagic brown crusts, organized in rupioid layers commonly on the face and scalp. The mucosa is involved in about one third of affected patients. Lues maligna gives rise to crateriform or shallow ulcers on the gingivae, palate or buccal mucosa, with multiple erosions on the hard and soft palates, tongue and lower lip.

Nodular Disease

Rarely, secondary syphilis can manifest as nodules alone. This nodular eruption of syphilis has a predilection for the face, mucous membranes, palms of the hands and soles of the feet. Lesions may occur on the vermillion, mimicking squamous cell carcinoma or keratoacanthoma.

Gumma Formation

Gummas tend to arise on the hard palate and tongue, although very rarely they may occur on the soft palate, lower alveolus, and parotid gland. A gumma manifests initially as 1 or more painless swelling. When multiple, they tend to coalesce, giving rise to serpiginous lesions. The swellings eventually develop into areas of ulceration, with areas of breakdown and healing. There may be eventual bone destruction, palatal perforation, and oro-nasal fistula formation. Rarely, a gumma may erode into blood vessels—e.g. the inferior alveolar artery. Gumma manifests radiologically as ill-defined radiolucencies that may resemble malignancy. The areas of ulceration eventually heal, although the resultant scarring can, at least on the tongue, cause fissuring.

Syphilitic Leukoplakia and Risk of Squamous Cell Carcinoma

Syphilitic leukoplakia would appear to be a homogenous white patch affecting large areas of the dorsum of the tongue. There are few good descriptions of syphilitic leukoplakia, and it is unclear whether this lesion truly reflects syphilis, or more likely a tobacco smoking habit—indeed this was observed by Hutchinson in the 19th century.

Neurosyphilis

Aside from the well-recognized Argyll Robertson pupil, tertiary syphilis can give rise to both unilateral and bilateral trigeminal neuropathy and facial nerve palsy.

21

RGUHS August 2007 (RS)

QUESTION PAPER
Long Essays

1. Discuss the conditions which cause pigmentations of the oral mucosa
2. Radiographic features of fibrosseous Lesions of the jaws

Short Essays

3. Juvenile periodontitis
4. Multilocular radiolucencies
5. Depapillation of tongue
6. Localization technique
7. Causes of bleeding in the oral cavity
8. Cherubism
9. Pemphigus vulgaris
10. Light radiograph
11. Hyperparathyroidism
12. Alkaline phosphatase

Short Answers

13. Nikolsky's sign
14. Paul-Bunnel test
15. Radiation caries
16. Lipoma
17. Draw a neat labeled diagram of an X-ray tube
18. Hereditary opalescent dentin
19. Koplik's spots
20. Cone-cut
21. Herpangina
22. Garre's osteomyelitis

SOLUTIONS

Long Essays

Q1 Discuss the conditions which cause pigmentations of the oral mucosa.

Ans.

Refer to Q1 of March 1999.

Q2 Radiographic features of fibro-osseous Lesions of the jaws.

Ans.

Fibro osseous Lesions of the jaws are benign bone tumor in which the normal osseous structures are replaced by fibrous tissues. It is commonly used term that includes the following bone dysplasias,as well as neoplasms and other lesions of the bone.

For radiographic features Refer to Q11 of September 2003.

Fibrous dysplasia

Refer Q11 Sept 2003 and Q9 sept 2004

Cemento Osseous Dysplasia

*   Periapical cemental dysplasia
    Refer Q4 March 2000
*   Florid osseous dysplasia

Location: Bilateral present in both the jaws, Mandible is more common, epicenter apical to teeth with in alveolar process and posterior to cuspid

Periphery: Well defined and has sclerotic border

Internal structure: Equal mixture of radiolucent and radiopaque regionsto almost complete radiopacity. Cysts may enlarge with time even beyond the boundary of the lesion into surrounding normal bone or may fill in with abnormal dysplastic cemento osseous tissue.

Radiopaque regions can vary from small oval to circular regions (cotton wool appearance)to large, irregular, amorphous areas of calcification.

Effects on the surrounding structure: Large FOD can displace the inferior alveolar nerve canal an an inferior direction.

Other Lesions of Bone

Cemento Ossifying Fibroma (ossifying fibroma)

Location: COF appears almost exclusively in the facial bones and most commonly in the mandible,typically inferior to the premolars and molars and superior to the inferior alveolar canal.In maxilla it occurs in the canine fossa and zygomatic arch area.

Periphery: Borders are well defined.A thin radiolucent line,representing a fibrous capsule ,may separate it from surrounding bone.

Internal structure: Mixed radiolucent-radiopaque density with apattern that depends on the amountand form of manufactured calcified material.

Effects on the surrounding structure: COF has tumour like behaviour which tends to be concentric within the medullary part of the bone with outward expansion approx equal in all directions. This results in displacement of teeth or of the inferior alveolar canal and expansion of the outer cortical plates of bone which is thinned but remains intact resorption of teeth may occur.

Central Giant Cell Granuloma

It is a reactive lesion to an as- yet-unknown stimulus and not a neoplastic lesion.

Location: Mandible twice as that of maxilla-epicenter is anterior to first molar. Large lesions can extend posterior to first molar.

Periphery: Produces well defined radiographic margin in the mabndible and ill defined in maxilla.

Internal structure: Subtle granular pattern of calcification that may require a bright light source behind the film for visualization. It is occasionally organized into ill-defined, wispy septa. In some instances the septa are better defined and divide the internal aspect into compartments, creating a multilocular appearance.

Effects on surrounding structure: It displace and resorb teeth. lamina dura of teeth within the lesion is missing.inferior alveolar canal may be displaced in inferior direction.

Aneurysmal Bone Cyst

Location: Mandible is involvedmore often than the maxilla (ratio 3:2), molar ramus region is involved

Periphery and shape: Well defined and shape is circular or "hydraulic."

Internal structure: Multilocular appearancesepta positioned at right angle to outer expanded border.

Effects on surrounding structures: Strong propensity for extreme expansion of the outer cortical plates

Cherubism

Refer to Q8

Paget's Disease (osteitis deformans)

Definition

Pagets disease/osteitis deformans; a generalized skeletal disease, frequently familial, of older persons in which bone resorption and formation are both increased, leading to thickening and softening of bones (e.g. the skull), and bending of weight-bearing bones.

It is a condition of abnormal resorption and apposition of osseous tissue in one or more bones.

Symptoms

Paget's disease can cause bone pain, deformity, fracture, and arthritis. The bone pain of Paget's disease is located in the affected bone. The most common bones affected by Paget's disease include the spine, the thigh bone (femur), the pelvis, the skull, the collar bone (clavicle), and the upper arm bone (humerus).

Radiographic Appearance

The disease is characterized by multiple stages. In the skull, the initial osteolytic phase of pagets is called "osteoporosis circumscripta" due to the presence of geographic lucent regions primarily within the frontal bone. This is followed by excessive new bone formation leading to cortical thickening and osteosclerotic changes in the inner table, diploe, and subsequently the inner surface of the outer table. In this phase, plain radiographs manifest a characteristic "cotton wool" appearance of sclerotic lesions surrounded by areas of demineralization. Ultimately, the disease results in diffuse sclerosis and enters an inactive stage.

General

- Early osteoporosis circumscripta
- Disease involvement usually seen at one end of the bone (generally proximal)
- The bone as a whole is thick and bent
- Density in the vascular stage is decreased and it is increased in the sclerotic stage
- Trabeculae are coarse and widely separated
- In vascular stage areas of porosis shaped like a candle flame are seen in the cortex (arrow or flame sign)
- Fine cracks may appear (stress fractures) which resemble Looser zones may be evident, but they occur on the convex surface
- Acetabular involvement may be protrusion
- Cortical thickening pelvic brim signs or framed picture appearance of vertebrae

- Remodelling of the skull base may result in its invagination by the cervical vertebrae platybasia
- Only 65% of the lesions seen on bone scan will be seen on X-rays
- *Bone scans:* Useful in determining the extent and activity of the condition.

Langerhan's cell histiocytosis

Location: Alveolar type of LCH lesions are multiple, whereas the intraosseous type usually is solitary Mandible ramus is more common site.

Periphery and shape:moderately to well defined but without cortication, periphery appears punched out bone destruction progress in a circular shape, and after it includes a portion of superior border of alveolar process,it gives the impression that the alveolar process is scoopedc out.

Internal structure: Totally radiolucent.

Effects on surrounding structures: LCH destroys bone.in alveolar lesions the bone around teeth,including the lamina dura ,is destroyed; as a result teeth appear to be standing in space. The lesion does not displace teeth,although teeth may move because they are bereft of bone support. Intraosseous type of lesion stimulate periosteal new bone formation.

SHORT ESSAYS

Q3 Juvenile Periodontitis

Ans.

Juvenile Periodontitis is an uncommon condition characterized by severe loss of attachment and destruction of alveolar bone around one or more permanent teeth in otherwise healthy adolescent. The disease has a predilection for first molars and incisors and when limited to these teeth is termed localized juvenile periodontitis. A generalized form of juvenile periodontitis has been described in which there is severe tissue destruction around many teeth. The generalized form may be preceded by localized juvenile peridontitis or arise spontaneously.

Definition

Localized juvenile periodontitis was described by Gottlieb as a chronic, degenerative, noninflammatory disease of the periodontal tissues, which he referred to as "diffuse atrophy of alveolar bone".

Clinical Features

Juvenile periodontitis becomes apparent about the time of puberty, usually between the ages of 10 and 15. The disease progresses rapidly at the mesial or distal surfaces of one or more first permanent molars or distal surfaces of one or more first permanent molars, and in most instances there is additional involvement of one or more incisors. As the disease progresses, the affected teeth may become increasingly mobile, with labial movement and spacing of incisors. Bleeding on probing of the periodontal pockets is also evident, reflecting ulceration of the crevicular epithelium. This has been confirmed by histologic examination of localized juvenile periodontitis lesions.

Localized juvenile periodontitis tends to occur among members of the same family and although an X linked inheritance has been suggested both sexes are affected and an autosomal recessive pattern of inheritance seems more likely.

Actinobacillus actinomycetemcomitans, a gram negative facultative anaerobic rod, plays a dominant role in the disease process.

Histologic Examination

Shows numerous areas of chronic inflammation containing polymorphonuclear leukocytes, lymphocytes and large numbers of plasma cells.

Unlike ordinary periodontitis which usually progresses at a slow rate, juvenile periodontitis progresses rapidly and this destructive from of periodontal disease frequently remain undetected in young individuals, until increased tooth mobility, drifting, and spacing of teeth, abscess formation occurs. This makes the treatment so difficult.

Etiology

A brief understanding of the etiologic agents in juvenile periodontitis may help clinicians provide a more efficient and effective therapy. A. actinomycetemcomitans is the mostly found organism in the mixed anaerobic pocket microflora of diseased sites in juvenile periodontitis. Culture studies of sulcular epithelium have comfirmed the histologic impression that, A. actinomycetemcomitans, invades and thrives within the periodontal soft tissues.

Treatment

Therapy should be directed at the total elimination of A. actinomycetemcomitans from the subgingival and supragingival plaque, from the subgingival microflora and from the periodontal soft tissues. Closed curettage and surgical curettage in conjunction with scaling and root planning should be done.

Q4 Multilocular radiolucencies
Ans.

Refer to Q13 of September 2001.

Q5 Depapillation of tongue
Ans.

Refer March 2006 (OS) Q17.

Q6 Localization technique
Ans.

Refer march 2006 (RS) Q6

Q7 Causes of bleeding in the oral cavity
Ans.

1. Carcinoma, squamous cell of head and neck
2. Dental caries
3. Gardner-Morrisson-Abbot syndrome
4. Hantavirosis
5. Hemophilia
6. Injury
7. Leukemia
8. Periodontitis
9. Sackey-Sakati-Aur syndrome
10. Stomatitis
11. Thrombocytopenic purpura, autoimmune
12. Viral hemorrhagic fevers

Bleeding gums may be due to:

- Injury or trauma, which may be caused by a blow, insertion of foreign substances, tooth picking, dentures, improper brushing, flossing. It may also get injured from irritation of chemicals and acids in foods, drinks, mouth fresheners, tooth whiteners and medicines.

- Disease - conditions can also cause bleeding gums. For example, there could be gum problems or infection of gums, retracted or receded gums, weak and spongy gums. It is also a common incidence of dental problems such as caries, excessive tartar or plaque formation, periodontitis.

- Mouth sores can also spread infection to gums to cause bleeding.

- Blood disorders, bleeding and clotting disorders, deficiency of coagulation factors, Thrombocytopenic purpura, hemophilia, and leukemia can cause bleeding as well.

- Systemic, such as liver disorders, kidney disorders, arterial or capillary diseases, diabetes, or heart disorder can also reflect as bleeding gums.

- Nutritional and physiological, such as vitamin C and K deficiency will lead to bleeding disorders.

- Pregnancy and hormonal changes can also cause gums to bleed occasionally, as well as poor oral hygiene, due to infection and weakness.
- Medications could also cause bleeding gums, because continuous usage of blood thinners, such as Aspirin, heparin therapy, pain-killers and treatment procedures like chemo-therapy, radiation therapy, can also cause bleeding from gums.
- Hot food and chemicals can end up burning the gums, further resulting in bleeding. For example, some people still follow the practice of placing pain relieving tablets on the gum adjacent to the painful tooth, which invariably causes burns. Certain rapidly spreading infections can damage the blood vessels of the gums resulting in bleeding as well.

Q8 Cherubism

Ans.

Cherubism is a rare genetic disorder that causes prominence in the lower portion in the face. The name is derived from the temporary chubby-cheeked resemblance to putti, often confused with cherubs, in Renaissance paintings.

Pathology

loss of bone in the mandible which the body replaces with excessive amounts of fibrous tissue. In most cases, the condition fades as the child grows, but in a few even rarer cases the condition continues to deform the affected person's face. Also causes premature loss of the primary teeth and uneruption of the permanent teeth.

Features (Fig. 21.1)

- Autosomal dominant disease of the maxilla and mandible believed to be traced to a genetic defect resulting from a mutation of the SH3BP2 gene from chromosome 4p16.3

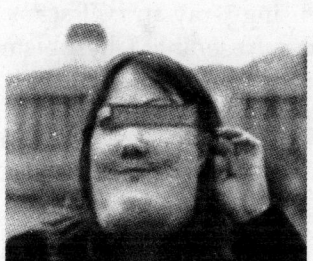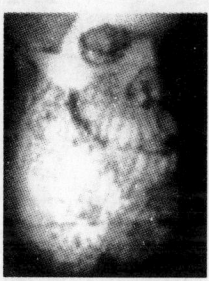

Fig. 21.1: Features of Cherubism

- Approximately 200 cases have been reported by medical journals with the majority being males
- Usually first diagnosed around age 7 and continues through puberty and may or may not continue to advance with age. The degrees of Cherubism vary from mild to severe.
- Osteoclastic and osteoblastic remodeling contributes to the change of normal bone to fibrous tissue and cyst formation
- The patients face becomes enlarged and disproportionate due to the fibrous tissue and atypical bone formation
- The sponge like bone formations lead to early tooth loss and permanent tooth eruption problems. The disease also affects the orbital area creating an upturned eye appearance.
- While the disease is rare and painless the afflicted suffer the emotional trauma of disfigurement. The affects of Cherubism may also interfere with normal jaw motion and speech.

Diagnosis

The disease is usually diagnosed when dental abnormalities like premature deciduous teeth and abnormal growth of permanent teeth due to displacement by cysts and lesions. The only definite way to correctly diagnose the disease is by sequence analysis of the SH3BP2 gene. The gene has been found to have mis-sense mutation in exon 9. Initial study of the patient is usually conducted using x-ray and CT scans. Neurofibromatosis may resemble Cherubism and may accompany the disease. Genetic testing is the final diagnosis tool.

Treatment

- Because Cherubism changes and improves over time the treatment should be individually determined
- Generally moderate cases are watched until they subside or progress into the more severe range
- Severe cases may require surgery to eliminate bulk cysts and fibrous growth of the maxilla and mandible
- Surgical bone grafting of the cranial facial bones may be successful on some patients. Surgery is preferred for patients ages 5 to 15.
- Orthodontic treatment is generally required to avoid permanent dental problems arising from malocclusive bite, misplaced, and unerupted permanent teeth
- In patients with orbital issues of diploia, globe displacement, and visual loss will require ophthalmologic treatment.

Prevention

Since this disease is genetically linked genetic counseling may be the only way to decrease occurrences of Cherubism. The lack of severity of symptoms of the parents may be cause for failure to recognize the disorder. The optimal time to be tested for mutations is prior to having children. The disease results from a genetic mutation and this gene has been found to spontaneously mutate. Therefore there may be no prevention techniques available.

Q9 Pemphigus vulgaris
Ans.
Refer to Q1 of September 2003.

Q10 Light Radiograph
Ans.
Refer Q4 of September 1998.

Q11 Hyperparathyroidism
Ans.
It is a condition of hyperactivity of parathyroid glands either due to a primary hyperplasia or due to secondary pathology.

Radiographic Features
Refer to Q20 of March 2002 solution.

Q12 Alkaline phosphatase
Ans.
Refer to Q12 of March 2001.

SHORT ANSWERS

Q13 Nikolsky's sign
Ans.
Refer to Q11 of march 2002.

Q14 Paul-Bunnell test
Ans.
Refer to Q13 of March 2002.

Q15 Radiation caries
Ans.
Refer to march 2000 Q19 solution.

Q16 Lipoma
Ans.
A lipoma is a benign tumor composed of fatty tissue. They are the most common form of soft tissue tumor. Lipomas are soft to the touch, usually movable, and are generally painless. Many lipomas are small (under one centimeter diameter) but can enlarge to sizes greater than six centimeters. There are several subtypes of lipoma

- Angiolipoleiomyoma
- Chondroid lipomas
- Corpus callosum lipoma

Lipomas are usually relatively small with diameters of about 1–3 cm, but in rare cases they can grow over several years into "giant lipomas" that are 10–20 cm across and weigh up to 4–5 kg. Hibernoma is a lipoma of brown fat.

- Intradermal spindle cell lipoma
- Neural fibrolipoma
- Pleomorphic lipomas
  - Spindle-cell lipoma
  - Superficial subcutaneous lipoma

Prevalence

Approximately one percent of the general population has a lipoma. These tumors can occur at any age, but are most common in middle age, often appearing in people from 40 to 60 years old.

Causes

The tendency to develop a lipoma is not necessarily hereditary although hereditary conditions, such as familial multiple lipomatosis, may include lipoma development.

Treatment

Usually, treatment of a lipoma is not necessary, unless the tumor becomes painful or restricts movement. They are usually removed for cosmetic reasons, if they grow very large, or for histopathology to check that they are not a more dangerous type of tumor such as a liposarcoma.

Lipomas are normally removed by simple excision. This cures the majority of cases, with about 1–2% of lipomas recurring after excision.

Liposuction is another option if the lipoma is soft and has a small connective tissue component. Liposuction typically results in less scarring; however, with large lipomas it may fail to remove the entire tumor, which can lead to re-growth.

Removal by the use of injection of compounds that trigger lipolysis, such as steroids or phosphatidylcholine.

Q17 Draw a neat labeled diagram of an X-ray tube

Ans.

Refer Q2 March 2004

Q18 Hereditary opalescent dentin

Ans.

It is also called as dentinogenesis imperfecta which is a rare inherited disorder affecting both the primary as well as the permanent dentitions. It affects the development of dentin and may be accompanied by similar disturbance in the bones (osteogenesis imperfecta). Three types

- Type I - dentinogenesis imperfect that always occurs in families with osteogenesis imperfecta. Deciduous teeth are more affected than permanent teeth
- Type II - not associated with osteogenesis imperfect and both teeth are affected equally
- Type III - this is a racial isolate in Maryland also known as Brandywine type. Multiple pulp exposures in deciduous teeth are a characteristic feature seen. Both types of teeth are equally affected.

Radiographically the teeth have bulbous crowns with cervical constriction and short pointed roots. The pulp chamber become obliterated which is more pronounced in the coronal segment.

The histologic features report that enamel is normal except for its shade which is actually a manifestation of the dentinal disturbance. The dentin is composed of irregular tubules with large areas of uncalcified matrix. The tubules are larger in diameter and hence less in number.

The treatment is focused on preserving the tooth structure severely affected by attrition. Overdentures have been made in order to establish aesthetics, function and vertical dimension. Cast crown and jacket crowns would be given in the permanent teeth when and if desired. All carious teeth should be restored and the proper oral hygiene instructions must be given.

Early diagnosis and treatment is essential as it leads to the rehabilitation of the somatognathic system and helps in building up the lost confidence of the child.

Q19 Koplik's spots

Ans.

Refer to Q9 of March 2005.

Q20 Cone-cut

Ans.

Refer Q4 March 1999

Q21 Herpangina

Ans.

Refer to Q8 March 2006

Q22 Garre's Osteomyelitis

Ans.

This condition was described in 1893 by Garre as a focal gross thickening of the periosteum of long bones with peripheral reactive bone formation due to mild infection or irritation.

- Occurs in young persons and usually involves the anterior surface of tibia.
- It also affects the jaws where it is more dangerous as there is more probability of the infection entering maxilla and mandible than any other bone in the body.

- In jaws it shows predilection to mandible and occurs in children and young adults.
- Toothache, jaw pain, bony hard swelling on the outer surface of jaw are the presenting complaints.

Radiographic Features

Intraoral radiographs reveal a carious tooth opposite a hard bony mass.

Occlusal radiographs reveal a focal overgrowth of bone on the outer surface of the cortex which may be described as a duplication of the cortical layer of bone.

Histologic Features

Reactive new bone and osteoid tissue with osteoblasts bordering many of the trabeculae which are oriented perpendicular to the cortex.

Differential Diagnosis

Caffey's disease, hypervitaminosis A, syphilis, leukemia, Ewing's sarcoma, metastatic neuroblastoma and even fracture callus.

Treatment

Removal of carious tooth with no surgical intervention for the periosteal lesion except for a biopsy.

22

RGUHS January 2008

QUESTION PAPER
Long Essays

1. Enumerate the autoimmune disorders of the oral cavity. Discuss the clinical features, diagnosis and management of Sjogren's syndrome
2. Describe in detail the bisecting angle technique of intra oral periapical radiography

Short Essays

3. Trismus
4. Burning mouth syndrome
5. Oral manifestations of HIV infection
6. Principles of projection geometry
7. Lupus erythematosus
8. Oblique lateral radiograph of mandible

Short Answers

9. Gorlin–Goltz syndrome
10. Diclofenac sodium
11. Cotton–wool appearance on radiograph
12. Ankyloglossia
13. Patch test
14. Cleidocranial dysplasia
15. Composition of internsifying screen
16. PDL-space
17. 'TENS' therapy
18. Dilaceration

SOLUTIONS

LONG ESSAYS

Q1 Enumerate the autoimmune disorders of the oral cavity. Discuss the clinical features, diagnosis and management of Sjogren's syndrome.

Ans.

For 1st part refer to Q1 September 2003.

Sjogren's syndrome is an autoimmune disease. Autoimmune diseases are characterized by the abnormal production of extra antibodies in the blood that are directed against various tissues of the body. This particular autoimmune illness features inflammation in certain glands of the body. Inflammation of the glands that produce tears (lacrimal glands) leads to decreased water production for tears and eye dryness. Inflammation of the glands that produce the saliva in the mouth (salivary glands, including the parotid glands) leads to dry mouthand dry lips.

Sjogren's syndrome with gland inflammation (resulting dry eyes and mouth, etc.) that is not associated with another connective tissue disease is referred to as primary Sjogren's syndrome. Sjogren's syndrome that is also associated with a connective tissue disease, such as rheumatoid arthritis, systemic lupus erythematosus, or scleroderma, is referred to as secondary Sjogren's syndrome.

Causes

- Scientific support for genetic (inherited) factors.It is also found more commonly in families that have members with other autoimmune illnesses, such as systemic lupus erythematosus, autoimmune thyroid disease, juvenile diabetes, etc. About 90% of patients with Sjogren's syndrome are female.

- Symptoms of Sjogren's syndrome can involve the glands, as above, but there are also possible affects of the illness involving other organs of the body (extraglandular manifestations).

- When the tear gland (lacrimal gland) is inflamed from Sjogren's, the resulting eye dryness can progressively lead to eye irritation, decreased tear production, "gritty" sensation, infection, and serious abrasion of the dome of the eye (cornea). Dry eyes can lead to infections of the eyes.

- Inflammation of the salivary glands can lead to mouth dryness, swallowing difficulties, dental decay, gum disease, mouth sores and swelling, stones and/or infection of parotid gland inside of the cheeks. Dry lips often accompany the mouth dryness.

- Other glands that can become inflamed, though less commonly, in Sjogren's syndrome include those of the lining of the breathing passages (leading to lung infections) and vagina (sometimes noted as pain during intercourse recurrent vaginal infections).

- Extraglandular (outside of the glands) problems in Sjogren's syndrome include joint pain or inflammation (arthritis), Raynaud's phenomenon, lung inflammation, lymph-node enlargement, kidney, nerve, and muscle disease. A rare serious complication of Sjogren's syndrome is inflammation of the blood vessels (vasculitis), which can damage the tissues of the body that are supplied by these vessels.

- A common disease that is occasionally associated with Sjogren's syndrome is autoimmune thyroiditis (Hashimoto's thyroiditis), which can lead to abnormal thyroid hormone levels detected by thyroid blood tests. Heartburn and difficulty swallowing can result from gastroeso-phageal reflux disease (GERD), another common condition associated with Sjogren's syndrome. A rare disease that is uncommonly associated with Sjogren's syndrome is primary biliary cirrhosis, an immune disease of the liver that leads to scarring of the liver tissue. A small percentage of patients with Sjogren's syndrome develop cancer of the lymph glands (lymphoma). This usually develops only after many years with the illness. Unusual gland swelling should be reported to the physician.

- The diagnosis of Sjogren's syndrome involves detecting the features of dryness of the eyes and mouth. The dryness of the eyes can be determined in the doctor's office by testing the eye's ability to wet a small testing paper strip placed under the eyelid (Schirmer's test using Schirmer tear test strips). More sophisticated eye testing can be done by an eye specialist (ophthalmologist). Salivary glands can become larger and harden or become tender. Salivary-gland inflammation can be detected by radiologic nuclear medicine salivary scans. Also, the diminished ability of the salivary glands to produce saliva can be measured with salivary flow testing. The diagnosis is strongly supported by the abnormal findings of a biopsy of salivary-gland tissue.
- The glands of the lower lip are often used to obtain a biopsy sample the salivary-gland tissue in the diagnosis of Sjogren's syndrome. The lower lip salivary-gland biopsy procedure is easily performed under local anesthesia with the surgeon making a tiny incision on the inner part of the lower lip to expose and remove a sample of the tiny salivary glands within.
- Patients with Sjogren's syndrome typically produce a myriad of extra antibodies against a variety of body tissues (autoantibodies). These can be detected through blood testing and include antinuclear antibodies (ANAs), which are present in nearly all patients. Typical antibodies that are found in most, but not all patients, are SS-A and SS-B antibodies, rheumatoid factor, thyroid antibodies, and others. Low red blood count (anemia) and abnormal blood testing for inflammation (sedimentation rate) are seen.

Q2 Describe in detail the bisecting angle technique of intraoral periapical radiography.

Ans.

Refer to Q5 of September 1998.

SHORT ESSAYS

Q3 Trismus

Ans.

Trismus is the inability to normally open the mouth due to one of many causes. It involves the trigeminal nerve

Causes

- Pericoronitis (inflammation of soft tissue around impacted third molar) is the most common cause of trismus.
- Inflammation of muscles of mastication. It is a frequent sequel to surgical removal of mandibular third molars (lower wisdom teeth). The condition is usually resolved on its own in 10–14 days, during which time eating and oral hygiene are compromised. The application of heat (e.g. heat bag extra-orally, and warm salt water intraorally) may help, reducing the severity and duration of the condition.
- Peritonsillar abscess, a complication of tonsillitis which usually presents with sore throat, dysphagia, fever, and change in voice.
- Temporomandibular joint disorder (TMD)
- Trismus is a common temporary side effect of many stimulants of the sympathetic nervous system. Users of the recreational drugs methylenedioxymethamphetamine

(MDMA), methamphetamine (meth), methyl-phenidate (Ritalin), mephedrone (4-MMC), amphetamine as well as many other pharmacological agents commonly report trismus as a side effect.

- *Submucousfibrosis:* Treatment requires treating the underlying condition with dental treatments, physical therapy, and passive range of motion devices. Additionally, control of symptoms with pain medications (NSAIDs), muscle relaxants, and warm compresses may be used. Splints have been used.

Q4 Burning Mouth Syndrome
Ans.
Refer Q9 March 2006 RS

Q5 Oral manifestations of HIV infection
Ans.
Refer 2002 March Q3

Q6 Principles of projection geometry
Ans.
Refer Q8 2004 september

Q7 Lupus erythematosus
Ans. Refer Q16 Feb 2007 (OS)

Q8 Oblique lateral radiograph of mandible
Ans.
Lateral Oblique Radiograph

A radiographic view of the mandible, revealing one side of the mandible form symphysis to condyle by displacing the other side upwards. mandibular

SHORT ANSWERS
Q9 Gorlin-Goltz syndrome
Ans. Also called as focal dermal hypoplasia syndrome, is an autosomal dominant transmitted disease with incomplete penetrance. Marked female preponderance is seen.

Clinical Features
- Relative focal absence of dermis with herniation of subcutaneous fat into the defects
- Skin atrophy, streaky pigmentation and telengiectesia
- Multiple papillomas of the mucosa and or skin
- Syndactyly or polydactyly or adactyly
- Asymmetrical face with pointed chin and notched nasal alae, asymmetrical ears, sunken eyes (eye anomalies include iris and choroid colobomata and strabismus)
- Mental retardation

Oral Manifestations
- Papillomas of lips, buccal mucosa or gingiva
- Defective teeth–microdontia, enamel hypoplasia

Q10 Diclofenac Sodium
Ans.
Diclofenac is a non-steroidal anti-inflamma-tory drug (NSAID) taken to reduce inflammation and as an analgesic reducing pain in conditions such as dental pain, arthritis or acute injury

Mechanism of Action
The primary mechanism responsible for its anti-inflammatory, antipyretic, and analgesicaction is inhibition of prosta-glandin synthesis by inhibition of cyclo-oxygenase (COX) and it appears to inhibit DNA synthesis.

Indications
Diclofenac sodium:It is used to relieve the inflammation, swelling, stiffness, and joint pain associated with rheumatoid arthritis, osteoarthritis and ankylosing spondylitis. Voltaren-XR, the extended-release form of Voltaren, is used only for long-term treatment.

Cataflam is also prescribed for immediate relief of pain and menstrual discomfort.

Diclofenac sodium is taken for long term.To minimize stomach upset and related side effects, medicine is taken along with with food, milk, or an antacid. However, this may delay onset of relief.

Diclofenac sodium is taken with a full glass of water and patient is advised not to Also, do not lie down for about 20 minutes after taking it. This will help to prevent irritation in upper digestive tract.

• *If missed dose:* This medicine is to be taken on a regular schedule. If a patient misses the dose and it is time for next dose, he instructed to skip the missed dose and continued at. Do not take 2 doses at once.

• *Storage instructions:* Store at room temperature. Keep the container tightly closed and protect from moisture.

Contraindications

• Hypersensitivity against diclofenac

• History of allergic reactions (bronchospasm, shock, rhinitis, urticaria) following the use of Aspirin or another NSAID

• Third-trimester pregnancy

• Active stomach and/or duodenal ulceration or gastrointestinal bleeding

• Inflammative intestinal disorders such as Crohn's disease or ulcerative colitis

Diclofenac is among the better tolerated NSAIDs. Though 20% of patients on long-term treatment experience side effects, only 2% have to discontinue the drug, mostly due to gastrointestinal complaints.

Side effects may include: Abdominal bleeding, abdominal pain or cramps, abdominal swelling, anemia, blood clotting problems, constipation, diarrhea, dizziness, fluid retention, gas, headache, heartburn, indigestion, itching, nausea, peptic ulcers, rash, ringing in the ears, vomiting.

Q11 Cotton-wool appearance on radiograph
Ans.
Refer to Q14 of Feb 2007 (RS)

Q12 Ankyloglossia
Ans.
Ankyloglossia, commonly known as tongue tie, is a congenital oral anomaly which may decrease mobility of the tongue tip and is caused by an unusually short, thick lingual frenulum, a membrane connecting the underside of the tongue to the floor of the mouth. Ankyloglossia varies in degree of severity from mild cases characterized by mucous membrane bands to complete ankyloglossia whereby the tongue is tethered to the floor of the mouth.

Ankyloglossia can affect feeding, speech, and oral hygiene as well as have mechanical/social effects. Ankyloglossia can also prevent the tongue from contacting the anterior palate. This can then promote an infantile swallow and hamper the progression to an adult-like swallow which can result in an open bite deformity

Ankyloglossia can result in mechanical and social effects

Treatment

Intervention for ankyloglossia sometimes includes surgery in the form of frenotomy. It is done by laser.

Q13 Patch test
Ans.
Refer to Q9 of July 2008

Q14 Cleidocranial dysplasia
Ans.
Cleidocranial dysostosis, also called Cleidocranial dysplasia, is a hereditarycongenital disorder due to haploinsufficiency caused by

mutations in the CBFA1gene, located on the short arm of chromosome.

It is usually autosomal dominant, but in some cases the cause is not known.

Presentation

Cleidocranial dysostosis is a general skeletal condition so named from the collarbone (cleido) and cranium deformities which people with it often have. Common features are:

- Partly or completely missing collarbones., this allows hypermobility of the shoulders including ability to touch the shoulders together in front of the chest.
- A soft spot or larger soft area in the top of the head where the fontanelle failed to close.
- Bones and joints are underdeveloped.
- The permanent teeth include supernumerary teeth. Unless these supernumeraries are reabsorbed before adolescence, they will crowd the adult teeth in what already may be an underdeveloped jaw.
- Permanent teeth not erupting
- Bossing (bulging) of the forehead
- Hypertelorism

Q15 Composition of internsifying screen
Ans.

Refer Q3 March 2004

Q16 PDL-space
Ans.

The interproximal alveolar bone level (BC-CEJ distance) was determined by measuring the distance from the lowest point of alveolar bone crest to the imaginary line connecting the two CEJs of the adjacent teeth. Both the radiographic signs of lamina dura and of the PDL space were graded to compose Lamina Dura Index (LDI) and periodontal ligament space index (PDLI). It is found that the average distance of BC to CEJ in periodontally healthy subjects is from 0.62 to 1.67 mm. Radiographic

signs such as disappearance of lamina dura on the alveolar bone crest, wedge-shaped widening of the periodontal ligament space at the bone crest are not uncommonly seen in clinically healthy periodontal sites.

Q17 'TENS' therapy
Ans.

Definition

TENS stands for Transcutaneous Electrical Nerve Stimulation. It is a method of pain relief.

Description

In TENS therapy, electrodes are placed on the skin, either directly over the painful area or more commonly, at key points along the nerve pathway. A small, battery-powered generator emits a milli-amp (one thousandth of an ampere) of electricity through lead wires to the electrodes.

TENS has been used for a wide variety of complaints. TENS has been applied to almost every type of pain, from mildly persistent problems (such as sore muscles) to acute postoperative pain. It is used in myofacial pain dysfunction syndrome, TMJ problems.

Safety

TENS electrodes should never be placed On or near the eyes, In the mouth, Transcerebrally (on each temple), On the front of the neck (due to the risk of acute hypotension through a vasovagal reflex), On or near the trigeminal nerve if history of herpes zoster induced trigeminal neuralgia, i.e. postherpetic neuralgia persists. TENS should not be used by people with an artificial cardiac pacemaker due to risk of interference and failure of their implanted device.

Q18 Dilaceration

- Dilaceration is a developmental disturbance in shape of teeth. It refers to an angulation, or a sharp bend or curve, in the root or crown of a formed tooth.

- The condition is thought to be due to trauma during the period in which tooth is forming. The result is that the position of the calcified portion of the tooth is changed and the remainder of the tooth is formed at an angle.

- The curve or bend may occur anywhere along the length of the tooth, sometimes at the cervical portion, at other times midway along the root or even just at the apex of the root, depending upon the amount of root formed when the injury occurred.

- Such an injury to a permanent tooth, resulting in dilaceration, often follows traumatic injury to the deciduous predecessor in which that tooth is driven apically into the jaw.

23

RGUHS January 2008 (RS)

QUESTION PAPER
Long Essays

1. Enumerate the various causes of cervico facial lymphadenopathy. Write the differential diagnosis of cervical lymphadenopathy.
2. Write the principles of imaging and discuss the bisecting angle technique.

Short Essays

3. Dentinogenesis imperfecta
4. Internal derangement of temporomandibular joint
5. Differential diagnosis of bald tongue
6. Sialolithiasis
7. Role of cortico steroids in auto immune diseases
8. Sturge-Weber syndrome
9. Periapical radiolucencies
10. Digital radiography
11. Applications of ultra sound in dentistry
12. Kaposis sarcoma

Short Answers

13. Cherubism
14. Window period
15. Hairy leukoplakia
16. Structure of HIV
17. Oncogenes
18. Scurvy
19. Storage of X-ray films
20. Bence jones proteins
21. Bleeding time
22. Lip prints

LONG ESSAY

Q1 Enumerate the various causes of cervico facial lymphadenopathy. Write the differential diagnosis of cervical lympha-denopathy.

Ans.

The principle causes of cervical lymphadeno-pathy are:

1. Tuberculosis

2. Carcinoma

3. Lymphoma

Tuberculous lymph node – in the Indian subcontinent this is the commonest cause of lymph node swelling in the neck. The pathology passes through various stages starting from the stage of solid enlargement or lymphadenitis. Then periadinitis develops and the glands become matted. Later on the matted mass liquefies and cold abscess develops.

Carcinomatous lymph node – usually the patient is above 50 yrs of age excepting the case of papillary carcinoma of thyroid where in the metastasis can occur at an earlier age. The sewlling is painless and relatively grows fast. New lumps may appear on the sides.

Lymphoma – the commonest members in this group are the Hodgkin's disease, lymphosarcoma and reticulosarcoma.

For differential diagnosis, swellings of the neck can be divided into

a. *Midline swellings of neck from above downwards:* Ludwig's angina ,enlarged submental lymph nodes, sublingual dermoid and lipoma in the submental region, thyroglossal cyst and subhyoid bursitis; goiter of the thyroid isthmus and pyramidal lobe, enlarged lymph nodes and lipoma in the suprasternal space of burns. Retrosternal goiter and thymic swelling. A demoid cyst may occur anywhere in the midline.

b. *Lateral swellings according to their site of origin.* Submandibular triangle: plunging ranula and extension of growth from jaw. Carotid triangle: Carotid artery aneurysm, carotid body tumor, branchial cyst, brachiogenic carcinoma. Thyroid swelling will be deep to the sternomastoid. Sternomastoid tumor may be seen in a new born. Posterior triangle: cystic hygroma, pharyngeal pouch, subclavian aneurysm, aberrant thyroid, cervical rib, lipoma.

Clinically the swellings can be divided into acute and chronic swellings. Acute include, cellulitis including Ludwig's angina, boil, carbuncle and acute lymphadenitis. Chronic swellings can be further divided into cystic and solid swellings. Cystic include the following: branchial cyst, thyroglossal cyst, dermoid cyst, cystic hygroma, sebaceous cyst, cystic adenoma of thyroid gland and cold abscess.

Solid swellings include the following: solid swellings from thyroid, branchigenic carcinoma, sternomastoid tumor.

Pulsatile swellings include aneurysm of carotid and subclavian artery

Q2 Write the principles of imaging and discuss the bisecting angle technique.

Ans.

Ref to Q5 of September 1998

SHORT ESSAYS

Q3 Dentinogenesis imperfecta

Ans.

Dentinogenesis imperfecta (hereditary Opalescent Dentin) is a genetic disorder of tooth development. This condition causes teeth to be discolored (most often a blue-gray or yellow-brown color) and translucent. Teeth are also weaker than normal, making them prone to rapid wear, breakage, and loss. These problems can affect both primary (baby) teeth and permanent teeth. This condition is inherited in anautosomal dominant pattern, which means one copy of the altered gene in each cell is sufficient to cause the disorder. Dentinogenesis imperfecta affects an estimated 1 in 6,000 to 8,000 people.

Types

Types of dentinogenesis imperfecta with similar dental abnormalities usually an autosomal dominant trait with variable expressivity but can be recessive if the associated osteogenesis imperfecta is of recessive type. This type is no I.

Type II: Occurs in people without other inherited disorders (i.e. Osteogenesis imperfecta). It is an autosomal dominant trait. A few families with type II have progressive hearing loss in addition to dental abnormalities.

Mutations in the *DSPP* gene have been identified in people with type II and type III dentinogenesis imperfecta. Type I occurs as part of osteogenesis imperfecta.

Clinical Features

Clinical appearance is variable. However, the teeth usually involved and more severely affected are deciduous teeth in type 1; whereas in type 2 both the dentitions are equally affected.

The teeth may be gray to yellowish brown. They exhibit transluscent or opalescent hue. Enamel is usually lost early due to loss of scalloping at DEJ. The teeth however are not more susceptible to dental caries than normal ones.

Radiographic Features

Type I and II show total obliteration of the pulp chamber.

Type III shows thin dentin and extremely enormous pulp chamber. These teeth are usually known as shell teeth.

Histology

Dentinal tubules are irregular and are bigger in diameter. Areas of uncalcified matrix are seen. Sometimes odontoblasts are seen in dentin.

Treatment

A common one is bonding, putting bleacher on the weakened enamel of the teeth and with lots of treatments of this bonding, the teeth appear whiter to the eye, but the teeth on the inside and under that cover are still the same.

Q4 Internal derangement of temporo mandibular joint

Ans.

The most frequent structural (as opposed to muscular) causes of temporomandibular joint dysfunction (TMD) are internal derangements, which involve progressive slipping or displacement of a component of the temporomandibular joint called the articular disc.

Tearing or stretching of the ligaments holding the disc in place often causes an internal derangement. The condition can be caused by an acute trauma, such as a blow to the face. It may also be caused by more chronic, micro-trauma, wear on the joint, such as from bruxism, a very bad bite (severe malocclusion) or repeated excessive jaw movements.

Internal derangements can be either or both soft-tissue or bony. There are two basic types of soft-tissue internal derangements. The more common is referred to as an internal derangement with reduction; the disc slides into and out of its normal functional position as the jaw opens or closes, causing the popping sound characteristic of TMD. In cases of internal derangement without reduction, the disc is permanently displaced or dislocated to an incorrect position, and the jaw's range of motion is limited.

Symptoms

- Pain in the jaw joints, especially associated with jaw movements. Dull aching, stabbing, or burning pain may also be felt in the surrounding muscles of the face. This pain can occasionally refer elsewhere, potentially leading to pain throughout the head and in the neck and shoulders.
- Earaches, tinnitus (ringing in the ear), or even the feeling of reduced hearing can sometimes occur.
- Loud and/or painful clicking or popping sounds when opening or closing the jaw often characterizes internal derangement disorders. Patients may have a limited range of jaw opening, and/or will periodically or permanently feel that the jaw is locked.

Diagnosis

Imaging techniques such as X-ray, CT or MRI scans, and arthroscopy are used to determine whether there is a structural problem at the TMJ.

Treatment

In early stages of the condition, treatment may involve eating a soft diet and reducing strain on the jaw with the use of a splint or bite guard. Non-steroidal anti-inflammatory drugs or muscle relaxants may be prescribed. Physical therapy and stress management may also be helpful in managing the condition. If the derangement becomes more severe or refractory (unresponsive) to conservative and non-surgical treatment, it may be necessary to surgically repair, reposition, or possibly remove and consider replacing, the disc and/or bony joint.

Q5 Differential diagnosis of bald tongue
Ans.

Differential diagnosis is as follows:

Electromagnetic, Physical, Trauma or Radiation Causes

- Radiation sickness/severe, acute
- Radiation stomatitis

Infectious Disorders (Specific Agent)

- Scarlet fever
- Infected organ, Abscesses
- Glossitis
- Allergic, Collagen, Auto-immune disorders
- Sjogrens sicca syndrome
- Metabolic, Storage disorders
- Amyloidosis, gut
- Amyloidosis, systemic
- Amyloidosis/tongue

Deficiency Disorders

- Vitamin deficiency/Hypovitaminosis
- Folic acid deficiency anemia
- Malnutrition/starvation
- Pellagra/niacin deficiency
- Water soluble vitamin deficiencies
- Usage, degenerative, necrosis, age related disorders
- Atrophic glossitis
- Reference to Organ System
- Stomatitis
- Pernicious anemia
- Plummer-Vinson syndrome
- Drugs
- Methotrexate (Rheumatrex) administration/Toxicity

Q6 Sialolithiasis
Ans.

Refer to Q7 of March 2001

Q7 Role of cortico steroids in autoimmune diseases

Ans.

Corticosteroids can be used to induce a remission or reduce the morbidity in autoimmune diseases. Although high doses can be given for short periods, the aim is to achieve specific targets with the minimum effective dose.

- *An autoimmune disorder is a malfunction of the body's immune system that causes the body to attack its own tissues.* Some of the more common autoimmune disorders include rheumatoid arthritis, systemic lupus erythematosus (lupus), and vasculitis, among others. Additional diseases that are believed to be due to autoimmunity include glomerulonephritis, Addison's disease, mixed connective tissue disease, polymyositis, Sjögren's syndrome, progressive systemic sclerosis, and some cases of infertility.

- Corticosteroids induce a transient lymphocytopenia by altering lymphocyte recirculation. They also induce lymphocyte death. The most important immuno-suppressive effect of corticosteroids is on T cell activation, by inhibition of cytokine and effector molecule production.

- Starting treatment with corticosteroids When prescribing steroids, an adequate dose must be used for long enough to achieve an effect. The patient must be aware of the risks of therapy and the potential benefits. Care must be taken to prevent, minimise and appropriately treat complications of steroid therapy. Giving high-dose corticosteroid therapy for a few days to a critically ill patient, or for a few weeks in a patient with a condition such as asthma which should settle, is relatively safe. Patients with chronic incurable diseases such as systemic lupus erythematosus or nephritis need a clear plan of when, how much and for how long corticosteroid therapy is required. Patients who require long-term treatment should be advised about the adverse effects of corticosteroids, particularly the risk of adrenal insufficiency, osteoporosis and cataracts.

- Reducing morbidity or inducing remission in chronic progressive diseases

- Minimising symptoms in chronic inflammatory conditions. Classical examples of this are rheumatoid arthritis and polymyalgia rheumatica.

- Saving lives and saving organs very high-dose therapy might be indicated for several days in critically ill patients with an aggressive acute presentation or a life- or organ-threatening relapse.

Q8 Sturge-Weber syndrome

Ans.

Refer Q13 March 2003

Q9 Periapical radiolucencies

Ans.

Refer Q2 2002 March

Q10 Digital radiography

Ans.

Digital radiography is a form of x-ray imaging, where digital X-ray sensors are used instead of traditional photographic film. Advantages include time efficiency through bypassing chemical processing and the ability to digitally transfer and enhance images. Also less radiation can be used to produce an image of similar contrast to conventional radiography.

- Digital radiography (DR) or (DX) is essentially filmless X-ray image capture. In place of X-ray film, a digital image capture device is used to record the X-ray image and make it available as a digital file that can be presented for interpretation and saved as part of the patient's medical record. The advantages of DR over film include immediate image preview and availability, a wider dynamic range which makes it more forgiving for over- and under-exposure as well as the ability to apply special image processing techniques that enhance overall display of the image

- Radiological examinations
- Dental
- The radiological examinations in dentistry may be classified in: intraoral - where the film or the sensor is placed in the mouth, the purpose being to visualize a limited region and extraoral where the film or the sensor is outside the mouth and the purpose is to visualize a wide region. In dentistry, extraoral imaging splits in: Panoramic X-ray (aka "panorex" or "pano") showing a section, curved following more or less mandible shape, of the whole maxillo-facial block and the Cephalometric X-ray showing a projection, as parallel as possible, of the whole skull.
- Digital radiographic systems
- One particular type of digital system uses a Memory Phosphor Plate (a.k.a. PSP— Photostimulable Phosphor) in place of the film. After X-ray exposure the plate (sheet) is placed in a special scanner where the latent formed image is retrieved point by point and digitized, using laser light scanning. The digitized images are stored and displayed on the computer screen.
- This method is halfway between old film-based technology and current direct digital imaging technology. It is similar to the film process because it involves the same image support handling but differs because the chemical development process is replaced by the scanning process. However, it has the clear advantage to be able to fit within any pre-existing equipment without modification because it replaces just the existing film.
- Also, sometimes the term "Digital X-rays" is used to designate the scanned film documents which are handled by further computer processing.
- Other types of digital imaging technologies use electronic sensors.

Q11 Applications of ultra sound in dentistry
Ans.

Ultrasonic is a branch of acoustics concerned with sound vibrations in frequency ranges above audible level. Ultrasound uses the transmission and reflection of acoustic energy. A pulse is propagated and its reflection is received, both by the transducer. For clinical purposes ultrasound is generated by transducers, which converts electrical energy into ultrasonic waves. This is usually achieved by magnetostriction or piezoelectricity.

- An ultrasonic descaler working at kHz frequencies is used in dentistry to remove attached deposits from the teeth. Such devices offer many advantages over conventional hand instruments by reducing both the work and time involved in the clinical descaling process. Diagnostic applications of MHz ultrasound is limited by the structure and arrangement of the dental tissues. Therapeutic ultrasound has been used to treat a variety of dentally related ailments, and ultrasonic cleaning baths are used to clean both dental instruments and materials.
- Instruments were used with abrasive slurry for preparation of tooth cavities prior to restoration. With advent of high-speed drills, technology was repositioned for ultrasonics and power scaling, which revolutionized mechanical debridment. Use of ultrasonic was first introduced in periodontal procedure and have undergone many changes, and since then, simple compact devices have replaced large, heavy units.

Q12 Kaposi's sarcoma
Ans.

Kaposi's sarcoma (KS) is a tumor caused by Human herpesvirus 8 (HHV8), also known as Kaposi's sarcoma-associated herpesvirus (KSHV)

Signs and Symptoms

KS lesions are nodules or blotches that may be red, purple, brown, or black, and are usually papular (i.e. palpable or raised).

They are typically found on the skin, but spread elsewhere is common, especially the mouth, gastrointestinal tract and respiratory tract. Growth can range from very slow to explosively fast, and is associated with significant mortality and morbidity

Mouth is involved in about 30%, and is the initial site in 15% of AIDS related KS. In the mouth, the hard palate is most frequently affected, followed by the gums. Lesions in the mouth may be easily damaged by chewing and bleed or suffer secondary infection, and even interfere with eating or speaking.

Skin commonly affected areas include the lower limbs, back, face, mouth and genitalia.

The gastrointestinal lesions may be silent or cause weight loss, pain, nausea/vomiting, diarrhea, bleeding (either vomiting blood or passing it with bowel motions), malabsorption, or intestinal obstruction.

Respiratory Tract

Involvement of the airway can present with shortness of breath, fever, cough, hemoptysis (coughing up blood), or chest pain, or as an incidental finding on chest X-ray.

Treatment

Kaposi's sarcoma is not curable (in the usual sense of the word) but it can often be effectively palliated for many years and this is the aim of treatment. In KS associated with immuno-deficiency or immunosuppression, treating the cause of the immune system dysfunction can slow or stop the progression of KS.

SHORT ANSWERS

Q13 Cherubism
Ans.
Refer Q8 Aug 2007(RS)

Q14 Window period
Ans.
In medicine, the window period for a test designed to detect a specific disease (particularly infectious disease) is the time between first infection and when the test can reliably detect that infection. In antibody-based testing, the window period is dependent on the time taken for seroconversion.

The window period is important to epidemiology and safe sex strategies, and in blood and organ donation, because during this time, an infected person or animal cannot be detected as infected but may still be able to infect others. For this reason, the most effective disease-prevention strategies combine testing with a waiting period longer than the test's window period.

Example: During the window period (or equivalence zone) of Hepatitis B, both serological markers HBsAg (Hepatitis B surface antigen) and Anti-HBs (antibody against HBsAg) are negative (which is due to the fact that, although there are Anti-HBs antibodies present, they are actively bound to the HBsAg). Other serological markers, IgM (antibody) against HBc can be positive at this point.

Window period in AIDS: There is usually a period of several weeks in which newly infected people have not yet produced enough HIV antibodies to be detected. Its a brief time after infection, people make too few antibodies for these tests to detect. As a result, their blood passes all the screening tests, even though it can transmit HIV. The "window period" for HIV-1 lasts about 22 days

Q15 Hairy leukoplakia
Ans.
Refer March 2002 Q3. and Q14 2001

Q16 Structure of HIV
Ans.
Outside of a human cell, HIV exists as roughly spherical particles (sometimes called virions). The surface of each particle is studded with lots of little spikes (Fig. 23.1).

An HIV particle is around 100–150 billionths of a metre in diameter. That's about the same as:

- 0.1 microns
- 4 millionths of an inch
- One twentieth of the length of an E. coli bacterium
- One seventieth of the diameter of a human CD4+ white blood cell.

In electron microscope, HIV particles surround themselves with a coat of fatty material known as the viral envelope (or membrane). Projecting from this are around 72 little spikes, which are formed from the proteins gp120 and gp41. Just below the viral envelope is a layer called the matrix, which is made from the protein p17.

The proteins gp120 and gp41 together make up the spikes that project from HIV particles, while p17 forms the matrix and p24 forms the core.

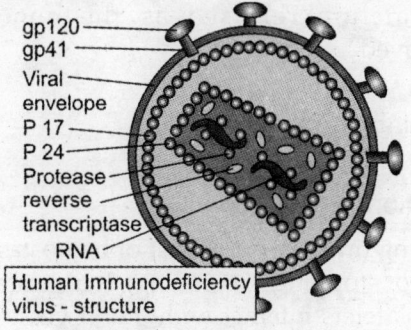

gp120
gp41
Viral envelope
P 17
P 24
Protease
reverse transcriptase
RNA

Human Immunodeficiency virus - structure

Fig. 23.1: Structure of HIV

The viral core (or capsid) is usually bullet-shaped and is made from the protein p24. Inside the core are three enzymes required for HIV replication called reverse transcriptase, integrase and protease. Also held within the core is HIV's genetic material, which consists of two identical strands of RNA.

Q17 Oncogenes
Ans.
An oncogene is a gene that, when mutated or expressed at high levels, helps turn a normal cell into a tumor cell.

Many abnormal cells normally undergo a programmed form of death (apoptosis). Activated oncogenes can cause those cells to survive and proliferate instead. Most oncogenes require an additional step, such as mutations in another gene, or environmental factors, such as viral infection, to cause cancer. Since the 1970s, dozens of oncogenes have been identified in human cancer. Many cancer drugs target those DNA sequences and their products.

A proto-oncogene is a normal gene that can become an oncogene due to mutations or increased expression. The resultant protein may be termed an oncoprotein.

Q18 Scurvy
Ans.
Scurvy is a disease resulting from a deficiency of vitamin C, which is required for the synthesis of collagen in humans. The chemical name for vitamin C, ascorbic acid.

Scurvy leads to the formation of spots on the skin, spongy gums, and bleeding from the mucous membranes. The spots are most abundant on the thighs and legs, and a person with the ailment looks pale, feels depressed, and is partially immobilized. In advanced scurvy there are open, suppurating wounds and loss of teeth. In infants, scurvy is sometimes referred to as Barlow's disease, named after Sir Thomas Barlow

Cause

Scurvy or subclinical scurvy is caused by the lack of vitamin C

Pathogenesis

Ascorbic acid is needed for a variety of biosynthetic pathways, by accelerating hydroxylation and amidation reactions. In the synthesis of collagen, ascorbic acid is required as a cofactor for prolyl hydroxylase and lysyl hydroxylase. Defective collagen fibrillogenesis impairs wound healing. Collagen is also an important part of bone, so bone formation is also affected. Defective connective tissue also leads to fragile capillaries, resulting in abnormal bleeding.

Prevention

Scurvy can be prevented by a diet that includes certain citrus fruits such as oranges or lemons. Other sources rich in vitamin Care fruits such as black currants, guava, kiwifruit, papaya, tomatoes, bell peppers, and strawberries. It can also be found in some vegetables, such as carrots, broccoli, potatoes, cabbage, spinach and paprika.

Q19 Storage of X-ray films
Ans.

Unexposed films awaiting exposure as well as exposed films awaiting processing are subjected to scattered radiation if kept unprotected in the dental X-ray clinic. It is concluded that if dental X-ray films not in use are kept at a distance of 200 cm from the X-ray source and protected by lead foil additional blackening due to scattered radiation is negligible and further protective precautions are unnecessary.

Storage

Dentix D and Dentix E should be stored in the original packing in a dry and cool place at a temperature from 10°C to 21°C and a relative humidity max. 60 % protected from damaging fumes, gazes and ionizing radiation. For long-term storage the film should be stored in a refrigerator. In such a case before use, the film in the intact original packaging should be allowed to adjust to room conditions for at least 2–4 hours.

For regular usage : Vinyl pocket mounts available in clear and black or green masking. All pocket styles offer the ultimate in film protection and easy storage

Classic open window film mounts provide excellent contrast for viewing, safely store your radiographs, and films load easily.

Q20 Bence Jones proteins
Ans.

Bence Jones protein is a monoclonal globulin protein found in the blood or urine, with a molecular weight of 22–24 kDa

Bence Jones proteins are particularly diagnostic of multiple myeloma in the context of end-organ manifestations such as malignant bone marrow cancer, renal failure, lytic bone disease, or anemia, or large numbers of plasma cells in the bone marrow of patients. Bence Jones Proteins are present in 2/3 of multiple myeloma cases

They are found in urine due to the kidneys' decreased filtration capabilities due to renal failure, often induced by hypercalcemia from the calcium released as the bones are destroyed.

Q21 Bleeding time
Ans.
Definition

Bleeding time is a crude test of hemostasis (the arrest or stopping of bleeding). It indicates how well platelets interact with blood vessel walls to form blood clots.

Purpose

Bleeding time is used most often to detect qualitative defects of platelets, such as Von Willebrand's disease. The test helps identify people who have defects in their platelet function. This is the ability of blood to clot following a wound or trauma. Normally, platelets interact with the walls of blood vessels to cause a blood clot. There are many factors in the clotting mechanism, and they are initiated by platelets. The bleeding time test is usually used on patients who have a history of prolonged bleeding after cuts, or who have a family history of bleeding disorders. Also, the bleeding time test is sometimes performed as a preoperative test to determine a patient's likely bleeding response during and after surgery.

Bleeding time is affected by platelet function, certain vascular disorders and von Willebrand Disease which is a platelet agglutination protein, not by other coagulation factors such as haemophilia.

Diseases that cause prolonged bleeding time include thrombocytopenia, disseminated intravascular coagulation (DIC), Bernard-Soulier disease, and Glanzmann's thrombas-thenia. Aspirin and other cyclooxy-genase inhibitors can prolong bleeding time significantly.

While warfarin and heparin also causes an increased bleeding time.

Q22 Lip prints

Ans.

Very few people know that just like fingerprints, even lip prints can be instrumental in identifying a person positively. Stand before a mirror and look at your lips carefully. You would find that they present several fissures and some other criss-cross lines. You may be surprised to know that these fissures and criss-cross lines are different in different people and at many times can form a very good basis of identification.

Dental surgeon has to actively involve in various objectives of forensic dentistry like age and sex determination ,personal identification of unknown deceased person ,identifying bite marks as evidence, participating in mass disaster,studying lip prints,giving evidence in child abuse and in civil and criminal litigation.

Process

A piece of paper has to be folded and the prints has to be taken on it by applying lipsticks on the lips. The furrows has to be observed which will be different in different individuals.

QUESTION PAPER
Long Essays

1. Classify anemias. Discuss in detail the oral manifestations diagnosis and management of pernicious anemia

2. Classify white lesion. Discuss in detail the etiopathogenesis – clinical features, diagnosis and management of oral submucous fibrosis

Short Essays

3. Xerostomia
4. Oral manifestations of diabetes
5. Significance of Haemogram
6. CT in dentistry
7. Production of X-rays
8. Mumps

Short Answers

9. Patch test
10. 'Onion – peel' appearance on a radiograph
11. Actinic chelitis
12. Garre's osteomyelitis
13. Periapical granuloma
14. Talon's cusp
15. Frictional Keratosis
16. Sialadenosis
17. Ranula
18. Inverse square law

SOLUTIONS

LONG ESSAY

Q1 Classify anemias. Discuss in detail the oral manifestations, diagnosis and manage-ment of pernicious anemia.

Ans.

Classification

Refer to Q2 of September 1998

Oral Manifestations

Refer Q2 sept 1998

Pernicious anemia (or pernicious anemia - also known as Biermer's anemia, Addison's anemia, or Addison–Biermer anemia) is one of many types of the larger family of megaloblastic anemias. It is caused by loss of gastric parietal cells, and subsequent inability to absorb vitamin B12.

Usually seated in an atrophic gastritis, the autoimmune destruction of gastric parietal cells leads to a lack of intrinsic factor, and since the absorption from the gut of normal dietary amounts of vitamin B12 is dependent on intrinsic factor, the loss of intrinsic factor leads to vitamin B12 deficiency.

Pernicious anemia presents insidiously, and many of the signs and symptoms are due to anemia itself, where anemia is present. While it may consist of the triad of paraesthesias, sore tongue and weakness, this is not the chief symptom complex.

The patient may complain of fatigue, depression, forgetfulness, difficulty concentrating, low-grade fevers, nausea and gastro-intestinal symptoms (heartburn), weight loss, Because PA may affect the spinal cord, the patient may also complain of impaired urination, loss of sensation in the feet, unsteady gait, weakness and clumsiness. Anemia may cause tachycardia (rapid heartbeat) and cardiac murmurs, along with a waxy pallor. In severe cases, the anemia may cause evidence of congestive heart failure.

Long term complications may include gastric cancer and carcinoids.

Signs and Symptoms

Many signs and symptoms are attributed to pernicious anemia: Fatigue, low blood pressure, rapid heart rate, high blood pressure, pallor, depression, muscle weakness and shortness of breath (known as 'the sighs')

Difficulty in Proprioception

- Mild cognitive impairment, including diffi-culty concentrating and sluggish responses, colloquially referred to as cognitive dysfunc-tion brain fog.
- Neuropathic Pain
- Frequent diarrhea
- Paresthesias, such as pins an needles sensations or numbness in fingers or toes, due to B12 deficiency affecting nerve function. Jaundice due to impaired formation of blood cells. Glossitis (swollen red tongue) due to B12 deficiency. May present with hyperthyroidism or hypo-thyroidism.
- Personality or memory changes

Diagnosis

The first step is always a thorough history and physical examination by a health care practi-tioner. The results of this examination are used to help direct further testing. A number of laboratory tests are available that can help diagnose pernicious anemia as well as other causes of vitamin B12 deficiency. These tests include:

Complete Blood Cell Count (CBC)

A diagnosis of pernicious anemia first requires demonstration of megaloblastic anemia (through a full blood count) which evaluates the mean corpuscular volume (MCV), as well the mean corpuscular hemoglobin concentration (MCHC). Pernicious anemia is identified with a high MCV and a normal MCHC (that is, it is a macrocytic, normochromic anemia). Ovalocytes are also typically seen on the blood smear, and a pathognomonic feature of megaloblastic anemias (which include pernicious anemia and others) is hyper-segmented neutrophils.

Blood Vitamin B12 Level Measurements

Tests for the presence of autoantibodies to intrinsic factor or stomach lining cells

Blood Levels of Iron and Iron-binding Capacity

Folate levels (which are often reduced when vitamin B12 levels are low)

Blood levels of methylmalonic acid or homocysteine, both of which may be sensitive indicators of vitamin B12 deficiency

The Schilling test, a measure of how well the body can absorb vitamin B12, is less commonly used today than in the past.

Finally, bone marrow aspiration or bone marrow biopsy may be recommended in some cases if bone marrow disorders are suspected

The diagnosis of atrophic gastritis Type A should be confirmed by gastroscopy and stepwise biopsy. Approximately 90% of individuals with PA have antibodies for parietal cells; however, only 50% of all individuals in the general population with these antibodies have pernicious anemia.

Treatment

- Repletion of vitamin B12 should be expected to result in a cessation of anemia-related symptoms, a halt in neurological deterioration, and (in cases where neurological problems not advanced) neurological recovery and a complete and permanent remission of all symptoms, so long as B12 is supplemented.

- Vitamin B12 is typically given as an intramuscular injection (shot). An injection of 1000 micrograms (1 mg) of vitamin B12 is generally given every day for one week, followed by 1 mg every week for four weeks and then 1 mg every month thereafter.

- Alternative treatments for pernicious anemia include high-dose oral vitamin B12, since a lower-efficiency absorption system for vitamin B12 exists in the intestine that does not require the presence of IF.

However, the oral dose required for this type of therapy (1 to 2 milligrams/day) is more than 200 times higher than the minimum daily vitamin B12 requirement for adults and is significantly higher than that available in most standard multivitamins and B12 supplements. Nasal spray and sublingual (under the tongue) preparations of vitamin B12 are also available and are under investigation.

Q2 Classify white lesion. Discuss in detail the etiopathogenesis–clinical features, diagnosis and management of oral submucous fibrosis.
Ans.

Classification

Refer to Q1 of October 1999.

Oral Submucous Fibrosis

Etiopathogenesis: Refer to Q5 September 2004. Clinical features, diagnosis and management: March 2003 Q1.

SHORT ESSAYS

Q3 Xerostomia

Ans.

Xerostomia is the medical term for the subjective complaint of dry mouth due to a lack of saliva.

Xerostomia can cause difficulty in speech and eating. It also leads to halitosis and a dramatic rise in the number of cavities, as the protective effect of salivas remineralizing the enamel is no longer present, and can make the mucosa and periodontal tissue of the mouth more vulnerable to infection

Causes

It may be a sign of an underlying disease, such as Sjögren's syndrome, poorly controll-ed diabetes, or Lambert-Eaton syndrome, but this is not always the case.

Other causes of insufficient saliva include anxiety, medications, or the consumption of alcoholic beverages, physical trauma to the salivary glands or their ducts or nerves, dehydration caused by lack of sufficient fluids, excessive breathing through the mouth, previous radiation therapy, and also a natural result of aging,

Xerostomia is a common side-effect of various drugs such as cannabis, amphetamines, antihistamines, and some antidepressants.

Treatment

Good oral hygiene maintainance. Sipping non-carbonated sugarless fluids frequently, chewing xylitol containing gum and using a carboxy-methyl cellulose saliva substitute as a a mouth-wash may help. Aquoral or pilocarpine may be prescribed to treat xerostomia.

Non-systemic relief can be found using an oxidized glycerol triesters treatment used to coat the mouth. Drinking water when there is another cause of the xerostomia besides dehydration may bring little to no relief and can even make the dry mouth more uncomfor-table

The use of an enzymatic product such as Biotene toothpaste, Biotene mouthwash, and Biotene dry mouth moisturizing liquid has been proven to reduce the rate of recurrence of dental plaque resulting from dry mouth.

Q4 Oral manifestations of diabetes

Ans.

Refer to Q6 of September 2004.

Q5 Significance of Haemogram

Ans.

A complete detailed record of the findings in a thorough examination of the blood, especially with reference to the numbers, proportions, and morphologic features of the formed elements.

Hemogram is useful in diagnosis of various diseases like: Typhoid fever, pernicious anemia, blood borne diseases.

Q6 CT in dentistry

Ans.

CAT Scans

- Computer technology in the field of dentistry now appears ready to offer a wonderful new benefit: less dental surgery. The "CAT scan" or "CT scan," named for "computed tomography" is a procedure that can create an x-ray film of very small "slices" of the body and head. It produces a picture so accurate that dentists can build an exact model of a jawbone from the computer data.
- CT scans are helpful in evaluation of mid facial trauma.
- Being able to determine the exact contours of the jaw means that the dentist no longer has to open the gums surgically and take an impression of the bone from which a plaster model is made. This is particularly important in placing dental implants under gums.

- These "subperiosteal" implants are used primarily in cases in which bone loss has created an intolerable situation for either removable dentures or for in-bone implants. The subperiosteal framework supports a permanently mounted artificial tooth, which is much more functional and stable than removable artificial teeth.

- The procedure for placing a subperiosteal implant now involves surgery to take an impression of the jawbone, construction of the implant framework and then a second surgery to implant it. With use of CT scans to determine the jaw contours, dentists and lab technicians obtain an accurate picture of the amount and thickness of bone in addition to its curves and valleys.

- Specialists in dental research are still developing the best techniques for using the CT scan and are devising ways to train more dentists and technicians in the procedure. Researchers must find the best ways, for instance, of making sure that patients don't move during the procedure — even a sigh could spoil the result. Special devices placed in the mouth put the upper and lower jaws in proper position and keep them steady while the computerized x-ray is being taken.

- Radiation exposure during the CT appears to be minimal, since the concentration is placed in very small areas which are then "layered" by the computer to give a complete picture. Preliminary studies indicate the process could cost patients about the same as a first surgery for the bone impression and possibly — eventually — even less.

- 3D Cone-Beam CT scans

- A regular X-ray can only show how "tall" the bone is; it can not show the "width." CT or "CAT" scans allow the width to be determined.

- So often times a regular X-ray, just doesn't show enough information to safely place a dental implant. A regular X-ray is a 2 dimensional image while the jaws and facial skeleton are 3-dimensional structures-therefore, they are unable to provide all the information sometimes required

- When an image has been transferred to paper, critical areas of anatomy cannot always be discerned adequately in order to safely plan. Transferring radiographic data from electronic media to paper can result in significant loss of image resolution and clarity. A dentist can plan the surgery in advance.

Q7 Production of X-rays.
Ans.
Refer to Q2 of March 2004

Q8 Mumps
Ans.
Mumps and epidemic parotitis is a viral disease of the human species, caused by the mumps virus. Before the development of vaccination and the introduction of avaccine, it was a common childhood disease worldwide, and is still a significant threat to health

Signs and symptoms
Parotid inflammation (or parotitis) in 60–70% of infections and 95% of patients with symptoms. Parotitis causes swelling and local pain, particularly when chewing. It can occur on one side (unilateral) but is more common on both sides (bilateral) in about 90% of cases
Fever

Headache
Orchitis, referring to painful inflammation of the testicle Males past puberty who develop mumps have a 30 percent risk of orchitis.
Other symptoms of mumps can include dry mouth, sore face and/or ears and occasionally in more serious cases, loss of voice. In addition, up to 20% of persons infected with the mumps

virus do not show symptoms, so it is possible to be infected and spread the virus without knowing it

Prodrome

Fever and headache are prodromal symptoms of mumps, together with malaise and anorexia.

Causes

Mumps is a contagious disease that is spread from person-to-person through contact with respiratory secretions such as saliva from an infected person. When an infected person coughs or sneezes, the droplets aerosolize and can enter the eyes, nose, or mouth of another person.

Mumps can also be spread by sharing food, sharing drinks, and kissing. The virus can also survive on surfaces and then be spread after contact in a similar manner.

A person infected with mumps is contagious from approximately 6 days before the onset of symptoms until about 9 days after symptoms start.

The incubation period (time until symptoms begin) can be from 14 to 25 days but is more typically 16 to 18 days.

Diagnosis

A physical examination confirms the presence of the swollen glands. Usually the disease is diagnosed on clinical grounds and no confirmatory laboratory testing is needed. If there is uncertainty about the diagnosis, a test of saliva, or blood may be carried out; a newer diagnostic confirmation, using real-time nested polymerase chain reaction (PCR) technology, has also been developed.

An estimated 20–30% of cases are asymptomatic. As with any inflammation of the salivary glands, serum amylase is often elevated.

Prevention

The most common preventative measure against mumps is immunization with a mumps vaccine

Treatment

- There is no specific treatment for mumps. Symptoms may be relieved by the application of intermittent ice or heat to the affected neck/testicular area and by acetaminophen/ paracetamol (Tylenol) for pain relief. Aspirin is not used due to a hypothetical link with Rayes. Salt water gargles may also help relieve symptoms.

- Patients are advised to avoid fruit juice or any acidic foods, since these stimulate the salivary glands, which can be painful.

Prognosis

- Death is very unusual. The disease is self-limiting, and general outcome is good, even if other organs are involved.

Complications of Mumps include

- Infection of other organ systems

- Mumps viral infections in adolescent and adult males carry an up to 30% risk that the testes may become infected (orchitis orepididymitis), which can be quite painful; about half of these infections result in testicular atrophy, and in rare cases sterility can follow.

- Spontaneous abortion in about 27% of cases during the first trimester of pregnancy.

- Mild forms of meningitis

- Oophoritis (inflammation of ovaries)

- Pancreatitis manifesting as abdominal pain and vomiting

- Encephalitis rare.

SHORT ANSWERS

Q9 Patch test

Ans.

A patch test is a method used to determine if a specific substance causes allergic inflammation of the skin. Any individual with eczema suspected of having allergic contact dermatitis and/or atopic dermatitis needs patch testing. A patch test relies on the principle of a type IV hypersensitivity reaction.

Process

- Prior to testing, avoid taking oral prednisone or other immuno suppressive medications for at least a week prior to testing. Steroid inhalers are OK to use. Avoid sunlight/sunburn for at least a week on the back as this may suppress positive reactions. Antihistamines such as diphenhydramine (Benadryl) or cetirizine (Zyrtec) are permissible prior to and during testing.

- Application of the patch tests will take about half an hour, though many times the overall appointment time will be longer as your provider will take an extensive history. Tiny quantities of 25 to ~150 materials (allergens) in individual square plastic or round aluminium chambers are applied to the upper back. They are kept in place with special hypoallergenic adhesive tape. The patches stay in place undisturbed for at least 48 hours. Getting the back wet during patch testing should be avoided. Vigorous exercise or stretching may disrupt the tests.

- At the second appointment, usually 48 hours later, the patches will be removed. Sometimes further patches are applied. The back is marked with an indelible black felt tip pen or other suitable marker to identify the test sites and a preliminary reading is done. These marks must be visible at the third appointment, usually 24–48 hours later (72–96 hours after application). The back

should be checked and if necessary re-marked on several occasions between the 2nd and 3rd appointments. In some cases, a reading at 7 days may be requested, especially if a special metal series is tested.

Q10 'Onion–peel' appearance on a radio graph

Ans.

Refer to Q15 of September 2004

Q11 Actinic chelitis

Ans.

Actinic cheilitis is a form of cheilitis which is the counterpart of actinic keratosis of the skin and can develop into squamous cell carcinoma. In actinic cheilitis, there is thickening whitish discoloration of the lip at the border of the lip and skin. There is also a loss of the usually sharp border between the red of the lip and the normal skin, known as the vermillion border. The lip may become scaly and indurated as actinic cheilitis progresses. The lesion is usually painless, persistent, more common in older males, and more common in individuals with a light complexion with a history of chronic sun exposure.

Causes

Actinic cheilitis is caused by chronic and excessive exposure to ultraviolet radiation in sunlight. Additional factors may also play a role, including tobacco use, lip irritation, poor oral hygiene, and ill-fitting dentures.

Treatment

This condition is considered premalignant because it may lead to squamous cell carcinoma (SCC) in about 10% of all cases. Treatment options include 5-fluorouracil, imiquimod, scalpel, vermillionetomy, chemical peel, electrosurgery, and carbon dioxide laser vaporization. These curative treatments attempt to destroy or remove the damaged epithelium. All methods are associated with some degree of pain, edema, and a relatively low rate of recurrence

Q12 Garre's osteomyelitis

Ans.

Refer Aug 2007 (RS) Q22.

Q13 Periapical granuloma

Ans.

Refer to Q4 of March 2001

Q14 Talon's cusp

Ans.

Refer to Q10 of March 2004

Q15 Frictional Keratosis

Ans.

Frictional keratosis is the oral counterpart of a callus on the skin. It is a common alteration, especially in areas of recurring, mild mechanical trauma or irritation from malposed teeth, dental prosthetics or patient habit, such as smokeless tobacco use (smokeless tobacco keratosis), exuberant toothbrushing with an overly firm brush (toothbrush keratosis), constant rubbing of the tongue against the teeth (tongue thrust keratosis), or the frequent clenching of the facial muscles, thereby pushing cheek and lips firmly against the dentition (chronic cheek bite keratosis, chronic lip bite keratosis)

Most patients with frictional keratosis are free of symptoms, with the exception of those with aggressive cheek and lip biting habits. In some individuals who repeatedly traumatize the tissues, tenderness, swelling, and a burning sensation may be presenting symptoms.

Q16 Sialadenosis

Ans.

Sialadenosis (or sialosis) has been defined as a non-inflammatory disease causing recurrent, bilateral swelling of the salivary glands, particularly the parotids which may or may not be associated with pain. The swelling is unrelated to meals and there is no particular sex predominance. The condition usually begins between the ages of 20 and 60 years, may persist for more than 20 years and may cause problems in diagnosis both clinically and histopathologically.

The aetiology is unknown but is thought to be due a peripheral neuropathy of the autonomic nerve supply of the salivary glands leading to disordered secretory activity in acinar cells. In 50% of cases the disease is associated with underlying systemic factors eluding endocrine disorders such as diabetes, malutritlon, alcohol abuse and drugs.

Differential Diagnosis

Includes sialadenitis, obstructlon due to salivary calculi, sarcoidosis, autoimune connective tissue diseases (such as Sjogren's syndrome) tumours and cysts. Sialadenosis could be associated with an underlying desease which may be endocrine, metabolic or neuronic in origin.

Surgery

A superficial parotidectomy must be performed because of the cosmetic deformity caused by the swollen gland.

Q17 Ranula

Ans.

A ranula is a type of mucocele found on the floor of the mouth. Ranulas present as aswelling of connective tissue consisting of collected mucin from a ruptured salivary gland duct, which is usually caused by local trauma.

An oral ranula is a fluctuant swelling with a bluish translucent color that somewhat resembles the underbelly of a frog Rana. If it is large (2 or more cm.), it may hide the salivary gland and affect the location of the tongue. Most frequently it stems from the sublingual salivary gland, but also from the submandibular gland.

Though normally above the mylohyoid muscle, if a ranula is found deeper in the floor of the mouth, it can appear to have a normal color. A ranula below the mylohyoid muscle is referred to as a "plunging or cervical ranula", and produces swelling of the neck with or without swelling in the floor of the mouth.

Symptoms

Ranulas may be asymptomatic, although they can fluctuate rapidly in size, shrinking and swelling, making most ranulas hard to detect. However, if it gets large enough it may interfere with swallowing. The overlying mucosa is usually intact. The swelling is not fixed and is non-painful unless it becomes secondarily infected.

Treatment of ranulas could involve either marsupialization or more often excision of both the gland and lesion. Ranulas are likely to reoccur if the sublingual gland or other gland causing them is not also removed with the lesion. There is little morbidity or mortality connected with treatment.

Q18 Inverse square law

Ans. In physics, an inverse-square law is any physical law stating that some physical quantity or strength is inversely proportional to the square of the distance from the source of that physical quantity (Fig. 24.1).

Radiographic Inspection - Formula Based on Newton's Inverse Square Law

In radiographic inspection, the radiation spreads out as it travels away from the gamma or X-ray source. Therefore, the intensity of the radiation follows Newton's Inverse Square

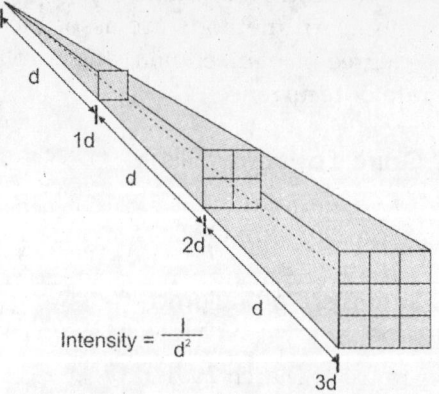

Intensity $= \frac{I}{d^2}$

Fig. 24.1: Inverse square law

Law. As shown in the image to the right, this law accounts for the fact that the intensity of radiation becomes weaker as it spreads out from the source since the same about of radiation becomes spread over a larger area. The intensity is inversely proportional to the distance from the source.

In industrial radiography, the intensity at one distance is typically known and it is necessary to calculate the intensity at a second distance. Therefore, the equation takes on the form of:

$$\frac{I_1}{I_2} = \frac{D2^2}{D1^2}$$

Where:

$I_1 =$ Intensity 1 at D_1
$I_2 =$ Intensity 2 at D_2
$D_1 =$ Distance 1 from source
$D_2 =$ Distance 2 from source

Note: This is the commonly found form of the equation. However, for some it is easier to remember that the intensity time the distance squared at one location is equal to the intensity time the distance squared at another location. The equation in this form is:

$$I_1 \times d_1^2 = I_2 \times d_2^2$$

25

RGUHS July 2008 (RS)

QUESTION PAPER
Long Essays

1. Classify oral white lesions, write the clinical features, differential diagnosis and management of oral submucous fibrosis
2. Discuss the differential diagnosis of periapical radiolucencies

Short Essays

3. Occlusal radiograph
4. Osteo radionecrosis
5. Brems strahlung radiation
6. Treatment of oral lichen planus
7. Dental considerations in pregnancy
8. Drug induced gingival hyperplasia
9. Mumps
10. Erythema multiforme
11. Management of myofacial pain dysfunction syndrome
12. Exfoliative cytology

Short Answers

13. Herpes labialis
14. Composition of developing solution
15. Decrotizing sialometaplasia
16. Pathergy test
17. Radiographic appearance of ameloblastoma
18. Mucocele
19. Plummer-Vinson syndrome
20. Median rhomboid glossitis
21. Filters
22. Ectodermal dysplasia

SOLUTIONS

LONG ESSAYS

Q1 Classify oral white lesions, white the clinical features, differential diagnosis and management of oral submucous fibrosis.
Ans.
Refer to Q2 of July 2008 old scheme.

Q2 Discuss the differential diagnosis of periapical radiolucencies.
Ans.
Refer to Q2 of March 2002.

SHORT ESSAYS

Q3 Occlusal radiograph
Ans.
Refer to Q2 of September 2003.

Q4 Osteo radionecrosis.
Ans.
Refer to Q5 of September 2000.

Q5 Bremsstrahlung radiation
Ans.
Refer to Q2 of March 2004.

Q6 Treatment of oral lichen planus.
Ans.
Refer to Q1 of October 1999.

Q7 Dental considerations in pregnancy.
Ans.
Refer Q6 Feb 2007 (RS)

Q8 Drug induced gingival hyperplasia.
Ans.
Refer Q18 Feb 2007 (OS) and Q17 2003 March

Q9 Mumps
Ans.
Refer July 2008 (OS) Q8

Q10 Erythema multiforme
Ans.
Refer to Q1 of March2004.

Q11 Management of myofacial pain dysfunction syndrome.
Ans.
Refer to March 2001 Q10

Q12 Exfoliative cytology
Ans.
Refer to September 2003 Q17.

SHORT ANSWERS

Q13 Herpes labialis
Ans.
Herpes labialis or "orolabial herpes" is an infection of the lip by herpes simplex virus. An outbreak typically causes small blisters or sores on or around the mouth commonly known as **cold sores** or **fever blisters**. The sores typically heal within 2–3 weeks, but the herpes virus remains dormant in the facial nerves, following orofacial infection, periodically reactivating (in symptomatic people) to create sores in the same area of the mouth or face at the site of the original infection

Herpes labialis infection occurs when the herpes simplex virus comes into contact with oral mucosal tissue or abraded skin of the mouth. Finger infection (herpetic whitlow) can occur when a child with cold sores or primary HSV-1 infection sucks his/her fingers.

Treatment

Acyclovir and penciclovir are used, although the shortening of duration of healing, pain and detectable virus is, at maximum, one day. Furthermore, Famciclovir and Docosanol are in use for treatment against Herpes labialis.

Laser therapy is a new option: A single 5 minute 1072 nm narrow waveband light application treatment has been shown to significantly reduce cold sore healing time by 4 days

Q14 Composition of developing solution
Ans.
Refer to Q6.2 of September 1998.

Q15 Necrotizing sialometaplasia
Ans.
Found mostly on the posterior hard palate, is due to necrosis of minor salivary glandsdue to trauma It is **a benign, self-limited lesion** (often palatal infiltrations of local anaesthetic or trauma duringintubation).

Etiology
May occur de novo after surgery or anesthesia in palatal region.

Clinical Features
It is rapidly growing self limioting lesion in the palate region .Often painless, condition is self limiting and should resolve in 6–10 weeks

Differential Diagnosis
Subacute necrotizing sialadenitis, squamous cell carcinoma or mucoepidermoid carcinoma

Q16 Pathergy test
Ans.
The pathergy test is helpful in diagnosing Behcet's Disease although not 100% specific. It is a simple test in which the forearm is pricked with a small, sterile needle. Occurrence of a small red bump or pustule at the site of needle insertion, 1 to 2 days after the test, constitutes a positive test. Although a positive pathergy test is helpful in the diagnosis of Behçet's disease, only a minority of Behçet's patients demonstrate the pathergy phenomenon (i.e., have positive tests).

Pathergy is a cutaneous phenomenon seen with both Behçet's disease and pyoderma gangrenosum

Q17 Radiographic appearance of amelo-blastoma
Ans.
Refer to Q2 of March 2000.

Q18 Mucocele
Ans.
An **oral mucocele**, is a clinical term that refers to two related phenomena: **mucus extravasation phenomenon**, and **mucus retention cyst**. The former is a swelling of connective tissue consisting of collected mucin due to a ruptured salivary gland duct usually caused by local trauma, in the case of mucus extravasation phenomenon, and an obstructed salivary duct in the case of a mucus retention cyst. The mucocele is a bluish translucent color, and is more commonly found in children and young adults. The size of oral mucoceles vary from 1 mm to several centimeters and they usually are slightly transparent with a blue tinge. On palpation, mucoceles may appear fluctuant but can also be firm. Their duration lasts from days to years, and may have recurrent swelling with occasional rupturing of its contents.

Locations
The most common location to find a mucocele is the surface of the lower lip. It can also be found on the inner side of the cheek (known as the buccal mucosa), on the anterior ventral tongue, and the floor of the mouth.

Microscopically, mucoceles appears as granulation tissue surrounding mucin. Since inflammation occurs concurrently, netrophils and foamy histiocytes usually are present.

Treatment
Some mucoceles spontaneously resolve on their own after a short time. Others are chronic and

require surgical removal. Recurrence may occur, and thus the adjacent salivary gland is excised as a preventive measure.

Q19 Plummer–Vinson syndrome
Ans.
Refer Q2 of September 1998.

Q20 Median rhomboid glossitis
Ans.
The embryonic tongue is formed by two lateral processes (lingual tubercles) meeting in the midline and fusing above a central structure from the first and second branchial arches, the tuberculum impar. The posterior dorsal point of fusion is occasionally defective, leaving a rhomboid-shaped, smooth erythematous mucosa lacking in papillae or taste buds.

- This median rhomboid glossitis (central papillary atrophy, posterior lingual papillary atrophy) is a focal area of susceptibility to recurring or chronic atrophic candidiasis, prompting a recent movement toward the use of posterior midline atrophic candidiasis as a more appropriate diagnostic term.
- Median rhomboid glossitis presents in the posterior midline of the dorsum of the tongue, just anterior to the V-shaped grouping of the circumvalate papillae. The long axis of the rhomboid or oval area of red depapillation is in the anterior-posterior direction. Most cases are not diagnosed until the middle age of the affected patient, but the entity is, of course, present in childhood. There appears to be a 3:1 male predilection.
- Lesions are typically less than 2 cm in greatest dimension and most demonstrate a smooth, flat surface, although it is not unusual for the surface to be lobulated.

Those lesions with atrophic candidiasis are usually more erythematous but some respond with excess keratin production and, therefore, show a white surface change. Infected cases may also demonstrate a midline soft palate erythema in the area of routine contact with the underlying tongue involvement; this is euphemistically referred to as a kissing lesion.

- No treatment is necessary for median rhomboid glossitis, but nodular cases are often removed for microscopic evaluation. Recurrence after removal is not expected

Q21 Filters
Ans.
One of the limitations of "**plain film**" radiography is that the X-ray beam is, for practical purposes, uniform in its intensity. A notable exception is the *anode heel effect*, but this is limited in its utility and effectiveness.

Using aluminium filters enables the utilisation of an X-ray beam which is graduated in its intensity. The shaped **aluminium filter** causes variable absorption of the X-ray beam across its change in thickness. The uses are only limited by the imagination of the radiographer.

Antero posterior mandible non-digital radiograph is taken using two identical aluminium filters. The filters are arranged with their thinnest edges touching at the midline in a *butterfly wing* configuration.

In comparison with the use of traditional aluminum filtration, a radiation dose reduction of 40% at 90 kVp and 25% at 70 kVp was found with the use of aluminum-yttrium (Al-Y) filtration for intraoral bitewing and periapical radiographs.

Advantages of Filters

Aluminium filters are one of the most useful aids available to the plain film radiographer. A selection of filters in different thicknesses , shapes and tapers allows the radiographer to select a filter whenever there is anatomy of significant varying thickness to be imaged with a single exposure. Aluminium filters are quick and easy to use. They are also long-lasting and they have the potential to save on unnecessary expenditure on film (one exposure instead of two).

The thicker the aluminium filter, the greater the beam hardening. This will reduce the radiation dose to the patient by absorbing some of the lower energy photons from the X-ray beam.

Disadvantages of Filters

The aluminium filter may produce an artifact if the edge of the filter is projected onto the film/receptor. In practice, this is of minimal concern as the image of the filter's edge is usually barely perceptible. If the radiographer is concerned that the artifact from the edge of the filter will be confusing to the radiologist, it should be labelled on the film/image.

The aluminium filter will remove lower energy photons from the X-ray beam. Whilst this will reduce the radiation dose to the patient, it will also cause a reduction in image contrast. This is not usually a problem, but is worthy of consideration when using thick filtration, and will be most noticeable when two filters are *"piggy backed"* together. Of course, patient anatomy is better displayed at reduced contrast rather than not at all.

Q22 Ectodermal dysplasia
Ans.
Refer Q14 2007 Feb

26

RGUHS January 2009

QUESTION PAPER
Long Essays

1. Classify the various causes of orofacial pain. Discuss in detail the clinical features, diagnosis and management of trigeminal neuralgia
2. Enumerate the causes of faulty radiographs. Discuss the measures to rectify them

Short Essays

3. Pindborg's tumour
4. Alkaline phosphatase
5. Herpes zoster
6. Radiation mucositis
7. Oral hairy leukoplakia
8. Significance of medical history

Short Answers

9. 'Hair on end' appearance
10. Gorlin Sign
11. Melkerson – Rosenthal syndrome
12. 'Jug handle' view
13. Mesiodens
14. Tzanck test
15. Leukoedema
16. 'Moth eaten' appearance
17. Tobacco pouch Keratosis
18. Osteoarthritis of TMJ

SOLUTIONS

LONG ESSAYS

Q1 Classify the various causes of orofacial pain. Discuss in detail the clinical features, diagnosis and management of trigeminal neuralgia.
Ans.

Classification causes of Orofacial Pain

Refer to Q1 of September 2004

Trigeminal Neuralgia

Q4 of March 2004 and Q1 of September 1998.

Q2 Enumerate the causes of faulty radiographs. Discuss the measures to rectify them.
Ans.
Refer Q4 of September 1998.

SHORT ESSAYS

Q3 Pindborg's tumor.
Ans.
Also called as calcifying odontogenic tumor first described by Pindborg in 1956.

Clinical Features

- Middle ages with a range from 8 yrs to 92 yrs. No sexual preponderance
- Mandible to maxilla ratio is 2:1 and prevalence in molar regions is 3 times the bicuspid region
- Painless swelling. 52% of the cases are associated with unerupted or impacted tooth
- Extraosseous C.O.T. occurrence, though rare has been reported to occur in the middle ages

Radiographic Features

- Early in the development the tumor reveals a radiolucent area around the crown of a mature unerupted tooth
- Periphery–well defined cyst like cortical border
- Internal–unilocular or multilocular with numerous scattered radiopaque foci of varying size and density. Radioopacity close to crown of embedded tooth is the characteristic finding.
- Histology shows – polyhedral epithelial cells in bland fibrous connective tissue stroma. Tumor cells have well outlined border with a fine granular eosinophillic cytoplasm and prominent intercellular bridges with polymorphic nuclei. Mitotic figures are rare.
- Clear cell variant exhibit a clear cytoplasm with round or oval nucleus in the centre.
- Presence of homogenous eosinophillic substance can lead to confusion with amyloid deposits.
- Sometimes there is presence of calcification in the form of Lisesegang rings.

Effects on Surrounding Structures

CEOT may displace a developing tooth or prevent its eruption. Associated expansion of the jaw with maintainence of a cortical boundary may also occur.

Differential Diagnosis

- Dentigerous cyst
- Ameloblastoma
- AOT
- Ameloblastic fibroodontoma
- Calcifying odontogenic cyst

Treatment

Local resection.

Q4 Alkaline phosphatase
Ans.
Refer to Q12 of March 2001.

Q5 Herpes zoster.

Ans.

Herpes zoster (or simply **zoster**), commonly known as **shingles** and also known as **zona**, is a viral disease characterized by a painful skin rash with blisters in a limited area on one side of the body, often in a stripe. The initial infection with varicella zoster virus (VZV) causes the acute (short-lived) illness chickenpox which generally occurs in children and young people.

Varicella zoster virus can become latent in the nerve cell bodies and less frequently in non-neuronal satellite cells of dorsal root, cranial nerve or autonomic ganglion, without causing any symptoms. Years or decades after a chickenpox infection, the virus may break out of nerve cell bodies and travel down nerve axons to cause viral infection of the skin in the region of the nerve. The virus may spread from one or more ganglia along nerves of an affected segment and infect the corresponding dermatome(an area of skin supplied by one spinal nerve) causing a painful rash.

Signs and Symptoms

The earliest symptoms of herpes zoster, which include headache, fever, and malaise, are nonspecific, and may result in an incorrect diagnosis. These symptoms are commonly followed by sensations of burning pain, itching, hyperesthesia(oversensitivity), or paresthesia ("pins and needles": tingling, pricking, or numbness). The pain may be mild to extreme in the affected dermatome, with sensations that are often described as stinging, tingling, aching, numbing or throbbing, and can be interspersed with quick stabs of agonizing pain.

In most cases, after 1–2 days (but sometimes as long as 3 weeks) the initial phase is followed by the appearance of the characteristic skin rash., herpes zoster causes skin changes limited to a dermatome, normally resulting in a stripe or belt-like pattern that is limited to one side of the body and does not cross the midline. Later, the rash becomes vesicular, forming small blisters filled with a serous exudate, as the fever and general malaise continue. The painful vesicles eventually become cloudy or darkened as they fill with blood, crust over within seven to ten days, and usually the crusts fall off and the skin heals; but sometimes, after severe blistering, scarring and discolored skin remain. *Herpes zoster oticus*, also known as Ramsay Hunt syndrome type II, involves the ear. *Herpes zoster ophthalmicus* involves the orbit of the eye

Prevention

A live vaccine for VZV exists, marketed as Zostavax

Treatment

The aims of treatment are to limit the severity and duration of pain, shorten the duration of a shingles episode, and reduce complications. Symptomatic treatment is often needed for the complication of postherpetic neuralgia.

Q6 Radiation mucositis.

Ans.

Refer Q4. October 1999

Q7 Oral hairy leukoplakia.

Ans.

Refer Q3 march 2002

Q8 Significance of medical history.

Ans.

The **medical history** or **anamnesis** of a patient is information gained by a physician by asking specific questions, either of the patient or of other people who know the person and can give suitable information (in this case, it is sometimes called **hetero-anamnesis**), with the aim of obtaining information useful in formulating a diagnosis and providing medical care to the patient. The medically relevant complaints reported by the patient or others familiar with the patient are referred to as symptoms, in contrast with clinical signs, which are ascertained by direct examination on the part of medical personnel

Gathering a patient's medical history and giving a physical examination can be important parts of both routine office visits and checkups as well as in emergency situations. Both aspects of routine patient care can help to diagnose any current injuries, illnesses or conditions. Knowing the different aspects of proper patient care, and being able to place in a doctor's office, medical history is usually collected in the waiting room using a form on which the patient records all previous allergies, ailments, conditions and surgeries. The more information that can accurately and efficiently be gathered about a patient, the greater the likelihood that a patient will receive successful treatment.

Patient Medical History

The patient's medical history is a list of pertinent history related to the patient. In the doctor's office, the medical history is gathered covering nearly all of the procedures or ailments that the patient has experienced during her lifetime.

Process

A practitioner typically asks questions to obtain the following information about the patient:

- Identification and demographics: name, age, height, weight.
- The "chief complaint (CC)" - the major health problem or concern, and its time course (e.g. chest pain for past 4 hours).
- History of the present illness
- Past medical history (PMH) (including major illnesses, any previous surgery/operations, any current ongoing illness, e.g. diabetes).

- Review of systems (ROS) Systematic questioning about different organ systems
- Family diseases-especially those relevant to the patient's chief complaint.
- Childhood diseases
- Social history (medicine) - including living arrangements, occupation, marital status, number of children, drug use (including tobacco, alcohol, other recreational drug use), recent foreign travel, and exposure to environmental pathogens through recreational activities or pets.
- Regular and acute medications
- Allergies - to medications, food, latex, and other environmental factors
- Sexual history, obstetric/gynecological history, and so on, as appropriate.

SHORT ANSWERS

Q9 'Hair on end' appearance
Ans.
Refer to Q3 of March 2001.

Q10 Gorlin Sign
Ans.
Unusual ease in touching the tip of the nose with the tongue; seen in Ehlers-Danlos syndrome.

A connective-tissue disorder characterised by hyperelasticity of skin, poor wound healing, hyperextensibility of joints, soft-tissue calcifications (spheroids), vascular lesions: aortic dissection, aneurysms, rarely: tortuous arch, ectatic pulmonary artery, tissue fragility most likely to be haematomas, aortic rupture after angiography, clinical types: Gravis, mitis, benign hypermobile, ecchymotic, X-linked, associated with medullary sponge kidney.
Inheritance: Autosomal dominant, X-linked.

Q11 Melkerson–Rosenthal syndrome.
Ans.
Melkersson–Rosenthal syndrome is a rare neurological disorder characterized by

recurring facial paralysis, swelling of the face and lips (usually the upper lip), and the development of folds and furrows in the tongue.

- Onset is in childhood or early adolescence. After recurrent attacks (ranging from days to years in between), swelling may persist and increase, eventually becoming permanent. The lip may become hard, cracked, and fissured with a reddish-brown discoloration.

- The cause of Melkersson-Rosenthal syndrome is unknown, but there may be a genetic pre-disposition. It can be symptomatic of Crohn's disease or sarcoidosis.

- Treatment is symptomatic and may include medication therapies with nonsteroidal anti-inflammatory drugs (NSAIDs) and corticosteroids to reduce swelling, as well as antibiotics and immunosuppressants. Surgery may be recommended to relieve pressure on the facial nerves and to reduce swollen tissue, but its effectiveness has not been established. Massage and electrical stimulation may also be prescribed

Q12 'Jug handle' view.
Ans.

A modified basal view of the skull used to visualize the zygomatic arches, of interest in evaluating midfacial fractures. Helpful in diagnosis of LeFort fracture,especially zygomatic arch fracture is diagnosed by submento vertex view which gives a excellent detail of zygomatic arch which resembles jug handle

Fractures of the zygoma usually result from a direct blow to the arch or to the zygomatic process.

The arch and the skull form a rigid bony ring. Just like a pretzel, it cannot be broken in only one place. The view that should be ordered if an arch fracture is suspected is the "jug handle" view. If only one fracture is seen in the arch, then films of the facial bones should be obtained to exclude a so-called tripod fracture. The tripod fracture results from a direct blow to the zygomatic process. It actually consists of four fractures, not three, as the name suggests. The fractures are of the zygomatic arch, lateral orbital rim, inferior orbital rim, and lateral wall of the maxillary sinus.

Refer Submentovertex projection for detail explanation. Q8 of March 2003

Q13 Mesiodens
Ans.

Supernumerary teeth are a relatively frequent disorder of odontogenesis characterized by an excess number of teeth. Mesiodens is the most common type of supernumerary tooth found in the premaxilla between the two central incisors. They can be supplemental (resembling natural teeth), conical, tuberculate or molariform.

They can be well formed or just little clumps of tooth like stuff. A related phenomenon is the odontoma. They are often discovered on a routine X-ray or perhaps if the teeth are not erupting in a normal manner.

Treatment options may include surgical extraction of the mesiodens. If the permanent teeth do not erupt in a reasonable period after the extraction, surgical exposure and orthodontic treatment may be required to ensure eruption and proper alignment of the teeth.

Q14 Tzanck test
Ans.
Refer to Q11 of September 2004.

Q15 Leukoedema
Ans.
Leukoedema is a normal variation of the buccal mucosa, or inside surface of the cheek. It presents as a white-bluish tinge of the buccal mucosa but the color disappears when the cheek is stretched

Clinical Feature

It appears as a filmy opaque, white to slate gray discoloration of mucosa, chiefly buccal mucosa. Redundancy of the mucosa may impart a folded or wrinkled appearance to the relaxed mucous membrane. It partially disappears when the mucosa is stretched. It is stated to be seen in 90% of Blacks and 40% of Whites.

Etiology

Leukoedema is a variation of normal which should not be confused with something ominous. Intracellular edema of the superficial epithelial cells coupled with retention of superficial parakeratin is thought to account for the white appearance. It is more prevalent in people who have dark skin and can be more intense in smokers.

Histologically, the white appearance is caused by water within the spinous cells causing the light to reflect back as whitish.

Treatment

None

Prognosis

Good

Differential Diagnosis

White sponge nevus, hereditary benign intraepithelial dyskeratosis, and dyskeratosis congenita. All are extremely rare. This aids to differentiate this lesion from other similar looking conditions which could be premalignant, such as leukoplakia.

Q16 'Moth eaten' appearance.
Ans.
Refer to Q3 of March 2001.

Q17 Tobacco pouch Keratosis.
Ans.
Smokeless tobacco keratosis (snuff pouch, snuff dipper's lesion, tobacco pouch) is a chronic white or gray/translucent mucosal macule localized in areas of direct contact with smokeless tobacco. The lesion cannot be scraped off, disappears with cessation of the tobacco habit, and is poorly demarcated from surrounding mucosa. Typically there is a soft, velvety feel to the altered mucosa and further palpation of a tobacco chewer's cheek will usually reveal a distinct "pouch" caused by flaccidity in the chronically stretched muscles in the area of tobacco placement. As tobacco is not in the mouth during a clinical examination the usually stretched mucosa appears folded or fissured. Induration, ulceration and pain are not associated with this lesion but occasional inflammatory erythema may be noted.

The development of smokeless tobacco keratosis in users is very much dependent on the type of habit popular in a society. Snuff appears to produce more keratoses, for example, than chewing tobacco, and persons who keep their quid in one site are more prone to keratoses than those using multiple sites. Other factors leading to high risk of keratosis include the specific brand of tobacco used, an extended duration of the habit, an excessive daily contact-hours of tobacco on oral mucous membranes, an increased amount of tobacco consumed daily, and a deficiency of beta-keratin or vitamin A.

Q18 Osteoarthritis of TMJ.
Ans.
Refer to Q7 of August 2007 (OS)

QUESTION PAPER

Long Essays

1. Classify salivary gland diseases. Describe the various causes, clinical features and the management of sialadenitis
2. Describe in detail technique, advantages and limitations of bisecting angle technique of periapical radiography

Short Essays

3. Oral manifestations of AIDS
4. Multilocular radiolucencies (rep in DEC 09- old scheme)
5. Osteo radionecrosis
6. Filtration
7. Localization of impacted canine in maxilla
8. Caries activity tests
9. Endogenous pigmentation of oral mucosa
10. Toluidine blue test
11. Corticosteroids in oral diseases
12. Hamartomas

Short Answers

13. Nutrient canals
14. Turner's hypoplasia
15. Onion skin radiographic appearance
16. Penny tests
17. Wickhams striae
18. Sturge-Weber syndrome
19. Pathergy test
20. Nikolsky's sign
21. Fordyce's granules
22. Kveim – siltz bach test

LONG ESSAYS

Q1 Classify salivary gland diseases. Describe the various causes, clinical features and the management of sialadenitis.

Ans.

Classification I

- Obstructive and Inflammatory disorders
  - Sialolithiasis
  - Bacterial sialadenitis
  - Sialodochitis
  - Autoimmune sialadenitis.
- Non inflammatory disorders
  - Sialadenosis
  - Cystic lesions
- Benign tumors
- Malignant tumours

Classification II

A. Reactive lesions
- Mucocele
- Mucus retention cysts
- Sialolitiasis
- Chronic sclerosing sialadenitis
- Necrotizing sialometaplasia

B. Salivary infections
- Acute parotitis
- Viral endemic parotitis(Mumps)
- Bacterial sialadenitis

C. Immune related diseases
- Lymphoepithelial sialadenitis
- Sjogren Syndrome.

D. Salivary gland tumors

Benign
- Pleomorphic adenoma
- Monomorphic adenoma
- Papillary cystadenoma
- Oncocytoma
- Other adenomas

Malignant
- Mucoepidermoid carcinoma.
- Adenoid cystic carcinoma
- Acinic cell carcinoma
- Polymorphous low grade adenocarcinoma
- Other adenocarcinomas

Classification III

Functional
- *Sialorrhea (increase in salivary flow):* Psychosis, mental retardation, neurological disorders, rabies
- *Xerostomia (decrease in salivary flow):* Mumps, sarcoidosis, sjogrens syndrome, lupus, post irradiation
- Mucocele
- Ranula

Obstructive
- Sialolithiasis: Submandibular gland 92%, parotid gland 6%

Non-neoplastic
- Acute sialadenitis
- Chronic sialadenitis
- Necrotising sialometaplasia is a benign inflammatory condition involving minor salivary gland

Neoplastic

Adenomas
- Pleomorphic adenoma
- Monomorphic adenoma
- Adenolymphoma adenoma
- Oxyphic adenoma
- Others

Salivary gland tumours
- Mucoepidermoid tumor
- Acinic cell tumor

Carcinomas
- Adenoid cystic carcinoma
- Adenocarcionoma
- Epidermoid carcinoma
- Undifferenciated cell carcinoma
- In pleomorphic adenoma

Non epithelial
- Malignant lymphoma
- Unclassified tumor

Allied conditions
- Benign lymphoepithelial lesion
- Sialosis
- Oncocytosis

Sialadenitis is inflammation of a salivary gland. It may be subdivided temporally into acute, chronic and recurrent forms.
Acute form

Causes

- Decreased flow (dehydration, post-op, drugs)
- Poor oral hygiene
- Exacerbation of low grade chronic sialadenitis

Clinical Features

- Painful swelling
- Reddened skin
- Oedema of the cheek, Periorbital region and neck
- Low grade fever
- Malaise
- Raised ESR, CRP, leucocytosis
- Purulent exudate from duct punctum

Chronic form Clinical Features

- Unilateral
- Mild pain/swelling

- Common after meals
- Duct orifice is reddened and flow decreases
- May or may not have visible/palpable stone.
- Parotid gland
- Recurrent painful swellings
- Submandibular gland
- Usually secondary to sialolithiasis or stricture

The first step in getting correct treatment is to get a correct diagnosis. Differential diagnosis list for Sialadenitis may include:
- Sialolithiasis
- Salivary gland tumour
- Facial cellulitis (*type of* Cellulitis)
- Dental abscess
- TMJ syndrome

Treatment

Supportive treatment for viral adenitis
- Bacterial sialoadenitis requires antibiotic therapy with warm compresses and sialogogues to help promote salivary flow; IV antibiotic therapy may be required in severe cases
- Sialolithiasis is treated with surgical excision of the stone or the gland
- Hemangiomas are simply observed unless rapid growth, functional impairment, infection, bleeding, or severe cosmetic deformity is present
- Tumors are treated surgically
  - Parotid neoplasms that are lateral are treated with superficial parotidectomy; submandibular neoplasms require total submandibular gland excision.
  - If malignancy is suspected, neck dissection is performed when palpable lymphadenopathy is present and considered for high-grade lesions.
  - Possible radiation therapy based on final pathology.

Radiation Exposure: Treatment

Treatment is essentially aimed at relieving symptoms and includes antiemetics to counter nausea and vomiting, fluid and electrolyte replacement, antibiotics, and possibly sedatives (if seizures occur). Transfusions of plasma, platelets, and red blood cells may be necessary. Bone marrow transplantation is a controversial treatment but may be the only recourse in extreme cases. When radiation exposure results from inhalation or ingestion of large amounts of radioactive iodine, potassium iodide or a strong iodine solution may be given to block thyroid uptake.

Q2 Describe in detail technique, advantages and limitations of bisecting angle technique of periapical radiography.
Ans.
Bisecting angle technique Refer to Q5 sept 1998.

Advantages

Bitewing radiography may still be used in individual caries diagnosis and clinical trials for detecting demineralization caused by microbial activity on the tooth surface: the caries lesion. Radiography plays a part in monitoring lesion development over time, since remineralization procedures can arrest or reverse progression of the lesion and lead to changes in mineral quality and quantity. The evidence for dental caries is not restricted to the levels of surface cavitation, and radiography can add information about many of the clinical stages of the caries process at approximal surfaces and the more advanced stages on occlusal surfaces. Refer March 1999 Q5

Limitations

- Periapical radiographs show one or two teeth in focus so the abscess formed near adjacent tooth may be missed and false diagnosis is possible.

- Overlapping of teeth may mimic concrescense,
- Interdental caries may be difficult to diagnose
- Occlusal caries may be overlapped
- Periapical radiographs are prone for cone cuts if angulation and centration of the X-ray.

SHORT ESSAYS

Q3 Oral manifestations of AIDS
Ans.
Refer to Q1 of September 2000.

Q4 Multilocular radiolucencies.
Ans.
Refer Q4 Aug 2007 (RS)

Q5 Osteo radionecrosis
Ans.
Refer to Q5 of September 2000 and 2002.

Q6 Filtration
Ans.
Refer to March 2002 Q8 solution.

Q7 Localization of impacted canine in maxilla.
Ans.
Refer Q6 Aug 2007 (RS)

Q8 Caries activity tests
Ans.
A test used to predict the probability of developing new or increased decay; may include assessments of saliva and plaque for the presence of certain designated micro-organisms or studies of salivary secretion and sugar clearance.

Requirements of Caries Activity Test

Test should be reproducible and valid. There should be good correlation between caries activity scores and actual caries development.

It should be simple. Results should be obtained within hours or few days. Should have measurement of mechanisms involved in caries process should be inexpensive, non invasive and applicable to clinical sitting.

Types of Tests

Snyder Test

Snyder test measures the ability of salivary microorganisms to form organic acid from the carbohydrate medium.

A calorimetric test for evaluating caries activity or susceptibility. Saliva is brought in contact with an acid agar to which is added glucose and bromcreosol green as indicator. Acid producing microorganisms (e.g. lactobacillus) in the saliva make the colour change from blue-green to yellow. A rapid change of colour indicates high caries activity.

Colour change to yellow:

- In 24 hours marked caries activity
- In 48 hours definite caries activity caries
- In 72 hours limited caries activity

Lactobacillus Colony Count Test

Saliva is collected by chewing paraffin before breakfast. Sample is shaken and 0.1 cc is withdrawn.

Diluted and undiluted samples are spread evenly over the SL rogosa's agar plate. The plate is incubated for 4 days and no. of colonies that are developed are counted.

No. of organisms	Symbolic designation suggested	Degree of caries activity
1–1000	+	Little or none
1000–5000	+	Slight
5000–10,000	++	moderate
More than 10,000	+++/++++	marked

Alben's Test

It's a modified snyder test. In this at the time of test the 5 ml semisolid agar is removed from refrigerator but not heated. The patient is asked to spit unstimulated saliva directly in to the tube and is incubated for 4 days

Swab Test

Advantage in no collection of saliva is necessary and is valuable in evaluating caries activity in very young children. The oral flora is sampled by swabbing the buccal surface of tooth with cotton.

Reductase Test

Measures the activity of reductase enzyme. Sample is mixed with equal amount of diazo-resorcinol. Change in colour after 15 mins is taken as a measure of caries activity.

Blue: 15 mins non conductive
Orchid: 15 mins slightly conductive
Red: 15 mins moderately conductive
Red: Immediately highly conductive
Pink: Immediately extremely conductive

Enamel solubility Test

Based on the fact that when glucose is added to saliva containing powdered enamel the organic acids are formed.

Organic acid decalcifies the enamel, resulting in the increase in the soluble calcium. The extent of increase of calcium is direct measure of caries activity.

Saliva Flow Test

Flow rate is determined and reduced rate indicates the caries susceptibility.

Q9 Endogenous pigmentation of oral mucosa
Ans.
Refer to September 2001 Q1 solution

Q10 Toluidine blue test

Ans.

Refer to March 2004 Q9 solution.

Q11 Corticosteroids in oral diseases

Ans.

Refer to Q5 of March 2004

Q12 Hamartomas

Ans.

Refer to Q12 of February 2007 (RS)

SHORT ANSWERS

Q13 Nutrient canals

Ans.

Nutrient canals appear in a small number of patients as radiolucent lines extending vertically from the inferior dental canal to the interdental space between the mandibular incisors. Occasionally the canals may appear as small round radiolucencies perpendicular to the cortex and can be mistaken for pathology.

The incidence of nutrient canals was very high in patients with periodontal disease, in patients of advanced age, and especially in endentulous patients. Nutrient canals appeared most frequently in radiographs demonstrating "above average" bone density with small diminutive trabecular spaces. Other factors influencing the presence of nutrient canals included the thickness of the alveolar bone, the quality of both cortical and cancellous bone, and the loss of mandibular teeth.

Q14 Turner's hypoplasia

Ans.

Enamel hypoplasia due to local infection or trauma is called as Turner's hypoplasia. Generally only a single tooth is involved and hence it is also called as Turner's teeth.

Most common tooth involved is permanent maxillary incisor or a maxillary or mandibular premolar. Pathogenesis involves carried deciduous tooth which leads to infection eating away the forming crown of the permanent tooth.

The severity of the hypoplasia depends upon the severity of the infection and the stage of the permanent tooth in formation.

Q15 Onion skin radiographic appearance

Ans.

Refer to Q15 of September 2004.

Q16 Penny tests

Ans.

One half of all hyperthyroids had clinically diagnosed anemia. Other half were also anemic but not diagnosed because they had copper-deficiency anemia and not iron-deficiency anemia.

Anemia is usually caused by a deficiency of hemoglobin which is the oxygen carrying molecule in the red blood cell. While many minerals are important in the body's manufacture of hemoglobin, iron and copper are the most important. A deficiency of either iron or copper will result in anemia, either iron-deficiency anemia or copper-deficiency anemia.

Anemia is often medically diagnosed by determining blood levels of iron and the iron-carrying protein ferritin. This test will determine anemia if the anemia is due to iron deficiency. However, this test will not show if the person has copper-deficiency anemia.

It seems that many doctors are unaware of copper-deficiency anemia and will try to correct all cases of anemia by prescribing very large doses of iron. Since the majority of cases of anemia are probably the result of iron deficiency, then this procedure usually works. However, in copper-deficiency anemia, taking excess amounts of iron will further deplete copper and cause the anemia to worsen.

Q17 Wickhams striae

Ans.

Oral lichen planus (OLP) may present in one of three forms. The reticular form is the most common presentation and manifests as white lacy streaks on the mucosa (known as Wickham's striae) or as smaller papules (small raised). The lesions tend to be bilateral and are asymptomatic. The lacy streaks may also be seen on other area parts of the mouth, including the gingiva (gums), the tongue, palate and lips.

Q18 Sturge–Weber syndrome

Ans.

Refer March 2003 Q13

Q19 Pathergy test

Ans.

Refer July 2008 (RS) Q16.

Q20 Nikolsky's sign

Ans.

Refer March 2002 Q11

Q21 Fordyce's granules

Ans.

Refer Aug 2005 Q11

Q22 Kveim-siltz bach test

Ans.

The Kveim test, Nickerson-Kveim or Kveim-Siltzbach test is a skin test used to detect sarcoidosis, where part of a spleen from a patient with known sarcoidosis is injected into the skin of a patient suspected to have the disease. If granulomas are found (4–6 weeks later), the test is positive. If the patient has been on treatment (e.g. glucocorticoids), the test may be false negative. The test is not commonly performed. There is a concern that certain infections, such as bovine spongiform encephalopathy, could be transferred through a Kveim test.

It is named for the Norwegian pathologist Morten Ansgar Kveim, who first reported the test in 1941 using lymph node tissue from sarcoidosis patients.

QUESTION PAPER

Long Essays

1. Classify red and white lesions. Describe etiology, clinical features and treatment plan of leukoplakia.
2. What is ionizing radiation? Describe the biological effects of excessive radiation on orofacial structures.

Short Essays

3. Congenital syphilis.
4. Radiographic features of ameloblastoma.
5. Position indicating device.
6. Oral manifestations of leukemia.
7. Sialolith.
8. X-ray film.
9. Bell's palsy.
10. Differential diagnosis of bald tongue.
11. Stevens-Johnson syndrome.
12. Manual film processing

Short Answers

13. Treatment of acute necrotizing ulcerative gingivitis.
14. ALARA principle.
15. Mesiodens.
16. Plummer-Vinson syndrome.
17. Café-au-lait pigmentation.
18. Composition of dental x-ray film.
19. Black hairy tongue.
20. Indications of bitewing radiographs.
21. Nikolsky's sign.
22. Globulomaxillary cyst.

SOLUTIONS

LONG ESSAYS

Q1 Classify red and white lesions. Describe etiology, clinical features and treatment plan of leukoplakia.

Ans.

Refer to Q3.1 of march 1999, Q1 of October 1999, Q8 of March 2000, Q2 of February 2002 (RS) and Q3 of March 2004.

Q2 What is ionizing radiation? Describe the biological effects of excessive radiation on orofacial structures.

Ans.

Ionizing radiation consists of subatomic particles or electromagnetic waves that are energetic enough to detach electrons from atoms or molecules, thus ionizing them. The occurrence of ionization depends on the energy of the individual particles or waves, and not on their number. An intense flood of particles or waves will not cause ionization if these particles or waves do not carry enough energy to be ionizing. Roughly speaking, particles or photons with energies above a few electron volts (eV) are ionizing (Fig. 28.1).

Examples of ionizing particles are energetic alpha particles, beta particles, and neutrons. The ability of an electromagnetic wave (photons) to ionize an atom or molecule depends on its frequency. Radiation on the short-wavelength end of the electromagnetic spectrum—high frequency ultraviolet, X-rays, and gamma rays—is ionizing.

Ionizing radiation comes from radioactive materials, X-ray tubes, particle accelerators, and

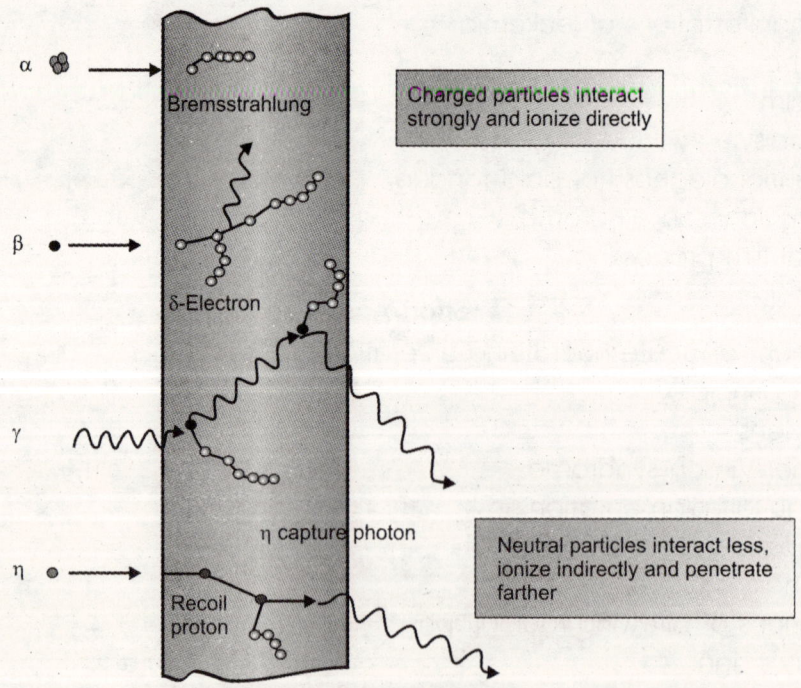

Fig. 28.1: Ionizing radiation

is present in the environment. It is invisible and not directly detectable by human senses, so instruments such as Geiger counters are usually required to detect its presence. In some cases it may lead to secondary emission of visible light upon interaction with matter, as in Cherenkov radiation and radioluminescence. It has many practical uses in medicine, research, construction, and other areas, but presents a health hazard if used improperly. Exposure to radiation causes damage to living tissue, resulting in skin burns, radiation sickness and death at high doses and cancer, tumors and DNA damage at low doses.

An ionization event normally produces a positive atomic ion and an electron. High-energy beta particles may produce bremsstrahlung when passing through matter, or secondary electrons (ä-electrons); both can ionize in turn. Energetic Beta-particles. like those emitted by 32P, are quickly decelerated when passing through matter. The energy lost to deceleration is emitted in the form of X-rays called "Bremsstrahlung" which translates "Braking Radiation". Bremsstrahlung is of concern when shielding beta emitters. The intensity of bremsstrahlung increases with the increase in energy of the electrons or the atomic number of the absorbing medium.

Refer to Q4 of October 1999 for the second part of the question.

SHORT ESSAYS

Q3 Congenital Syphilis
Ans.

Congenital syphilis is syphilis present in utero and at birth, and occurs when a child is born to a mother with secondary syphilis. Untreated syphilis results in a high risk of a bad outcome of pregnancy, including Mulberry molars in the fetus. Syphilis can cause miscarriages, premature births, stillbirths, or death of newborn babies. Some infants with congenital syphilis have symptoms at birth, but most develop symptoms later. Untreated babies can have deformities, delays in development, or seizures along with many other problems such as rash, fever, swollen liver and spleen, anemia, and jaundice. Sores on infected babies are infectious. Rarely, the symptoms of syphilis go unseen in infants so that they develop the symptoms of late-stage syphilis, including damage to their bones, teeth, eyes, ears, and brain.

According to the CDC, 40% of births to syphilitic mothers are stillborn, 40–70% of the survivors will be infected, and 12% of these will subsequently die in infancy.

Manifestations of Congenital Syphillis

- Abnormal X-rays.
- Hutchinson's triad, a set of symptoms consisting of deafness, Hutchinson' teeth (centrally notched, widely-spaced peg-shaped upper central incisors); and interstitial keratitis (IK), an inflammation of the cornea which can lead to corneal scarring and potentially blindness.
- Mulberry molars (sixth year molars with multiple poorly developed cusps).
- Frontal bossing.
- Poorly developed maxillae.
- Enlarged liver.
- Enlarged spleen.
- Petechiae.
- Other skin rash.
- Sabre shins.
- Anemia.
- Lymph node enlargement.
- Jaundice.
- Pseudoparalysis.
- Snuffles, the name given to rhinitis in this situation. When chronic, this can lead to saddle nose deformity.
- Rhagades, linear scars at the angles of the mouth and nose result from bacterial infection of skin lesions.

- Higoumenakis sign, enlargement of the sternal end of clavicle in late congenital syphilis.

Death from congenital syphilis is usually through pulmonary hemorrhage.

Treatment

If a pregnant mother is identified as being infected with syphilis, treatment can effectively prevent congenital syphilis from developing in the unborn child, especially if she is treated before the sixteenth week of pregnancy. The child is at greatest risk of contracting syphilis when the mother is in the early stages of infection, but the disease can be passed at any point during pregnancy, even during delivery (should the child have not contracted it already). However, a woman in the secondary stage of syphilis decreases her child's risk of developing congenital syphilis by 98% if she receives treatment before the last month of pregnancy. An afflicted child can be treated using antibiotics much like an adult, however any developmental symptoms are likely to be permanent.

Q4 Radiographic features of ameloblastoma.
Ans.
Refer to Q2 of March 2000.

Q5 Position indicating device.
Ans.
A position indicating device for dental X-ray machines is a device comprising of a lead lined tubular member having an X-ray receiving end and an X-ray emitting end, with the tubular member at its X-ray receiving end being in the form of a hub portion in which the collimator is mounted. This hub portion is journaled in an adapter member that is formed for securement to the specific X-ray machine to which the positioning indicating device is to be applied. The journaling of the PID relative to the adapter member is such that the PID makes no movement axially thereof, relative to the adapter member, or the X-ray machine, on adjustment of same about the axis of the cone.

The tip of the PID or aiming cylinder should be closely aligned with the X-ray beam so as to keep the field diameter for dental intraoral X-ray machines no greater than 2.75 inches. This may be evaluated by making a star pattern with dental films, marking them with pinholes and centering the aiming cylinder over the pattern. Then expose the films using bitewing values, process the films and reconstitute the star pattern. The size and alignment of the beam can then be determined.

Q6 Oral manifestations of leukemia.
Ans.
Common oral findings in leukemia include spontaneous gingival hemorrhaging and small petechial hemorrhages or bruising of the oral soft tissue secondary to thrombocytopenia. Leukemic patients are more prone to oral candidiasis, herpetic infections, and neutropenic ulceration. These ulcers are typically deep, punched-out lesions with a gray-white necrotic base. They occur most commonly after chemotherapeutics, related to mucosal trauma or opportunistic infections. Acute leukemias, particularly acute monocytic and myelogenous subtypes, cause infiltration of leukemic cells into oral soft tissue, especially gingival tissue, resulting in swollen, boggy hyperplastic gingivitis.

Q7 Sialolith.
Ans.
Refer to Q7 of March 2001.

Q8 X-ray film.
Ans.
Refer to Q16 of September 2002.

Q9 Bell's palsy.

Ans.

Refer to Q4 of September 2003.

Q10 Differential diagnosis of bald tongue.

Ans.

Refer to Q5 of January 2008 (RS).

Q11 Stevens-Johnson syndrome.

Ans.

Refer to Q8 of September 2000.

Q12 Manual film processing

Ans.

Refer to Q6 of February 2007 (OS).

SHORT ANSWERS

Q13 Treatment of acute necrotizing ulcerative gingivitis.

Ans.

Refer to Q10 of September 2000.

Q14 ALARA principle.

Ans.

"ALARA" is an acronym for "As Low As Reasonably Achievable". ALARA is a basic radiation protection concept or philosophy. It is an application of the "Linear No Threshold Hypothesis," which assumes that there is no "safe" dose of radiation. Under this assumption, the probability for harmful biological effects increases with increased radiation dose, no matter how small. Therefore, it is important to keep radiation doses to affected populations (for example, radiation workers, minors, visitors, students, members of the general public, etc.) as low as is reasonably achievable. ALARA is not a dose limit, but rather a goal. It exemplifies a mind set to achieve radiation exposures which are as far below the applicable limits as is reasonably achievable.

Implementing the ALARA concept involves six basic principles. These are:

- Eliminating or reducing the source of radiation—Source reduction is a reduction in the dose rate
- Containing the source—Containment involves using leak-tight or controlled-opening enclosures to prevent radioactive materials from migrating to areas where we don't want them
- Minimizing the time spent in a radiation field—the less time spent in a radiation field, the lower the dose
- Maximizing the distance from a radiation source—the further away from a radiation source you are, the lower the dose
- Using radiation shielding—Shielding involves the use of different materials placed between the worker and the source to absorb the radiation optimization analyses - cost-benefit analyses are performed to balance economic considerations with the expected benefits.

Q15 Mesiodens.

Ans.

Refer to Q13 of January 2009.

Q16 Plummer-Vinson syndrome.

Ans.

Refer to Q6 of September 2000.

Q17 Café-au-lait pigmentation.

Ans.

Refer to Q11 of March 2001.

Q18 Composition of dental X-ray film.

Ans.

Refer to Q16 of September 2002.

Q19 Black hairy tongue.

Ans.

Refer to Q15 of March 2001.

Q20 Indications of bitewing radiographs.

Ans.

Refer to Q14 of March 2003.

Q21 Nikolsky's sign.

Ans.

Refer to Q11 of March 2002.

Q22 Globulomaxillary cyst.

Ans.

The globulomaxillary cyst is a cyst that appears between a maxillary lateral incisor and the adjacent canine. It exhibits as an "inverted pear-shaped radiolucency" on radiographs, or X-ray films. However, all regional teeth will be vital.

It often causes the roots of adjacent teeth to diverge. It is believed to be odontogenic.

Treatment is by enucleation, or surgical removal.

RGUHS December 2009 (OS)

QUESTION PAPER

Long Essays

1. Classify temporomandibular joint disorders. Discuss the etiopathogenesis, clinical features, diagnosis and management of myofacial pain dysfunction syndrome.

2. Elaborate the various effects of radiation on oral tissues.

Short Essays

3. Radioghraphic appearance of fibrous dysplasia.

4. Dosimetry.

5. Hereditary ectodermal dysplasia.

6. Orthopantomograph.

7. Salivary scintigraphy.

8. Multilocular radiolucencies.

Short Answers

9. Epstein's pearls.

10. Taurodontism.

11. Pindborg's tumor

12. Radigraphic appearance of ameloblastoma.

13. Lamina dura

14. Medial rhomboid Glossitis.

15. Carbamazepine.

16. Rickets.

17. Cervical burn out.

18. Position-distance rule.

SOLUTIONS

LONG ESSAYS

Q1 Classify temporomandibular joint disorders. Discuss the etiopathogenesis, clinical features, diagnosis and management of myofacial pain dysfunction syndrome.

Ans.

Refer to Q10 of March 2001.

Q2 Elaborate the various effects of radiation on oral tissues.

Ans.

Refer to Q19 of March 2000.

SHORT ESSAYS

Q3 Radioghraphic appearance of fibrous dysplasia.

Ans.

Refer to Q11 of September 2003.

Q4 Dosimetry

Ans.

Refer to Q9 of March 2002.

Q5 Hereditary ectodermal dysplasia.

Ans.

Refer to Q14 of February 2007 (OS).

Q6 Orthopantomograph.

Ans.

Refer to Q8 of September 2004.

Q7 Salivary scintigraphy.

Ans.

- It is a specialized investigative modality which uses radiopharmaceuticals. It is also called as positron emission tomography.
- It provides a functional study of the salivary glands, taking advantage of the selective concentration of specific radionuclides in the salivary glands.
- Provides the only means of assessing physiologic change that is a direct result of biochemical alteration.
- Gamma emitting radioisotopes like iodine (^{131}I), gallium (^{67}Ga), selenium (^{74}Se) and technetium (^{99m}Tc) are used in radionuclide imaging.
- The radiations emitted by these isotopes is captured by the gamma scintillation camera, which use scintillation crystal that has the ability to fluoresce on interaction with gamma rays.
- This fluorescence is detected by a photomultiplier tube that magnifies and amplifies the signal which is then digitized and used to produce an image by computer algorithm.
- ^{99m}Tc-pertechnetate is injected intravenously and it gets concentrated in and excreted by the glandular structures, including the salivary, thyroid and mammary glands.
- In salivary glands the radionuclide appears within minutes and reaches its maximum concentration within 30–45 mins.
- To evaluate the secretory capacity, a sialogogue is then administered.
- All major salivary glands can be studied at once.
- This technique lacks specificity and morphology is not demonstrated properly.
- Pathosis may be demonstrated by increased, decreased or no uptake of the radionuclide.
- Warthin tumor and oncocytoma demonstrate increased uptake.

Q8 Multilocular radiolucencies.

Ans.

Refer to Q13 of September 2001.

SHORT ANSWERS

Q9 Epstein's pearls.

Ans.

Epstein's pearls are small white or yellow cystic papules (1 to 3 mm in size) often seen in the median palatal raphe of the mouth of newborn infants (occur in 65–85% of newborns). They are typically seen on the roof of the mouth (palate) and are filled with fluid. They are caused during the development of the palate by entrapped epithelium (fissural cyst).

They do not require treatment because they resolve spontaneously over the first few weeks of life.

Similar cysts that are scattered over the hard palate are referred to as Bohn's nodules come from minor salivary glands.

Q10 Taurodontism.

Ans.

Refer to Q13 of August 2007.

Q11 Pindborg's tumor

Ans.

Refer to Q3 of January 2009.

Q12 Radigraphic appearance of amelo-blastoma.

Ans.

Refer to Q2 of March 2000.

Q13 Lamina dura

Ans.

Refer to Q2 of March 2002.

Q14 Medial rhomboid Glossitis.

Ans.

Refer to Q20 of July 2008 (RS).

Q15 Carbamazepine.

Ans.

This is a very detailed explanation beneficial for long answers type. For short answers type questions, write a very 'to the point' answer.

Carbamazepine (CBZ) is an anticonvulsant and mood stabilizing drug used primarily in the treatment of epilepsy and bipolar disorder, as well as trigeminal neuralgia. It is also used off-label for a variety of indications, including attention-deficit hyperactivity disorder (ADHD),schizophrenia, phantom limb syndrome, paroxysmal extreme pain disorder, and post-traumatic stress disorder.

Indications for carbamazepine use are epilepsy (including partial seizures and tonic-clonic seizures), trigeminal neuralgia, and manic and mixed episodes of bipolar I disorder.

Pharmacokinetics

Carbamazepine exhibits autoinduction: it induces the expression of the hepatic microsomal enzyme system CYP3A4, which metabolizes carbamazepine itself. Upon initiation of carbamazepine therapy, concentra-tions are predictable and follow their respective baseline clearance/half-life values that have been established for the specific patient. However, after enough carbamazepine has been presented to the liver tissue, the CYP3A4 activity increases, speeding up drug clearance and shortening the half-life. Autoinduction will continue with subsequent increases in dose but will usually reach a plateau within 5–7 days of a maintenance dose. Increases in dose at a rate of 200 mg every 1–2 weeks may be required to achieve a stable seizure threshold. Stable carbamazepine concentrations occur usually within 2–3 weeks after initiation of therapy.

Other Uses for this Medicine

Carbamazepine is also sometimes used to treat mental illnesses, depression, posttraumatic stress disorder, drug and alcohol withdrawal, restless legs syndrome, diabetes insipidus, certain pain syndromes, and a disease in children called chorea.

Side Effects

Carbamazepine may cause the following side effects.drowsiness

- Dizziness
- Unsteadiness
- Nausea
- Vomiting
- Headache
- Anxiety
- Memory problems
- Diarrhea
- Constipation
- Heartburn
- Dry mouth
- Back pain
- Confusion
- Loss of contact with reality
- Chest pain
- Yellowing of the skin or eyes
- Vision problems

Symptoms of Overdose may include

- Unconsciousness
- Seizures
- Restlessness

- Muscle twitching
- Abnormal movements
- Shaking of a part of your body that you cannot control
- Unsteadiness
- Drowsiness
- Dizziness
- Blurred vision
- Irregular or slowed breathing
- Rapid or pounding heartbeat
- Nausea
- Vomiting
- Difficulty urinating.

Q16 Rickets.

Ans.

Refer to Q7 of March 2002.

Q17 Cervical burn out.

Ans.

Refer to Q22 of January 2009 (RS2).

Q18 Position-distance rule.

Ans.

This is a safety precaution for the operator against the radiations. This rule is the most

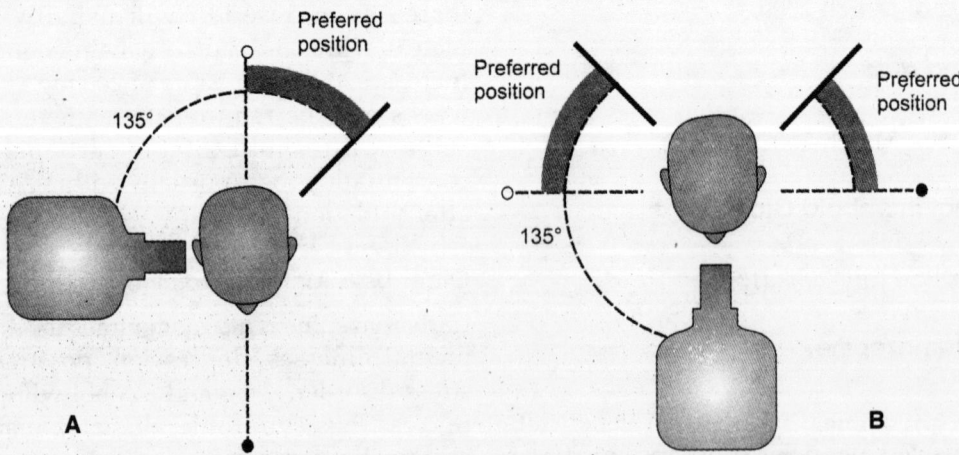

Fig. 29.1: Preferred position for A. posterior and B. anterior radiographs.

effective way of reducing the operator exposure. The rule states that–the operator should stand atleast 6 feet away from the patient in a quadrant that is at an angle between 90° and 135° from the primary beam (Fig. 29.1)

If the operator cannot satisfy these figures, then he should stand behind an appropriate protective barrier or outside the area behind a wall.

The tube head should never be held or stabilized by hand during the exposure.

QUESTION PAPER
Long Essays

1. Classify white lesions and discuss in detail about the clinical features and management of leukoplakia.
2. What are the radiation hazards and write about the protective measures to be taken by the operator and the patient.

Short Essays

3. Properties of X-rays.
4. Xerostomia.
5. Exfoliative cytology.
6. Amelogenesis imperfecta.
7. Intensifying screens.
8. Herpes zoster
9. Grids
10. Short cone technique.
11. Sialography
12. Occlusal film

Short Answers

13. Stomatitis nicotina
14. Hutchinson triad
15. Angular stomatitis
16. Café-au-lait spots
17. Radiographic features of chronic periodontitis.
18. Eagle's syndrome
19. Sclerosing osteitis
20. Papillon-Lefevre syndrome
21. Cleidocranial dysplasia
22. Tzanck tests

SOLUTIONS

LONG ESSAYS

Q1 Classify white lesions and discuss in detail about the clinical features and management of leukoplakia.

Ans.

Refer to Q3.1 of march 1999, Q1 of October 1999, Q8 of March 2000, Q2 of February 2002 (RS) and Q3 of March 2004.

Q2 What are the radiation hazards and write about the protective measures to be taken by the operator and the patient.

Ans.

Refer to Q2 of September 2004.

SHORT ESSAYS

Q3 Properties of X-rays.

Ans.

Refer to Q5 of September 2001.

Q4 Xerostomia.

Ans.

Refer to Q3 of July 2008.

Q5 Exfoliative cytology.

Ans.

Refer to Q17 of September 2003.

Q6 Amelogenesis imperfecta.

Ans.

Amelogenesis imperfecta presents with abnormal formation of the enamel or external layer of teeth. Enamel is composed mostly of mineral, that is formed and regulated by the proteins in it. Amelogenesis imperfecta is due to the malfunction of the proteins in the enamel: ameloblastin, enamelin, tuftelin and amelogenin.

People afflicted with amelogenesis imperfecta have teeth with abnormal color: yellow, brown or grey. The teeth have a higher risk for dental cavities and are hypersensitive to temperature changes. This disorder can afflict any number of teeth.

Mutations in the AMELX, ENAM, MMP20, and KLK-4 genes have been found to cause amelogenesis imperfecta. These genes provide instructions for making proteins that are essential for normal tooth development. These proteins are involved in the formation of enamel, which is a hard, calcium-rich material that forms the protective outer layer of each tooth. Mutations in any of these genes alter the structure of these proteins or prevent the genes from making any protein at all. As a result, tooth enamel is abnormally thin or soft and may have a yellow or brown color. Teeth with defective enamel are weak and easily damaged.

Amelogenesis imperfecta can have different inheritance patterns depending on the gene that is altered. Most cases are caused by mutations in the ENAM gene and are inherited in an autosomal dominant pattern. Amelogenesis imperfecta is also inherited in an autosomal recessive pattern; this form of the disorder can result from mutations in the ENAM or MMP20 gene. Symptoms include:

- Brown discoloration of teeth
- Yellow discoloration of teeth
- Thin tooth enamel
- Soft tooth enamel
- Easily damaged (fragile) teeth
- Smooth tooth enamel
- Rough tooth enamel
- Pitted tooth enamel
- Missing teeth
- Small teeth.

Treatment

Crowns are sometimes being used to compensate for the soft enamel. Usually stainless steel crowns are used in children which may be replaced by porcelain once they reach adulthood. In the worst case scenario, the teeth may have to be extracted and implants or dentures are required.

Q7 Intensifying screens.
Ans.
Refer to Q6.2 of October 1999.

Q8 Herpes zoster
Ans.
Refer to Q5 of January 2009.

Q9 Grids
Ans.
Refer to Q6 of September 2002.

Q10 Short cone technique.
Ans.
It is also called as the bisecting angle technique. Refer to Q5 of September 1998.

Q11 Sialography
Ans.
Refer to Q2 of September 2002.

Q12 Occlusal film
Ans.
Refer to Q2 of September 2003.

SHORT ANSWERS

Q13 Stomatitis nicotina.
Ans.
Stomatitis nicotina (also known as "Nicotine stomatitis," "Smoker's keratosis," and "Smoker's patches") is an oral pathological condition that appears in the hard palate as a white lesion. It is not considered to be premalignant and results from tobacco smoking (especially pipes or cigars) or long-term drinking of very hot beverages. Nicotine stomatitis should not be confused with reverse smoker's palate, which is a severe form of palatal keratosis and caused from smoking a cigarette with the lit end inside the mouth.

The cause of nicotine stomatitis stems from the palate being exposed to very hot conditions. Pipe smoking produces more heat on the palate than any other form of smoking. The frequency of this condition depends on a society's use of consuming hot beverages and of smoking in its various forms. More commonly found in men over 45 years of age, it is characterized as a "fissured" or "dried mud" appearance from excess keratin production by cells. The palate may appear gray or white and contain many papules that are slightly elevated with red in their center. Furthermore, the teeth may be stained brown or black from tobacco smoke.

Microscopically, epithelial cells of the palate exhibit signs of hyperkeratosis and acanthosis. There may be metaplasia of excretory ducts, which results in the visible papules if the ducts become hyperplastic.

There is usually no treatment since there is no increased risk of cancer. Immediate cessation of smoking may be advised in order to monitor lesion. Nicotine stomatitis should completely resolve on its own after 1–2 weeks upon termination of smoking. If the lesion persists, a biopsy may be done to confirm diagnosis.

Q14 Hutchinson triad
Ans.
Refer to Q12 of March 2003.

Q15 Angular stomatitis
Ans.
Refer to Q3.1 of October 1999.

Q16 Café-au-lait spots
Ans.
Refer to Q11 of March 2001.

Q17 Radiographic features of chronic periodontitis.

Ans.

Chronic periodontitis is a common disease of the oral cavity of chronic inflammation of the periodontal tissues that is caused by accumulation of profuse amounts of dental plaque. The radiographic features are as follows:

1. Changes in the morphology of the alveolar supporting bone–loss of interproximal crestal bone and bone overlapping the buccal or lingual aspects of the tooth roots.

Changes to the internal density and trabecular pattern–reduction (radiolucency) or increase (sclerosis) in the bone structure. Generally sclerotic changes are common in chronic disease.

Q18 Eagle's syndrome

Ans.

Refer to Q7 of September 2001.

Q19 Sclerosing osteitis

Ans.

Refer to Q6.3 of March 1999.

Q20 Papillon-Lefevre syndrome

Ans.

Refer to Q14 of August 2007.

Q21 Cleidocranial dysplasia

Ans.

Refer to Q14 of January 2008.

Q22 Tzanck tests

Ans.

Refer to Q10 of August 2005.

QUESTION PAPER
Long Essays

1. Define a white lesion. What are its different causes? Describe the etiology, clinical features and treatment of oral lichen planus.
2. Enumerate the techniques for imaging the temporomandibular joint. Describe any two in detail.

Short Essays

3. Cyclic neutropinea.
4. Differential diagnosis of multiple punched out radiolucencies of the jaw.
5. Periapical cemental dysplasia.
6. Oral manifestations of HIV infection.
7. Intensifying screens.
8. Lazy leukocyte syndrome.
9. Hemangioma.
10. Adenomatoid odontogenic tumour.
11. Eagle's syndrome.
12. Formation of latent image.

Short Answers

13. Epulis.
14. Radiographic appearance of mandibular canal.
15. Etiology of median rhomboid Glossitis.
16. Condensing osteitis.
17. Focused grid.
18. Define a vesicle and pustule
19. Define an ideal radiograph.
20. Leakage radiation
21. Linea alba
22. Static electricity.

SOLUTIONS

LONG ESSAYS

Q1 Define a white lesion. What are its different causes? Describe the etiology, clinical features and treatment of oral lichen planus.

Ans.

Refer to Q1 of October 1999.

Q2 Enumerate the techniques for imaging the temporomandibular joint. Describe any two in detail.

Ans.

Refer to Q5 of October 1999. Refer to Q8 of September 2004 for panoramic radiograph.

SHORT ESSAYS

Q3 Cyclic neutropinea.

Ans.

- Cyclic neutropenia is a benign, hematologic disorder characterized by recurrent episodes of severe neutropenia at 21 day intervals and lasting three to six days at a time due to changing rates of cell production by the bone marrow. There are associated cyclical variations in other blood cells.
- Patients with this disease have malaise, stomatitis, cervical lymphadenopathy and fever during the recurrent neutropenic periods.
- The exact cause of cyclic neutropenia is unknown. About one third of human cases appear to be inherited in autosomal dominant mutations in ELA2, the gene encoding neutrophil elastase. In the other cases, the disease appears to arise spontaneously with symptoms usually beginning in infancy or early childhood.
- In adult patients, the disease may be acquired and occur in association with a clonal proliferation of large granular lymphocytes.

- Treatment includes G-CSF (Granulocyte colony stimulating factor) and usually improves after puberty.

Q4 Differential diagnosis of multiple punched out radiolucencies of the jaw.

Ans.

- Metastatic carcinoma
- Osteomyelitis
- Inflamatory lesions and infections
- Simple bone cysts occurring bilaterally
- Hyperparathyroidism
- Thalassamia
- Gaucher's disease or oxalosis.........

Q5 Periapical cemental dysplasia.

Ans.

Refer to Q4 of March 2000.

Q6 Oral manifestations of HIV infection.

Ans.

Refer to Q1 of September 2000.

Q7 Intensifying screens.

Ans.

Refer to Q4 of September 2001.

Q8 Lazy leukocyte syndrome.

Ans.

A severe form of neutropenia which results from neutrophils that are incapable of moving properly. It is charecterised by:

- Severe neutropenia
- Recurring infection
- Increased risk of serious infections

The lazy leukocyte syndrome was first described by Miller et al. in 1971 in two children with recurrent infection. They had normal humoral and cellular immunity with a neutropenia, but adequate numbers of neutrophils in the bone marrow. Intracellular killing and phagocytosis were intact, the defect being in the mobilization of functionally normal neutrophils in response to chemical and inflammatory stimuli.

Q9 Hemangioma
Ans.

A hemangioma is an abnormal buildup of blood vessels in the skin or internal organs.

Causes

About 30% of hemangiomas are present at birth. The rest appear in the first several months of life. The hemangioma may be:
- In the top skin layers (capillary hemangioma)
- Deeper in the skin (cavernous hemangioma)
- A mixture of both

Symptoms

- A red to reddish-purple, raised sore (lesion) on the skin
- A massive, raised tumor with blood vessels Most hemangiomas are on the face and neck.

Hemangiomas are diagnosed by a physical examination. In the case of deep or mixed lesions, a CT or MRI scan may be performed.

Treatment

Superficial or "strawberry" hemangiomas often are not treated. When they are allowed to disappear on their own, the result is usually normal-appearing skin. In some cases, a laser may be used to remove the small vessels.

Cavernous hemangiomas that involve the eyelid and block vision are generally treated with steroid injections or laser treatments. These quickly reduce the size of the lesions, allowing vision to develop normally. Large cavernous hemangiomas or mixed hemangiomas may be treated with oral steroids and injections of steroids directly into the hemangioma.

Recently, lasers have been used to reduce the size of the hemangiomas. Lasers that emit yellow light damage the vessels in the hemangioma without damaging the skin over it. Some physicians use a combination of steroid injection and laser therapy.

Possible Complications

- Bleeding (especially if the hemangioma is injured)
- Problems with breathing and eating
- Psychological problems, from skin appearance
- Secondary infections and sores
- Visible changes in the skin
- Vision problems (amblyopia, strabismus)

Hemangiomas are associated with the following syndromes:
- Rendu-Osler-Weber syndrome
- Sturge-Weber-Dimitri syndrome
- Kasabach-Merritt syndrome
- Maffucci syndrome Klippel-Trenaunay-Weber syndrome
- PHACE(S) posterior fossa brain malformations, hemangiomas of the face (large or complex), arterial anomalies, cardiac anomalies, and eye abnormalities.

Q10 Adenomatoid odontogenic tumour.
Ans.
Refer to Q12 of February 2007 (OS).

Q11 Eagle's syndrome.
Ans.
Refer to Q7 of September 2001.

Q12 Formation of latent image.
Ans.
A latent image is an image that has been created on the film due to the interaction of radiation with the material making up the film. A latent image is an invisible image produced by the

exposure of the film to light. When the film is developed, the area that was exposed darkens and forms a visible image. This latent image is not visible to the naked eye until further processing has taken place. To make the latent image visible the film is processed by exposure to chemicals similar to that of photographic film. The parts of an X-ray film are:

1. The base
2. The emulsion
3. Protective coating

The protective layer has the important function of protecting the softer emulsion layers below. It is simply a very thin skin of gelatin protecting the film from scratches during handling. It offers very important properties to film manufacturers, which include shrinkage (during drying that forms glassy protective layers) and dissolving in warm water. It will absorb the water and swell if it is dissolved in cold water.

During manufacturing of the film, silver bromide is added to the solution of dissolved gelatin. When the gelatin hardens the silver bromide crystals are held in suspension throughout the emulsion. Upon exposure of the film to radiation, the silver bromide crystals become ionized in varying degrees forming the latent image. Each grain or crystal of silver bromide that has become ionized can be reduced or developed to form a grain of black metallic silver. This is what forms the visible image on the radiograph. This visible image is made up of an extremely large number of silver crystals each is individually exposed to radiation but working together as a unit to form the image.

SHORT ANSWERS

Q13 Epulis.

Ans.

Epulis fissuratum (also known as "Granuloma fissuratum") is an oral pathologic condition that appears in the mouth as an overgrowth of fibrous connective tissue. Also referred to less commonly as inflammatory fibrous hyperplasia, denture epulis, and denture induced fibrous hyperplasia, it is associated with the edges of a denture that does not fit well.

Epulis fissuratum appears as a single or multiple fold of tissue that grown in excess around the alveolar vestibule, which is the area where the gums meet the inner cheek. Usually, the edge of the denture rests in between two of the folds. The excess tissue is firm and fibrous, and ulcerations may be present. The size of the affected tissue varies widely, since almost the entire length of tissue around a denture can be affected. More commonly found in women, it can appear in either the mandible or maxilla (upper jaw) but is more commonly found in the anterior portions of the mouth rather than in the posterior. Women during pregnancy can also present with an epulis, which will resolve after birth. Fibroepithelial polyps, pedunculated lesions of the palate beneath an upper denture, are associated with this condition. An epulis fissuratum in a patient without dentures can also be diagnostic of Crohn's disease.

The appearance of an epulis fissuratum microscopically is an overgrowth of cells from the fibrous connective tissue. The epithelial cells are usually hyperkeratotic and irregular, hyperplastic rete ridges are often seen.

Treatment consists of surgical removal with the fixing of a denture in a process called a "reline" or with making a new denture.

Q14 Radiographic appearance of mandibular canal.

Ans.

Refer Q1 of February 2007 (OS).

Q15 Etiology of median rhomboid Glossitis.

Ans.

Refer to Q20 of July 2008 (RS).

Q16 Condensing osteitis.

Ans. Refer march 1999 Q6.3.

Q17 Focused grid.

Ans.

Refer September 2002 Q6

Q18 Define a vesicle and pustule

Ans.

Vesicle: A vesicle is a circumscribed, fluid-containing, epidermal elevation generally considered less than either 5 or 10 mm in diameter at the widest point

Pustule: A pustule is a small elevation of the skin containing cloudy or purulent material usually consisting of necrotic inflammatory cells.

Q19 Define an ideal radiograph.

Ans.

HM worth's definition; An ideal radiograph is one which has desired density and overall blackness and which shows the part completely without distortion with maximum details and has the right amount of contrast to make the details fully apparent.

Characteristics of an ideal Radiograph

A. Visual characteristics
   i. Density
   ii. Contrast
B. Geometric
   i. Sharpness, detail, resolution or definition
   ii. Magnification
   iii. Distortion
C. Anatomical accuracy of radiographic images
D. Adequate coverage of the anatomic region of interest

Density: Overall darkness/blackness of dental radiograph.

Q20 Leakage radiation

Ans.

The radiation, exclusive of the primary beam, that is emitted through the housing of equipment used in radiation therapy and radiography.

Q21 Linea alba

Ans.

It is a horizontal streak on the inner surface of the cheek, level with the biting plane. It usually extends from the commissure to the posterior teeth and can extend to the inner lip mucosa and corners of the mouth.

It is a common finding and most likely associated with pressure, frictional irritation, or sucking trauma from the facial surfaces of the teeth. It may be found in individuals who chew tobacco, and may be mistaken for a lesion requiring treatment.

Clinical Considerations

- The linea alba is usually present bilaterally.
- It is restricted to dentulous areas.
- It presents an asymptomatic, linear elevation, with a whitish colour, at the level of the occlusal line of the teeth.

Q22 Static electricity

Ans.

Static electricity refers to the build up of electric charge on the surface of objects. Xeroradiography is the technique in which electrostatically charged plates sensitive to X-rays are used in diagnostic radiology in place of conventional film. Comparison between these different types of radiographs of both lateral skull and lateral oblique mandibular projections shows xeroradiography to have many advantages. Hard and soft tissue details are more clearly defined and visible on the same picture. Radiation dosage is slightly less and this, combined with the need for fewer exposures, reduces the incident skin dose to the patient. The plates are re-usable and the process requires no silver.

These factors strongly suggest that xeroradiography may be of great value in routine dental radiology and further investigation is in progress.

QUESTION PAPER
Long Essays

1. Classify vesicobullous lesions and discuss the etiopathogenesis, clinical features and management of erythema multiformae.
2. Describe the parts of an x-ray tube and add a note on the properties of x-rays.

Short Essays

3. Radiographic accessories.
4. Digital radiography.
5. Grids.
6. Leukoplakia.
7. Radiographs to evaluate mandibular third molars.
8. Faulty radiographs.
9. Oral thrush.
10. Periapical cyst.
11. Differential diagnosis of oral pigmentation.
12. Broad spectrum antibiotics.

Short Answers

13. Adverse effects of brufen.
14. Name three specific infections of oral cavity.
15. Indications fro extraoral radiographs.
16. Café-au-lait spots.
17. Radigraphic densities.
18. Storage of X-ray films.
19. Gardner's syndrome.
20. Radiopaque landmarks in maxilla
21. Mesiodens.
22. Indications for bitewing radiographs.

SOLUTIONS

LONG ESSAYS

Q1 Classify vesicobullous lesions and discuss the etiopathogenesis, clinical features and management of erythema multiformae.

Ans.

Refer to Q1 of March 2000 and March 2004.

Q2 Describe the parts of an X-ray tube and add a note on the properties of X-rays.

Ans.

Refer to Q2 of March 2004 and Q5 of September 2001.

SHORT ESSAYS

Q3 Radiographic accessories.

Ans.

The radiographic accessories are the materials that are used while taking a radiographs and those that are used to reduce the radiation exposure. The accessories are as follows:

- Lead intensifying screens - Lead Intensifying Screens are thin sheets of lead foil mounted on card for ease of handling. One is placed on each side of an X-ray film and in close contact with it, inside a cassette or film-holder before exposure. They are used in most radiographic techniques, excluding some of those employing low kilovoltages, because they reduce the exposure required and improve the quality of the image.

- All indicators have a serial number for Quality Assurance purposes. From this, measured wire diameters and date of manufacture can be traced.

- Sharp face markers are generally used for X-radiography and produce a well-defined, clean image on the film. The flat face style has a greater bulk for use with the more penetrating gamma radiations. Markers are supplied either unmounted or mounted to

0.73 mm thick, rigid white PVC for easy handling. The charcters available are arrows (sharp face only), capital letters and numerals. Sharp face markers are measured with reference to the front, sharp face of the character. Flat face markers are measured on the back of the character. Sharp face markers are always, therefore, larger than the flat face characters of the same nominal size.

- Cassettes with film and plastic cassettes.

- Radiation warning signs–to warn about harmful radiations etc.

- Interleaving paper–The paper is white, 70 gsm and has a pH of 6.9 - as near to neutral as it is possible to get in practice. This ensures the paper will have no affect on the film, even after prolonged contact.

- Magnetic marker tapes

- Dosimetry

- Pair of gloves which have 0.5mm of lead equivalence.

Q4 Digital radiography.

Ans.

Refer to Q10 of January 2008 (RS).

Q5 Grids.

Ans.

Refer to Q6 of September 2002.

Q6 Leukoplakia.

Ans.

Refer to Q1 of August 2007.

Q7 Radiographs to evaluate mandibular third molars.

Ans.

The following radiographs can be taken for evaluating mandibular third molar:

1. Paralleling Technique

a. Mandibular molar projection–Image field–distal half of the second premolar and three mandibular permanent molars. Film placement–nearly horizontal plain inside the mouth. Rotate the inferior edge downward, beneath the lateral border of the tongue displacing it medially. Anterior edge of the film should be at about middle of second premolar (Fig. 32.1).

Projection of the central ray–the ray should be directed through the second molar. Adjust the horizontal angulation to project the beam through the contact areas.

b. Mandibular distal oblique molar projection–Image field–third molar and the retromolar area of the mandible that usually is not included in the molar radiograph. It is intended for detection or examination of impacted teeth and pathological conditions in bone (Fig. 32.2). Film placement–floor of the mouth between the tongue and alveolar process, parallel with the long axis of the molars. Position the instrument as far posteriorly as possible and rotate the film holding device distally moving the posterior margin of the film towards the midline.

Projection of the central ray–the ray should project more posteriorly through the third molar.

2. Molar Bitewing Radiograph

Image field– distal surface of the most posterior erupted molar and equally the crowns of the maxillary and the mandibular molars.

Film placement–place the film between the tongue and the teeth as far lingual as practical to avoid contacting the sensitive attached gingival. Distal margin of the film should extend 1–2 mm beyond the most posterior erupted molar.

Projection of central ray–the ray should project to the centre of the film and through the contact of the 1st and 2nd maxillary molars. Angle the central ray slightly from the anterior because the molar contacts are usually not oriented at right angles to the buccal surfaces of these teeth. Vertical angulation of +10° is recommended.

3. Lateral Mandibular Occlusal Projection

Refer to Q8 of January 2008.

Q8 Faulty radiographs.
Ans.
Refer to Q4 of September 1998.

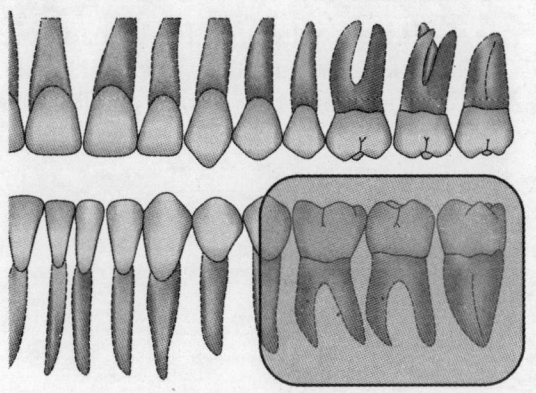
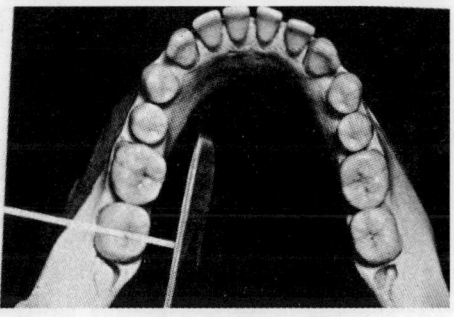

Fig. 32.1: Parallelling technique-Mandibular molar projection

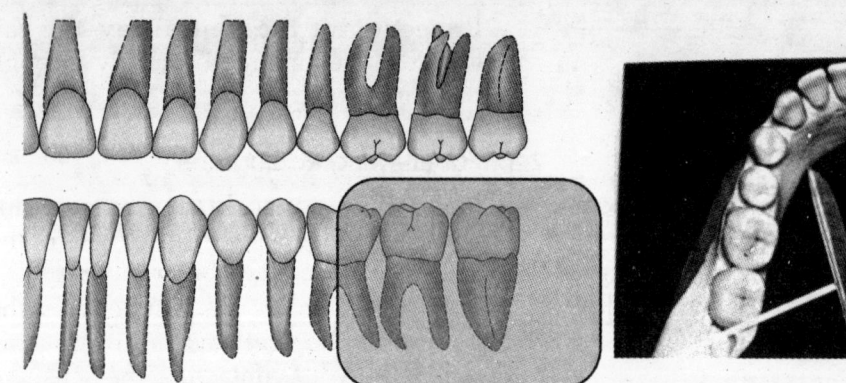
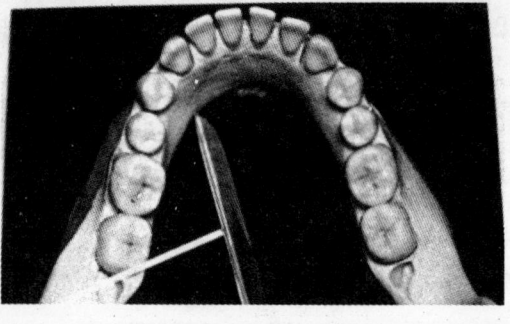

Fig. 32.2: Parallelling technique-Mandibular distal oblique molar

Q9 Oral thrush.
Ans.
Refer to Q3 of September 2002.

Q10 Periapical cyst
Ans.
Refer to Q2 of September 2000.

Q11 Differential diagnosis of oral pigmentation.
Ans.
Refer to Q1 of March 1999.

Q12 Broad spectrum antibiotics.
Ans.
The term broad-spectrum antibiotic refers to an antibiotic with activity against a wide range of disease-causing bacteria. It is also means that it acts against both Gram-positive and Gram-negative bacteria. This is in contrast to a narrow-spectrum antibiotic which is effective against only specific families of bacteria.

Broad-spectrum antibiotics are properly used in the following medical situations:
- Empirically prior to identifying the causative bacteria when there is a wide differential and potentially serious illness would result in delay of treatment. This occurs, for example, in meningitis, where the patient can become so ill that he/she could die within hours if broad-spectrum antibiotics are not initiated.
- For drug resistant bacteria that do not respond to other, more narrow-spectrum antibiotics.
- In super-infections where there are multiple types of bacteria causing illness, thus warranting either a broad-spectrum antibiotic or combination antibiotic therapy.

Advantages
- Broader Spectra of Activity
- A clear advantage to the use of broad-spectrum antibiotics is that there is less of a need (as compared with narrow-spectrum antibiotics) to identify the infecting pathogen with real certainty before commencing treatment.

Disadvantages
- Children who receive broad-spectrum antibiotics during their first year of life are at increased risk of developing childhood asthma.
- Broad Spectrum antibiotics may give rise to drug resistance.
  Examples
  - Amoxicillin
  - Levofloxacin
  - Gatifloxacillin
  - Streptomycin
  - Tetracycline
  - Chloramphenicol

SHORT ANSWERS

Q13 Adverse effects of brufen.

Ans.

Common side effects of Brufen may include, abdominal pain, diarrhea, constipation, dizziness, fluid retention and swelling, heartburn, indigestion, nausea, nervousness, rash, and vomiting. Rare side effects of Brufen may include, abdominal bleeding, hematuria, blurred vision, changes in heartbeat, confusion, depression, dry eyes, hives, inability to sleep, kidney or liver damage, severe allergic reactions, shortness of breath, sleepiness, stomach ulcer, vomiting blood, painful urination. It interacts with the following drugs.

- Aspirin
- Blood pressure medications
- Beta-blockers such as Atenolol
- Blood-thinning drugs
- Diuretics
- Lithium
- Methotrexate

Symptoms of Brufen overdose may include acute depression (crying spell), abdominal pain, short breath, drowsiness, irregular heartbeat, kidney failure, low blood pressure, nausea, seizures, and vomiting.

Q14 Name three specific infections of oral cavity.

Ans.

The three specific infections of oral cavity are:

- Scarlet fever–streptococcal–causes stomatitis scarlatina, strawbwrry tongue
- Diphtheria–cornybacterium diphtheriae–patchy diphtheritic membrane
- Actimomycosis–Actinomyces Israeli–abscesses discharging sulphur granules
- Tuberculosis–M. tuberculae–irregular ulcers.

Q15 Indications for extraoral radiographs.

Ans.

The following are a few indications for extraoral radiography

1. When large areas of the skull or jaw must be examined
2. When patients are unable to open their mouths for film placement
3. If a patient has swelling or severe pain and is unable to tolerate the placement of intraoral films
4. Patients who are uncooperative and may refuse to open their mouths.

Q16 Café-au-lait spots.

Ans.

Refer to Q11 of March 2001.

Q17 Radiographic densities.

Ans.

Radiographic or film density is a measure of the degree of film darkening. Technically it should be called "transmitted density" when associated with transparent-base film since it is a measure of the light transmitted through the film. Density is a logarithmic unit that describes a ratio of two measurements. Specifically, it is the log of the intensity of light incident on the film (I_0) to the intensity of light transmitted through the film (I_t).

$$D = \log \frac{I_0}{I_t}$$

Using the log of the ratio allows ratios of various sizes to be described using easy to work with numbers. The following table shows the relationship between the amount of transmitted light and the calculated film density.

Transmittance(I_0/I_t)	Percent Transmittance	Film Density Log(I_0/I_t)
1.0	100%	0
0.1	10%	1
0.01	1%	2
0.001	0.1%	3
0.0001	0.01%	4
0.00001	0.001%	5
0.000001	0.0001%	6
0.0000001	0.00001%	7

A density reading of 2.0 is the result of only one percent of the incident light making it through the film. At a density of 4.0 only 0.01% of transmitted light reaches the far side of the film. Industrial codes and standards typically require a radiograph to have a density between 2.0 and 4.0 for acceptable viewing with common film viewers. Above 4.0, extremely bright viewing lights is necessary for evaluation. Contrast within a film increases with increasing density, so in general the higher the density the better. When radiographs will be digitized, densities above 4.0 are often used since digitization systems can capture and redisplay for easy viewing information from densities up to 6.0.

Q18 Storage of X-ray films.
Ans.
Refer to Q19 of January 2008 (RS).

Q19 Gardner's syndrome.
Ans.
Gardner described a syndrome consisting of hereditary intestinal polyposis with osteomas and multiple cutaneous and subcutaneous lesions in 1953. This syndrome has since been modified by the addition of other features such as osteomas, supernumerary teeth, dental abnormalities, fibrous dysplasia of the skull, fibromas, desmoid tumours, epidermoid cysts and a number of malignant tumors.

The most important feature of the Gardner's syndrome is the association of multiple colonic polyps (familial adenomatous polyposis coli - FAP) with sebaceous cysts and jaw osteomas. The significance of this dominantly inherited condition to the dentist is that the colonic polyps usually undergo malignant change by the fourth decade and the extra-intestinal lesions may be apparent before those in the bowel. Although these are often subclinical oral manifestations could be diagnostical. As such, early detection of multiple jaw osteomas and/

or multiple sebaceous cysts (particularly on the scalp) may lead to appropriate further investigation and treatment which might be life saving. As the syndrome is genetically inherited, diagnosis of this condition also has implications for other family members.

Dental abnormalities are present in around 30% of patients with Gardner syndrome, and may include supernumerary teeth, compound odontomas, hypodontia, abnormal tooth morphology and impacted or unerupted teeth. The highest incidence of dental abnormalities is found in patients with multiple osteomas, but dental changes may be determined in the absence of skeletal lesions, and the dental anomalies are not secondary to bony changes.

These osteomas and adontomas, must be resected under general anesthesia, because of the unreachable regions like paranasal sinuses, condylar and angular region. Also, recurrence of osteomas and odontomas after inadequate surgery could be seen and to eliminate possible occurrence, several surgeries could be performed. Orthodontic treatment is not a valuable option for these patients because osteomas and the increased density of the bone would inhibit tooth movement. The density of the bone is so dense to erupt impacted tooth so surgical extraction would be the most suitable alternative. After extraction of all impacted tooth conventional partial or total prosthetic rehabilitation must be performed.

Q20 Radiopaque landmarks in maxilla.
Ans.
1. *Maxillary tuberosity:* The maxillary tuberosity is the convex distal inferior border of the maxilla, curving upward from the alveolar process and distal of the third molar. An extension of the maxillary sinus is occasionally seen within the maxillary tuberosity.
2. Coronoid process of the mandible. The coronoid process of the mandible sometimes

appears on maxillary molar films as a triangular opaque area located in the region of or distal to the maxillary tuberosity.

3. Zygomatic process (Malar Bone). The zygomatic arch commonly appears as a well-defined radiopaque area that may be superimposed over the molar roots. Additional radiographs are sometimes made at adjusted angulation to provide a better view of the molar root area.

4. Nasal septum. The nasal septum is usually seen as a white ridge extending above and between the central incisors.

Q21 Mesiodens.

Ans.
Refer to Q13 of January 2009.

Q22 Indications for bitewing radiographs.
Ans. Refer to Q11 of March 2000.

QUESTION PAPER
Long Essays

1. Classify white lesions. Describe in detail the etiology, clinical features and management of leukoplakia.
2. Discuss in detail the various causes of faulty radiographs and the measures to rectify them.

Short Essays

3. Herpetic gingivostomatitis.
4. Erythroplakia.
5. Infectious mononucleosis.
6. Oral manifestations of diabetes.
7. Diagnosis of pernicious anaemia.
8. Erythrocyte sedimentation rate.
9. Antifungal drugs in oral medicine.
10. Grids.
11. Internal derangement of temporomandibular joint.
12. Properties of X-rays

Short Answers

13. Nikolsky' sign
14. Hutchinson's triad.
15. Dosimetry
16. Angular chelitis
17. Examination of ulcer.
18. Ankyloglossia
19. ALARA concept
20. Onion peel radiographic appearance
21. Periapical radioopacities.
22. Vasovagal syncope.

SOLUTIONS

LONG ESSAYS

Q1 Classify white lesions. Describe in detail the etiology, clinical features and management of leukoplakia.

Ans.

Refer to Q2 of August 2005.

Q2 Discuss in detail the various causes of faulty radiographs and the measures to rectify them.

Ans.

Refer to Q4 of September 1998.

SHORT ESSAYS

Q3 Herpetic gingivostomatitis.

Ans.

Refer to Q1 of March 2002.

Q4 Erythroplakia.

Ans.

- Originally was described by Queyrat under the name "erythroplasia", as a lesion occurring on the glans penis of a syphilitic person.

- Similar lesions occur on the oral and the vulval mucosa.

- It is a clinical entity and represents a lesion of mucous membrane which exhibits epithelial changes ranging from mild dysplasia to carcinoma – in – situ and even invasive carcinoma.

- Three different forms have been described by Shear. They are as follows:

  1. The homogenous form–appears as bright red, soft velvety lesion, with straight or scalloped well demarcated margins, often extensive found on the buccal mucosa, soft palate and rarely on the tongue and flor of mouth.

  2. Erythroplakia with leokoplakic patches – in which erythematous ares are irregular, less brighter that the homogenous variety and found on tongue or floor of the mouth.

  3. Spekled erythroplakia–or sometimes called spekled leokoplakia exhibit soft, red lesions that are slightly elevated with an irregular outline and a granular or finely nodular surface spekeled with tiny white plaques, occurring anywhere in the oral cavity.

- Histologically, majority of the lesions are either invasive epidermoid carcinoma, carcinoma in-situ or epitheliai dysplasia at the time of biopsy.

- Connective tissue pegs are found to extend very high into the epithelium and the epithelium over the tips of these pegs is often very thin.

- Capillaries in these superficial pegs are often dialated.

- Absence of significant amount (or presence of very little if any) of surface orthokeratin or parakeratin also contributes to the red hue of these lesion.

Treated in the same way as invasive epidermoid carcinoma.

Q5 Infectious mononucleosis.

Ans.

Infectious mononucleosis (IM) is also known as EBV infectious mononucleosis or Pfeiffer's disease or Filatov's disease and colloquially as kissing disease, from its oral transmission, or as mono in North America and as glandular fever in all other English-speaking countries.

It is an infectious, very widespread viral disease caused by the Epstein-Barr virus (EBV), one type of herpes virus, to which more than

90% of adults have been exposed. Most people are exposed to the virus as children, when the disease produces no noticeable symptoms or only flu-like symptoms. In developing countries, people are exposed to the virus in early childhood more often than in developed countries, which is why the disease in its observable form is more common in developed countries. It is most common among adolescents and young adults.

Pathophysiology

Infectious mononucleosis occurs with infection by the Epstein-Barr virus. The infection is spread via saliva and has an incubation period of 4–7 weeks. Symptoms usually persist for 2–3 weeks, but fatigue is often more prolonged. A person can spread the infection for many months after the symptoms are completely gone—some studies show as long as 18 months.

The virus replicates first within epithelial cells in the pharynx, and later primarily within B cells (which are invaded via their CD21). The host immune response involves cytotoxic (CD8-positive) T cells against infected B lymphocytes, resulting in enlarged atypical lymphocytes (Downey cells).

Signs and Symptoms

The classical symptoms of mononucleosis are a sore throat, fever, fatigue, weight loss, malaise, pharyngeal inflammation, petechiae and loss of appetite. Common signs include lymphadenopathy, splenomegaly, hepatitis and hemolysins. Rarer signs and symptoms include thrombocytopenia, with or without pancytopenia, splenic rupture, splenic hemorrhage, upper airway obstruction, pericarditis and pneumonitis. Another rare manifestation of mononucleosis is erythema multiforme. Mononucleosis is sometimes accompanied by secondary cold agglutinin disease—an autoimmune disease in which abnormal circulating antibodies directed against red blood cells can lead to a form of autoimmune hemolytic anemia.

Diagnosis

The most commonly used diagnostic criterion is the presence of 50% lymphocytes with at least 10% atypical lymphocytes (large, irregular nuclei), while the person also has fever, pharyngitis and adenopathy. Furthermore, it should be confirmed by a serological test.

The heterophile antibody test which involves testing heterophile antibodies by agglutination of guinea pig, sheep and horse red blood cells. The newer tests are the Immunoglobulin G (IgG) and Immunoglobulin M (IgM) tests. IgG, when positive, reflects a past infection, whereas IgM reflects a current infection. When negative, these tests are more accurate in ruling out infectious mononucleosis. However, when positive, they feature similar sensitivities to the heterophile antibody test.

Differential Diagnosis

Diagnosis of acute infectious mononucleosis should also take into consideration acute cytomegalovirus infection and Toxoplasma gondii infections. These diseases are clinically very similar by their signs and symptoms. Because their management is much the same it is not always helpful, or possible, to distinguish between EBV mononucleosis and cytomegalovirus infection. However, in pregnant women, differentiation of mononucleosis from toxoplasmosis is associated with significant consequences for the fetus. Acute HIV infection can mimic signs similar to those of infectious mononucleosis and tests should be performed for pregnant women for the same reason as toxoplasmosis. Other conditions from which to distinguish infectious mononucleosis include leukemia, tonsillitis, diphtheria, common cold and influenza (the flu).

Treatment

Self care - Infectious mononucleosis is generally self-limiting and only symptomatic and/or supportive treatments are used. Rest is recommended during the acute phase of the infection, but activity should be resumed once acute symptoms have resolved. Nevertheless heavy physical activity and contact sports should be avoided to mitigate the risk of splenic rupture, for at least one month following initial infection or splenomegaly has resolved, as determined by a treating physician.

Medications - NSAIDs like ibuprofen may be used to reduce fever and pain. Prednisone, a corticosteroid, is commonly used as an anti-inflammatory to reduce symptoms of pharyngeal pain, odynophagia, or enlarged tonsils, although its use remains controversial due to the rather limited benefit and the potential of side effects. The antibiotics ampicillin and later the related amoxicillin are relatively contraindicated in the case of any coinciding bacterial infections during mononucleosis because their use precipitates a non-allergic rash close to 99% of the time.

Q6 Oral manifestations of diabetes.
Ans.
Refer to Q6 of September 2004.

Q7 Diagnosis of pernicious anaemia.
Ans.
Refer to Q1 of July 2008.

Q8 Erythrocyte sedimentation rate.
Ans.
Refer to Q3.3 of March 1999.

Q9 Antifungal drugs in oral medicine.
Ans.
The following antifungals are used in oral medicine
- Amphotericin–B for histoplasmosis, coccydiomycosis, candidiasis, mucormycosis
- Nystatin for candidiasis
- Clotimazoles for candidiasis
- Iconazoles for candidiasis.

Q10 Grids.
Ans.
Refer to Q6 of September 2002.

Q11 Internal derangement of temporo-mandibular joint.
Ans.
Refer to Q4 of January 2008 (RS).

Q12 Properties of X-rays.
Ans.
Refer to Q5 of September 2001.

SHORT ANSWERS

Q13 Nikolsky' sign
Ans.
Refer to Q11 of March 2002.

Q14 Hutchinson's triad.
Ans.
Refer to Q12 of March 2003.

Q15 Dosimetry
Ans.
Refer to Q9 of March 2002.

Q16 Angular chelitis
Ans.
Refer to Q3.1 of October 1999.

Q17 Examination of ulcer.
Ans.
Inspection
- Size and shape
- Location
- Numbers of ulcers
- Margin–healing, inflamed and fibrosed
- Edge – sloping, punched out, undermined, everted and raised

- Floor of the ulcer
- Surrounding area

Palpation

- Sorrounding area for rise of temperature and tenderness
- Edge and floor of the ulcer–soft, firm or hard
- Fixity to underlying tissue
- Palpation of local lymph nodes.

Q18 Ankyloglossia

Ans. Refer to Q12 of January 2008.

Q19 ALARA concept

Ans. Refer to Q14 of June/July 2009 (RS2).

Q20 Onion peel radiographic appearance

Ans. Refer to Q15 of September 2004.

Q21 Periapical radioopacities.

Ans. Refer to Q2 of March 2001.

Q22 Vasovagal syncope.

Ans. This is a very detailed explanation which can be written as a short note. For short answer, please write only specific points.

A vasovagal episode or vasovagal response or vasovagal attack (also called neurocardiogenic syncope) is a malaise mediated by the vagus nerve. When it leads to syncope or "fainting", it is called a vasovagal syncope, which is the most common type of fainting.

Signs and Symptoms

Prior to losing consciousness, the individual frequently experiences a prodrome of symptoms such as lightheadedness, nausea, sweating, ringing in the ears (tinnitus), uncomfortable feeling in the heart, weakness and visual disturbances such as lights seeming too bright, fuzzy or tunnel vision. These last for at least a few seconds before consciousness is lost (if it is lost), which typically happens when the person is sitting up or standing. When sufferers pass out, they fall down (unless this is impeded); and when in this position, effective blood flow to the brain is immediately restored, allowing the person to wake up. Short of fainting a person may experience an almost undescribable weak feeling resulting from a lack of oxygen to the brain due to a sudden drop in blood pressure. Tabor's describes this as the "feeling of impending death" caused by expansion of the aorta, drawing blood from the head and upper body.

Diagnosis

The core of the diagnosis of vasovagal syncope rests upon a clear description by the patient of a typical pattern of triggers, symptoms, and time course. It is also pertinent to differentiate lightheadedness, seizures, vertigo and hypoglycemia as other causes.

In patients with recurrent vasovagal syncope, or defecation syncope, diagnostic accuracy can often be improved with one of the following diagnostic tests:

1. A tilt table test
2. Implantation of an insertable loop recorder
3. A Holter monitor or event monitor
4. An echocardiogram
5. An electrophysiology study

Treatment

Treatment for vasovagal syncope focuses on avoidance of triggers, restoring blood flow to the brain during an impending episode, and measures that interrupt or prevent the pathophysiologic mechanism described above.

- The cornerstone of treatment is avoidance of triggers known to cause syncope in that person. However, new development in psychological research has shown that patients show great reductions in vasovagal syncope through exposure-based exercises with therapists.

- Because vasovagal syncope causes a decrease in blood pressure, relaxing the entire body as a mode of avoidance isn't favorable. A patient can cross his/her legs and tighten leg muscles to keep blood pressure from dropping so drastically before an injection.

- Before known triggering events, the patient may increase consumption of salt and fluids to increase blood volume. Sports and energy drinks may be particularly helpful.

- Discontinuation of medications known to lower blood pressure may be helpful, but stopping antihypertensive drugs can also be dangerous. This process should be managed by an expert.

- Patients should be educated on how to respond to further episodes of syncope, especially if they experience prodromal warning signs: they should lie down and raise their legs; or at least lower their head to increase blood flow to the brain. If the individual has lost consciousness, he or she should be laid down with his or her head turned to the side. Tight clothing should be loosened. If the inciting factor is known, it should be removed if possible (for instance, the cause of pain).

- Wearing graded compression stockings may be helpful.

- There are certain orthostatic training exercises which have been proven to improve symptoms in people with recurrent vasovagal syncope.

- Certain medications may also be helpful:

- Beta blockers (β-adrenergic antagonists) were once the most common medication given; however, they have been shown to be ineffective in a variety of studies and are thus no longer prescribed.

- Other medications which may be effective include: fludrocortisone, midodrine, SSRIs such as paroxetine or sertraline, disopyramide, and, in health-care settings where a syncope is anticipated, atropine.

QUESTION PAPER
Long Essays

1. Define premalignant lesions and conditions. Describe oral lichen planus in detail.
2. What are the hazards of radiation. Describe the protective measures for patient and operator against such hazards.

Short Essays

3. Burning mouth syndrome
4. Biopsy
5. Steroids in dentistry
6. Subepithelial dermatosis
7. Management of cardiac patient in dental clinic
8. Gingival enlargement
9. Orthopantomograph
10. X-ray tube
11. Object localization
12. Differential diagnosis of periapical radioopacities

Short Answers

13. Patterson–Kelly syndrome
14. Herpetic whitlow
15. Alarm clock headache
16. Compound odontome
17. Mucocoel
18. Keratoacanthma
19. Density of a radiograph
20. Properties of X-ray.
21. Composition of X-ray film.
22. Filteration.

LONG ESSAYS

Q1 Define premalignant lesions and conditions. Describe oral lichen planus in detail.

Ans.

Refer to Q1. of March 2003 for part 1 of the Q and Q1. of October 1999 for part 2.

Q2 What are the hazards of radiation. Describe the protective measures for patient and operator against such hazards.

Ans.

Refer to Q2. of September 2004.

SHORT ESSAYS

Q3 Burning mouth syndrome.

Ans.

Refer to March 2006 (RS) Q9.

Q4 Biopsy.

Ans.

Refer to Q16 of September 2004 and Q8. Of August 2007 (Old Scheme).

Q5 Steroids in dentistry.

Ans.

Refer to Q5. Of March 2004.

Q6 Subepithelial dermatosis.

Ans.

They are a group of mucocutaneous blistering diseases that are characterized by an autoimmune reaction that weakens a structural component of the basement membrane. The disease in this group include bullous pemphigoid, mucous membrane pemphigoid, linear IgA disease, epidermolysis bullosa aquisita and chronic bullous dermatosis of childhood (Table 34.1).

Subsets of patients diagnosed with subepithelial bullous disease have been found to have an underlying malignancy and this should be considered during the early phases of management.

Q7 Management of cardiac patient in dental clinic.

Ans.

History has to be taken prior to the beginning of the surgery, and consent is to be taken by medical personnel. Prophylactic antibiotics to be started (1 gm of penicillin to be administered.) Patient has to be regularly monitored for vital statistics throughout surgical procedure. Pulse oxymeter, life saving kit, etc. have to be kept stand by as well as contact of nearby emergency unit.

The extent of treatment by the dentist requires preparation, prevention and then management, as necessary. Prevention is accomplished by conducting a thorough medical history with appropriate alterations to dental treatment as required. The most important aspect of nearly all medical emergencies in the dental office is to prevent, or correct, insufficient oxygenation of the brain and heart. Therefore, the management of all medical emergencies should include ensuring that oxygenated blood is being delivered to these critical organs. This is consistent with basic cardiopulmonary resuscitation, with which the dentist must be competent. Dentist must be prepared to manage medical emergencies which may arise in practice and should be well versed with the ABCs of CPR(cardiopulmonary resuscitation), i.e. airway, breathing and circulation.

Drugs that should be promptly available to the dentist can be divided into two categories. The first category represents those which may be considered essential. The second category

Table 34.1

Entity	Etipathogenesis	Clinical manifestations	Oral findings	DD/Lab	Management
Bullous pem.	In age group above 60 yrs.	Blister on an inflamed area.	30–50% of the cases have oral lesions	Erosive lichen planus and pemphigus.	High potency topical steroids such as clobetasol or beta-methasone for localized lesions.
	Selflimiting, few months to 5 yrs	Pruritis is common	Small, form more slowly than Pem. Vulgaris.	Histopathology reveals separation of epithelium from the connective tissue at the basement membrane zone and inflammatory infilterate that is usually rich in eosinophills	For more extensive lesion systemic corticosteroids are required alone or along with immunosuppres-sants.
	Asso. With multiple sclerosis and malignancy also with use of diuretics

Autoantibodies against specific antigens inlamina lucida | Death from sepsis or CVS failure may occur | Desquamative gingivitis is reported to be the commonest manifestation Gingival lesions consist of oedema, inflammation and dequamation with localized areas of discrete vesicle formation. | | |
Mucous mem-brane pem (Cicatrical pemphigoid)	Above 50 yrs	Oral mucosa frequently involved after which the conjunctiva is the commonest site leading to scarring and adhesions	90% of the patients	Erosive lichen planus and pemphigus	When lesions are confined to oral cavity alone, short-term systemic corticosteroids are sufficient
	Chronic auto-immune	Corneal damage is common	Desquamatie gingivitis is the commonest lesion	Positive fluores-cense for IgG and complement C3 in basement membrane zone	Nt afatal disease
	F:M=2:1	Genital mucosa also may be involved			Desquamative lesions can be managed with topical steroids
Linear IgA disease	Deposition of IgA rather than IgG in the basement membrane	Skin lesion similar to dermatitis herpetiformis	70% of the cases	Histopath is similar to MMP but DIF study will show deposition of IgA instead of IgG	Topical steroids alone are not very helpful and may need supplemen-tation form systemic steroids as well as immuno-suppressants

Contd...

Table 34.1 *Contd...*

Entity	Etipathogenesis	Clinical manifestations	Oral findings	DD/Lab	Management
	Asso. with hemato-logic malignancies or connective tissue disorders like dermatomyositis	Bullous lesions similar to BP can also be seen	Clinically very similar to MMP with blisters and erosions freq. accompanied by desquamative gingivitis		
	Antibodies against lamina	Oral mucosa and conjunctiva commonly involved			

contains drugs which are also very helpful and should be considered as part of the emergency kit.

Essential Emergency Drugs

1. *Oxygen*–It is indicated in every emergency other than hyperventilation syndrome. Oxygen should be available in a portable manner, ideally in an E-size cylinder that holds over 600 litres

2. *Epinephrine*–is drug of choice for emergency treatment of anaphylaxis and asthma does not respond to its drug of first choice, albuterol or salbutamol. As a drug, epinephrine has a very rapid onset and short duration of action, usually 5 to 10 minutes when given intravenously. For emergency purposes, epinephrine is available in two formulations. It is prepared as 1 : 1,000, which equals 1 mg per ml, for intramuscular, including intralingual, injections. More than one ampule or pre-filled syringe should be present as multiple administrations may be necessary. It is also available as 1 : 10,000, which equals 1 mg per 10 mL for intravenous injection.

3. *Nitroglycerin*–This drug is indicated for acute angina or myocardial infarction. It is characterized by a rapid onset of action. For emergency purposes it is available as sublingual tablets or a sublingual spray. One important point to be aware of is that the tablets have a short shelf-life of approxi-mately 3 months once the bottle has been opened and the tablets exposed to air or light. The spray has the advantage of having a shelf-life which corresponds to that listed on the bottle.

4. *Injectable antihistamine*–An antihistamine is indicated for the management of allergic reactions. Whereas mild non-life threatening allergic reactions may be managed by oral administration, life-threatening reactions necessitate parenteral administration.

   Two injectable agents may be considered, either diphenhydramine or chlorphenira-mine. They may be administered as part of the management of anaphylaxis or as the sole management of less severe allergic reactions, particularly those with primarily dermato-logic signs and symptoms such as urticaria. Recommended doses for adults are 25 to 50 mg of diphenhydramine or 10 to 20 mg of chlorpheniramine.

5. *Albuterol (Salbutamol)*–A selective beta-2 agonist such as albuterol (salbutamol) is the first choice for management of bronchospasm. When administered by means of an inhaler, it provides selective bronchodilation with minimal systemic cardiovascular effects. It has a peak effect in 30 to 60 minutes, with a duration of effect of 4 to 6 hours. Adult dose is 2 sprays, to be repeated as necessary. Pediatric dose is 1 spray, repeated as necessary.

6. *Aspirin*–or acetylsalicylic acid is one of the more newly recognized life-saving drugs, as it has been shown to reduce overall mortality from acute myocardial infarction.

The purpose of its administration during an acute myocardial infarction is to prevent the progression from cardiac ischemia to injury to infarction.

7. *Oral carbohydrate*–An oral carbohydrate source, such as fruit juice or non-diet soft-drink, should be readily available. Whereas this is not a drug, and perhaps should not be included in this list, it should be considered essential. If this sugar source is kept in a refrigerator it may not be appreciated that it is a key part of the emergency equipment. Therefore, consideration should be given to making this part of the emergency kit. Its use is indicated in the management of hypoglycemia in conscious patients.

Additional Emergency Drugs

1. Glucagon

The presence of this drug allows intramuscular management of hypoglycemia in an unconscious patient. The ideal management of severe hypoglycemia in a diabetic emergency is the intravenous administration of 50% dextrose. Glucagon is indicated if an intravenous line is not in place and venipuncture is not expected to be accomplished, as may often be the case in a dental office. The dose for an adult is 1 mg. If the patient is less than 20 kg, the recommended dose is 0.5 mg. Glucagon is available as 1 mg formulation, which requires reconstitution with its diluent immediately prior to use.

2. Atropine

This anti-muscarinic, anti-cholinergic drug is indicated for the management of hypotension, which is accompanied by bradycardia. The dose recommended is 0.5 mg initially, followed by increments as necessary until one reaches a maximum of 3 mg. Paradoxically, doses of less than 0.4 mg have been associated with induction of a bradycardia, likely due to atropine's central nervous system's actions.

3. Ephedrine

This drug is a vassopressor which may be used to manage significant hypotension. It has similar cardiovascular actions compared with epinephrine, except that ephedrine is less potent and has a prolonged duration of action, lasting from 60 to 90 minutes. Similar precautions as noted with epinephrine administration should be considered when given to a patient with ischemic heart disease. For the treatment of severe hypotenson, it is ideally administered in 5 mg increments intravenously. Intramuscularly it should be given in a dose of 10 to 25 mg.

4. Corticosteroid

Administration of a corticosteroid such as hydrocortisone may be indicated for the prevention of recurrent anaphylaxis. Hydrocortisone may also play a role in the management of an adrenal crisis. The notable drawback in their use in emergencies is their relatively slow onset of action, which approaches one hour even when administered intravenously. This is the reason why these drugs are not considered essential, as they are of minimal benefit in the acute phase of the emergency. There is low likelihood of an adverse response with one dose. The prototype for this group is hydrocortisone, which may be administered in a dose of 100 mg as part of the management of these emergencies.

5. Morphine

Morphine is indicated for the management of severe pain which occurs with a myocardial infarction. Advanced Cardiac Life support recommendations list morphine as the analgesic of choice for this purpose. The dose involves titration in one to three mg increments intravenously until pain relief is accomplished. This should be guided by a decrease in blood pressure and respiratory depression. Extreme caution should be used in the elderly. If an intravenous is not in place, consideration can be given to administering morphine in a dose of approximately 5 mg intramuscularly. Again, lower doses need to be considered for the older patient.

6. Naloxone

If either morphine is included in the emergency kit, or opioids are used as part of a sedation regimen, then naloxene should also be present for the emergency management of inadvertent overdose. Doses should ideally be titrated slowly in 0.1 mg increments to effect.

7. Nitrous Oxide

Nitrous oxide is a reasonable second choice if morphine is not available to manage pain from a myocardial infarction. For management of pain associated with a myocardial infarction, it should be administered with oxygen, in a concentration approximating 35%, or titrated to effect.

8. Injectable Benzodiazepine

The management of seizures which are prolonged or recurrent, also known as status epilepticus, may require administration of a benzodiazepine. In most dental practices, it would not be realistic to assume that the dentist could achieve venipuncture in a patient having an active seizure. This leads to the need for a water-soluble agent such as midazolam or lorazepam. Lorazepam has been reported as the drug of choice for status epilepticus and can be administered intramuscularly. Midazolam, however, is another alternative which is water

soluble and could be considered. Sedation would be an expected side effect and patients should be appropriately monitored. Adult doses to consider for lorazepam are 4 mg intramuscularly, or midazolam 5 mg intramuscularly. If an intravenous is in place, these drugs should be slowly titrated to effect.

9. Flumazenil

The benzodiazepine antagonist flumazenil should be part of the emergency kit when oral or parenteral sedation is used, as these techniques are usually based on effective use of benzodiazepines. Dosage is 0.1 to 0.2 mg intravenously, incrementally.

In addition to having drugs available, a small amount of basic equipment should be readily available. This includes a stethoscope, blood pressure cuff, an oxygen delivery system, syringes and needles. Dentists should also consider having an automated external defibrillator (AED), as a means to treat cardiac arrest. Usage of this latter piece of equipment is easily learned and only requires strong knowledge of basic CPR with a small amount of additional training.

Q8 Gingival enlargement.
Ans.
Refer to Q5 of February 2007(RS).

Q9 Orthopantomograph.
Ans.
Refer to Q8 of September 2004.

Q10 X-ray tube.
Ans.
Refer to Q2 of March 2004.

Q11 Object localization.
Ans.
Refer to Q8 of September 2003.

Q12 Differential diagnosis of periapical radioopacities.

Ans.

Refer to Q2. Of March 2001.

SHORT ANSWERS

Q13 Patterson–Kelly syndrome.

Ans.

Refer to Q2 of September 1998.

Q14 Herpetic whitlow.

Ans.

A herpetic whitlow is a lesion (whitlow) on a finger or thumb caused by the herpes simplex virus. It is a painful infection that typically affects the fingers or thumbs. Occasionally infection occurs on the toes or on the nail cuticle. Herpes whitlow can be caused by infection by HSV-1 or HSV-2. HSV-1 whitlow is often contracted by health care workers that come in contact with the virus; it is most commonly contracted by dental workers and medical workers exposed to oral secretions. It is also often observed in thumb-sucking children with primary HSV-1 oral infection (autoinoculation) prior to sero conversion, and in adults aged 20 to 30 following contact with HSV-2-infected genitals.

Causes

In children the primary source of infection is the orofacial area, and it is commonly inferred that the virus (in this case commonly HSV-1) is transferred by the chewing or sucking of fingers or thumbs.

In adults it is more common for the primary source to be the genital region, with a corresponding preponderance of HSV-2. It is also seen in adult health care workers such as dentists because of increased exposure to the herpes virus.

Treatment

Although it is a self-limited illness, antiviral treatments applied to the infected skin, particularly topical acyclovir, have been shown to be effective in decreasing the duration of symptoms. Lancing or surgically debriding the lesion may make it worse by causing a superinfection or encephalitis.

Q15 Alarm clock headache

Ans.

This is a very detailed explanation. For short answers, write only what is necessary.

It is also called as sphenopalatine neuralgia. Also known as Cluster headache, nicknamed "suicide headache", is a neurological disease that involves, as its most prominent feature, an immense degree of pain. "Cluster" refers to the tendency of these headaches to occur periodically, with active periods interrupted by spontaneous remissions. The cause of the disease is currently unknown. It affects approximately 0.1% of the population, and men are more commonly affected than women.

Signs and Symptoms

Cluster headaches are excruciating unilateral headaches of extreme intensity. The duration of the common attack ranges from as short as 15 minutes to three hours or more. The onset of an attack is rapid, and most often without the preliminary signs that are characteristic of a migraine. However, some sufferers report preliminary sensations of pain in the general area of attack, often referred to as "shadows", that may warn them an attack is lurking or imminent. Though the headaches are almost exclusively unilateral, there are some documented as cases of "side-shifting" between cluster periods, or, even rarer, simultaneously (within the same cluster period) bilateral headache. Trigeminal neuralgia can also bring on headaches with similar qualities. However, with trigeminal neuralgia the pain is mostly located around the "cheek" area and is described as being more lance-like in quality.

Pain

The pain of cluster headaches is markedly greater than in other headache conditions, including severe migraines.

The pain is lancinating or boring/drilling in quality, and is located behind the eye (periorbital) or in the temple, sometimes radiating to the neck or shoulder. Analogies frequently used to describe the pain are a red-hot poker inserted into the eye, or a spike penetrating from the top of the head, behind one eye, radiating down to the neck, or sometimes having a leg amputated without any anaesthetic.

The cardinal symptoms of the cluster headache attack are the severe or very severe unilateral orbital, supraorbital and/or temporal pain lasting 15–180 minutes, if untreated, and the attack frequency of one to 16 attacks in 48 hours. The headache is accompanied by at least one of the following autonomic symptoms: ptosis (drooping eyelid), miosis (pupil constriction) conjunctival injection (redness of the conjunctiva), lacrimation (tearing), rhinorrhea (runny nose), and, less commonly, facial blushing, swelling, or sweating, all appearing on the same side of the head as the pain. The attack is also associated with restlessness, the sufferer often pacing the room or rocking back and forth. Less frequently, he or she will have an aversion to bright lights and loud noise during the attack. Nausea rarely accompanies a cluster headache, though it has been reported. The neck is often stiff or tender in the aftermath of a headache, with jaw or tooth pain sometimes present. Some sufferers report feeling as though their nose is stopped up and that they are unable to breathe out of one of their nostrils.

Secondary effects are inability to organize thoughts and plans, exhaustion (in response to such extreme stress, body shuts down and only wants to sleep/repair), and depression. Patients tend to dread facing another headache, and may adjust their physical activities or ask for help to accomplish normal tasks, and may hesitate to schedule plans in reaction to the clock-like regularity of the pain schedule leading to social isolation.

Medications to treat cluster headaches are classified as either abortives or prophylactics (preventatives). In addition, short-term transitional medications (such as steroids) may be used while prophylactic treatment is instituted and adjusted. With abortive treatments often only decreasing the duration of the headache and preventing it from reaching its peak rather than eliminating it entirely, preventive treatment is always indicated for cluster headaches, to be started at the first sign of a new cluster cycle.

Oxygen

During the onset of a cluster headache, some people respond to inhalation of 100% oxygen (12–15 litres per minute in a non-re-breathing mask). When used at the onset this can abort the attack in as little as 1 minute or as long as 10 minutes. Once an attack is at its peak, oxygen therapy appears to have little effect so many people keep an oxygen tank close at hand. An alternative first-line treatment is subcutaneous or intranasal administration of sumatriptan. Hyperbaric oxygen therapy has been used successfully in treating cluster headaches though it was not shown to be more successful than surface oxygen.

Triptans

Sumatriptan and zolmitriptan have both been shown to improve symptoms during an attack.

Other

Some non-narcotic treatments that have shown mixed levels of success are botox injections along the occipital nerve, as well as sarapin (pitcher plant extract) injections.

Lidocaine and other topical anesthetics sprayed into the nasal cavity may relieve or stop the pain, normally in a few minutes, but long term use is not suggested due to the side effects and possible damage to the nasal cavities.

Previously, vaso-constrictors such as ergot compounds were also used, and sufferers report a similar relief by taking strong cups of coffee immediately at the onset of an attack. Cafergot, a cheap off-the-shelf vasoconstrictor, has been shown to stop cluster headaches within 40 minutes of ingestion. BOL (2-bromo lysergic acid diethylamide), a non-psychedelic form of the ergot-derived psychedelicLSD, has shown promise in the treatment of cluster headaches.

Other abortive remedies that work for some include ice, hot showers, cool or lukewarm water sprayed on the face around the sinus, temple, and ear areas, breathing cold air, application of White Flower analgesic balm beneath the nostrils, caffeine, and drinking large amounts of water in the early stages of an attack. Vigorous exercise has been shown in some cases to be very effective in relieving and aborting an acute attack by increasing the levels of oxygen within the body. This could also be due to an increase in adrenaline and changes in blood pressure. Some people report that sexual intercourse and specifically orgasm may terminate an attack possibly by acutely modulating hypothalamic function. Concentrating one's thoughts to a remote part of one's anatomy, such as the opposite little toe, reduced the length of attacks. Headaches are self-perpetuating by concentrating the mind on the symptoms.

Q16 Compound odontome.

Ans.

This is a very detailed explanation. For short answers, write only what is necessary.

It is a tumor of odontogenic origin, a growth in which both the epithelial and the mesenchymal cells exhibit complete differentiation, with the result that functional ameloblasts and odontoblasts form enamel and dentin. This enamel and dentin are laid down in an abnormal pattern. Most odontomas represent a hamartomatous malformation rather than a neoplasm. This lesion is composed of more than one type of tissue, and for this reason has been called a composite odontoma. They have been termed

• Compound composite odontomas when there is at least superficial anatomic similarity to normal teeth.

• Complex composite odontoma: calcified dental tissues are irregular mass bearing no morphologic similarity even to rudimentary teeth.

Etiology

Local trauma or infection

Clinical Features

Occur at any age

At any location maxillary or mandibular

Most odontomas are asymptomatic, although occasionally signs and symptoms relating to their presence do occur. They are unerupted or impacted teeth, retained deciduous teeth, swelling and evidence of infection.

X – ray features: Often situated between the roots of the teeth

Appear as an irregular mass of calcified material surrounded by a narrow radiolucent band with a smooth outer periphery or as a variable number of tooth like structures with the same peripheral outline.

Histology

Normal appearing enamel or enamel matrix, dentin, pulp tissue or cememtum which may or may not exhibit a normal relationship to one another.

There may be presence of ghost cells in odontomas.

Treatment

Surgical removal is the treatment of choice and the recurrence rate is also very low.

Q17 Mucocoel.

Ans.

Refer to Q18 of July 2008(RS).

Q18 Keratoacanthoma.

Ans.

Again, this is a very detailed explanation. For short answers like these, write only what is necessary.

Keratoacanthoma (KA) is a common low grade (unlikely to metastasize or invade) skin cancer that is believed to originate from the neck of the hair follicle. Many pathologists consider it to be a form of squamous cell carcinoma (SCC). The pathologist often labels KA as "well-differentiated squamous cell carcinoma, keratoacanthoma variant", due to the fact that about 6% of KA manifests itself as squamous cell carcinoma when left untreated. KA is commonly found on sun exposed skin, and often is seen on the face, forearms and hands. The defining characteristic of KA is that it is dome shaped, symmetrical, surrounded by a smooth wall of inflamed skin, and capped with keratin scales and debris. It always grows rapidly, reaching a large size within days or weeks, and if untreated will starve itself of nourishment, necroses (die), slough, and heal with scarring.

Keratoacanthomas may be divided into the following types:

- Giant keratoacanthoma
- Keratoacanthoma centrifugum marginatum
- Multiple Keratoacanthomas (Ferguson Smith type of multiple self-healing keratoacanthomas, Multiple kerato-acanthomas of the Ferguson-Smith type)
- Generalized eruptive keratoacanthoma (Generalized eruptive keratoacanthoma of Grzybowski)
- Subungual keratoacanthoma

Etiology

The tumors usually occur in older individuals (mean age 64 years old). Like squamous cell cancer, data suggests ultraviolet light from the sun causes the development of KA. Just like its close relative, the squamous cell cancer, sporadic cases have been found co-infected with the human papilloma virus (HPV).

Diagnosis

Diagnosis is best done with clinical exam and history. It presents as a fleshy, elevated and nodular lesion with an irregular crater shape and a characteristic central hyperkeratotic core. Usually the patient will notice a rapidly growing dome-shaped tumor on sun-exposed skin.

Treatment

On the trunk, arms, and legs, electrodesiccation and curettage often suffice. Excision of the entire lesion is often required if one wants to confirm the clinical diagnosis of keratoacanthoma. On the nose and face, Mohs surgery allows for good margin control with minimal tissue removal; unfortunately, many insurance companies require the correct diagnosis of a malignancy before allowing such procedure. Recurrence after electrodesiccation and curettage is common, and usually can be identified and treated promptly with either further curettage or surgical excision. Allowing the KA to grow and necrose spontaneously is not acceptable in today's standard of care.

Q19 Density of a radiograph
Ans.
Refer to Q17 of June/July 2010 (RS)

Q20 Properties of X-ray
Ans.
Refer to Q5 of September 2001

Q21 Composition of X-ray film
Ans.
Refer to Q16 of August 2007 (Old scheme)

Q22 Filtration
Ans.
Refer to March 2002 Q8